CREATIVE INTERVENTIONS
WITH TRAUMATIZED CHILDREN

Creative Interventions

with Traumatized Children

edited by
Cathy A. Malchiodi

Foreword by Bruce D. Perry

THE GUILFORD PRESS
New York   London

Library of Congress Cataloging-in-Publication Data

Creative interventions with traumatized children / edited by Cathy A. Malchiodi ;
foreword by Bruce D. Perry.
  p. ; cm.
  Includes bibliographical references and index.
  ISBN-13: 978-1-59385-615-1 (hardcover : alk. paper)
  ISBN-10: 1-59385-615-6 (hardcover : alk. paper)
  1. Psychic trauma in children—Treatment.   2. Post-traumatic stress disorder in
children—Treatment.   3. Art therapy for children.   I. Malchiodi, Cathy A.
  [DNLM: 1. Stress Disorders, Post-Traumatic—therapy. 2. Child.
3. Creativeness.   4. Sensory Art Therapies—methods.
WM 170 C912 2008]
  RJ506.P66C74 2008
  618.92'8521—dc22

                                                              2007043168

To Shirley, who always transforms my traumas

About the Editor

Cathy A. Malchiodi, ATR-BC, LPCC, CPAT, is a licensed clinical mental health counselor, art therapist, and expressive arts therapist, and is also a faculty member at the National Institute for Trauma and Loss in Children and at Lesley University. She has more than 25 years of clinical experience in working with people of all ages and has worked as an art therapist with survivors of traumatic experiences, including domestic violence, physical and sexual abuse, disaster, and serious or life-threatening illnesses. Ms. Malchiodi is a frequent presenter on art and health care throughout the United States, Canada, Asia, and Europe, and has given more than 250 invited presentations. She is the only person to have received all three of the American Art Therapy Association's highest honors: Distinguished Service Award (1991), Clinician Award (2000), and Honorary Life Member Award (2002). The author or editor of numerous books, including *The Art Therapy Sourcebook*, *Understanding Children's Drawings*, and the *Handbook of Art Therapy*, she has also published over 70 peer-reviewed papers on the use of art therapy and arts medicine with trauma survivors, survivors of child physical and sexual abuse, people with psychiatric disorders, and those with physical illness.

Contributors

Ann Cattanach, PhD, MSc, private practice, Inverness-shire, United Kingdom, and Department of Social Policy and Social Work, University of York, York, United Kingdom

Lennis G. Echterling, PhD, Counseling Psychology Program, Department of Graduate Psychology, James Madison University, Harrisonburg, Virginia

Deanne Ginns-Gruenberg, BSN, MA, LPC, RPT-S, National Institute for Trauma and Loss in Children, Grosse Pointe Woods, Michigan, and Self-Esteem Shop, Royal Oak, Michigan

Craig Haen, MA, RDT, CGP, LCAT, Kids in Crisis, Cos Cob, Connecticut, and private practice, White Plains, New York

Russell E. Hilliard, PhD, LCSW, LCAT, MT-BC, Seasons Hospice and Palliative Care, Des Plaines, Illinois

Roger J. Klein, PsyD, private practice, Family Resources Associates, Inc., Watertown, Wisconsin, and Rogers Memorial Hospital, Oconomowoc, Wisconsin

P. Gussie Klorer, PhD, Art Therapy Counseling Program, Southern Illinois University, Edwardsville, Illinois

Caelan Kuban, LMSW, National Institute for Trauma and Loss in Children, Grosse Pointe Woods, Michigan

Laura V. Loumeau-May, MPS, ATR-BC, LPC, Journeys Program, Valley Home Care, Paramus, New Jersey, and Department of Psychology, Caldwell College, Caldwell, New Jersey

Cathy A. Malchiodi, ATR-BC, LPCC, CPAT, National Institute
for Trauma and Loss in Children, Grosse Pointe Woods, Michigan,
and Department of Expressive Therapies, Lesley University,
Cambridge, Massachusetts

Elizabeth Sanders Martin, ATR-BC, LPCC, Department of Expressive
Therapies, Kosair Children's Hospital, Louisville, Kentucky

Diane S. Safran, MS, LMFT, ATR-BC, Attention Deficit Disorders
Institute, Westport, Connecticut

Elysa R. Safran, PsyD, private practice, and William Alanson White
Psychoanalytic Institute, New York, New York

William Steele, MSW, PsyD, National Institute for Trauma and Loss in
Children, Grosse Pointe Woods, Michigan

Anne Stewart, PhD, Department of Graduate Psychology, James Madison
University, Harrisonburg, Virginia

Foreword

Childhood is, and always has been, a vulnerable time. Every generation from the Stone Age through thousands of cultures to the modern era has been challenged with war, famine, plague, murder, and rape—and always the most vulnerable, particularly children, have suffered the most. In early generations, trauma was pervasive; in many cases it was more pervasive than in the relatively safe and stable world we try to create for our children today. Yet while we like to think we protect, nurture, educate, and enrich our children better than our ancestors did, in actuality, many children's lives are still filled with threat, violence, loss, and trauma, as seen in domestic violence, the death of a loved one, physical abuse, sexual abuse, or natural disasters. Today, fully one-third of adults have experienced multiple forms of significant adverse childhood events—often traumatic in nature. And we are now more aware that these adverse and traumatic experiences change us in many ways; after trauma our bodies and minds, our hearts and souls are seared and then twisted and modified to help us survive.

The cost of childhood trauma is enormous, not only economically in the hundreds of billions of dollars spent in treating it each year, but also in the lost potential of creativity and productivity when a child's humanity is shattered. All too often children are diminished by the trauma they have experienced. Yet this need not be. A traumatized child *can* heal and grow stronger and wiser by facing, coping with, and overcoming trauma and its aftermath. This is the promise of effective healing from trauma, of true therapeutic experience.

Unfortunately, in our compartmentalized, "evidence-based practice," buzzword world of therapies, dominated by a reductionist medical model, we are not providing the majority of our traumatized

ix

children with true therapeutic experiences. The small percentage of traumatized children being served by our mental health system is a national disgrace. Those who enter the system receive fragmented, ineffective, often impersonal services. We are decidedly not helping traumatized children effectively cope and heal.

While much of the field looks ahead for solutions to these challenges, hoping that we will find the right neurobiological system to target with the right prophylactic drug to prevent posttraumatic stress disorder; or that we will find the subset of the most genetically vulnerable individuals to target with our interventions; or that we will be able to put all traumatized children into a one-size-fits-all, easy-to-export, 20-session group treatment protocol, I would suggest that, instead, we look back. There is something to be learned from our ancestors.

Our ancestors had to learn to cope with trauma in order to survive; somehow traumatized people had to find ways to continue to sustain family, community, and culture and move forward. What did they do to cope with trauma? Are there clues in what they did that may help us today? Examination of the known beliefs, rituals, and healing practices for loss and trauma that remain from aboriginal cultures reveal some remarkable principles. Healing rituals from a wide range of geographically separate, culturally disconnected groups converge into a set of core elements related to adaptation and healing following trauma. These core elements include an overarching belief system—a rationale, a belief, a reason for the pain, injury, loss; a retelling or reenactment of the trauma in words, dance, or song; a set of somato-sensory experiences—touch, the patterned repetitive movements of dance, and song—all provided in an intensely relational experience with family and clan participating in the ritual.

The most remarkable quality of these elements is that together they create a total neurobiological experience influencing cortical, limbic, diencephalic, and brainstem systems (not unlike the pervasive neurobiological impact of trauma):

Retell the story.
Hold each other.
Massage, dance, sing.
Create images of the battle, hunt, and death.
Fill literature, sculpture, and drama with retellings.
Reconnect to loved ones and to community.
Celebrate, eat, and share.

These aboriginal healing practices are repetitive, rhythmic, relevant, relational, respectful, and rewarding; they are experiences known to be effective in altering neural systems involved in the stress response in both animal models and humans. The remarkable resonance of these practices with the neurobiology of trauma is not unexpected. These practices emerged because they worked. People felt better and functioned better, and the core elements of the healing process were reinforced and passed on. Cultures separated by time and space all converged on the same general approach.

The beauty of this book, *Creative Interventions with Traumatized Children*, is that it draws on these ancient practices. It describes modern versions of the most effective, time-honored, and biologically respectful therapeutic practices created by our ancestors. It is important, however, that these innovative therapeutic practices now carry forward and refine these time-honored principles. While these therapeutic practices may not at first seem "biological," be assured that they are not only likely to change the brain, but they will assuredly provide the patterned, repetitive stimuli required to specifically influence and modify the impact of trauma, neglect, and maltreatment on key neural systems. The neural systems altered by trauma originate in the lower parts of the brain (e.g., dopaminergic, serotonergic, and noradrenergic neural networks). These brainstem and midbrain systems will only be modified effectively by patterned repetitive neural activity that gets to the brainstem and midbrain from primary somatosensory experiences—rhythmic auditory, tactile, visual, and motor–vestibular stimulation—such as massage, music, dance, and repetitive visual and tactile stimuli (e.g., eye movement desensitization and reprocessing).

Amid the current pressure for "evidence-based practice" parameters, we should remind ourselves that the most powerful evidence is that which comes from hundreds of separate cultures across thousands of generations independently converging on rhythm, touch, storytelling, and reconnection to community as the core ingredients to coping with and healing from trauma—all which are included in this book.

BRUCE D. PERRY, MD, PhD
Senior Fellow
The ChildTrauma Academy
Houston, Texas

Preface

In her seminal book *Trauma and Recovery*, Judith Herman (1992) notes,

> The ordinary response to atrocities is to banish them from consciousness. Certain violations of the social compact are too terrible to utter aloud: this is the meaning of the word unspeakable. Atrocities, however, refuse to be buried. . . . Remembering and telling the truth about terrible events are prerequisites both for the restoration of the social order and for the healing of individual victims. (p. 1)

Herman underscores that when an individual experiences a psychologically traumatizing event, there is simultaneously a need to articulate the unspeakable and an inability to verbally express or describe what has occurred. Yet in order to recover from trauma, it must be expressed in some way in order for it to be positively transformed.

For some children, a traumatizing event can mean a death of a parent or sibling, divorce, foster care, relocation, an accident, or a medical illness. For others, it can mean exposure to bullying, domestic violence, physical or sexual abuse, a catastrophic natural disaster, or terrorism and war. Unfortunately, some children may encounter multiple events and repetitive stressful circumstances throughout their lives, increasing their susceptibility to psychosocial and developmental problems. Depending on the child, the degree of exposure to distressing events, and other factors, trauma can be an experience that is not only unspeakable, but also mentally and physically exhausting, terrifying, and confusing for young people.

When I began working as an art therapist and mental health counselor for children from violent homes, I had very little knowledge about the effects of psychological trauma. At that time, very little literature and research on traumatized children were available, in contrast to the current interest in the effects of trauma on individuals of all ages and the now widespread acceptance that children do indeed suffer short- and long-term effects from adverse events. In fact, as recently as a decade ago many helping professionals still believed that directly addressing trauma events in therapy could be counterproductive, emotionally harmful, and retraumatizing, and that it was best to let children "forget about it."

Children relive their traumas not only in their minds but also through their actions. The premise that most children intuitively use art and play to act out what they are reliving and what they may find unspeakable is at the heart of this book. The contributing authors in this volume, each of whom uses action-oriented, creative interventions in their work with traumatized children, all agree on one thing: sensory, hands-on methods are an essential part of effective treatment in cases of trauma. For many children, the use of creative interventions provides the opportunity to immediately engage in experiences of mastery over the events that have disrupted their lives. For those children who are withdrawn or fear disclosure of abuse or violence, the sensory nature of creative activities allows expression of the unspeakable and circumvents "talk" that may be difficult or temporarily impossible. For helping professionals, these methods capitalize on metaphor and symbol as ways to help even the most troubled child clients depict, regulate, and control what cannot be told with words alone.

While children have always been exposed to crises, recently there has been global attention to understanding the effects of trauma on children who have experienced frightening events in their homes, neighborhoods, schools, and communities. High-profile incidents such as Hurricane Katrina and the Southeast Asia tsunami, war in Iraq, terrorism threats, and the shootings at Virginia Tech receive intense media coverage, as well as public and professional interest. Even children not directly exposed to these incidents have been affected by these crises, especially those who have previously experienced trauma or loss. Many of those who experienced these recent traumatic events are still struggling with reactions such as anxiety, depression, or post-traumatic stress disorder.

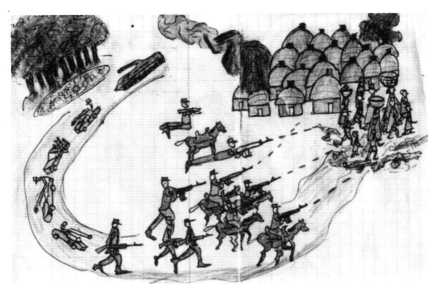

Bakhid was 8 when his village was attacked. He is now 11. This illustration shows tanks and sophisticated pickup trucks from the Sudanese army coming in support of the Janjaweed militia. The Janjaweed militia fires on civilians and sets the houses aflame. From Waging Peace (2007).

During the final months of completing this book, I became intrigued by the emerging story about children in Darfur (Waging Peace, 2007). In June and July 2007, peace campaigner and researcher Anna Schmitt went on a mission to Eastern Chad to assess the humanitarian efforts, human rights, and security in the region and to collect testimonies from Darfuri refugees and displaced people. While collecting testimonies from adults in the region, women told Schmitt how their children witnessed horrendous scenes when their villages were attacked. Schmitt decided to talk to the children but also gave them paper and pencils to draw two pictures: what their dreams were for the future and what their strongest memories were.

When Schmitt saw the children's drawings, she was shocked by the details of the memories of the attacks represented in the pictures. The majority of the images illustrated Sudanese government forces and Janjaweed militia killing, bombing, shooting, beating, and torturing Darfuri men, women, and children. The approximately 500 drawings collected now form part of a submission of evidence to the International Criminal Court that is investigating crimes taking place in Darfur. The atrocities depicted in the drawings directly contradict the Sudanese government's version of the events over the last 4 years, corroborating what was known to be taking place.

This story is a testament to the impact of creative intervention with children, underscoring that something as simple as pencils and paper can give a voice to those who may not be otherwise heard. Being able to communicate what has happened through pictures, play, and other media allows for emotions, events, and memories to be witnessed by others and is the powerful first step in addressing the needs of any trauma survivor. In the foreword, Bruce D. Perry observes that "the most powerful evidence is that which comes from hundreds of separate cultures across thousands of generations" (p. xi). In considering the Darfuri children and the numerous case examples in this book, it is impossible to ignore the possibility that creative expression can make a profound difference in the lives and recovery of traumatized children.

For the last 25 years, I have been studying how trauma impacts children and their families and assisting individuals of all ages overcome its effects. Professionals and students often ask me how I have continued to work with traumatized populations, particularly children who have experienced domestic violence, abuse, and loss, for so many years. My response to this question is simple: Witnessing how children use their creative potential to express, explore, and transform their traumatic experiences is deeply rewarding. It not only has sustained my work but also has provided a fascinating window into why expressive modalities enhance trauma recovery and restore children's health and well-being.

We all endure trauma at one point or another as adults; unfortunately, many of the children we see in treatment have had to endure the suffering that trauma brings throughout their young lives. A belief that has guided my work is found in the third noble truth of Buddhism: Human suffering can be ultimately transformed and healed. In more pragmatic terms, this means that recovery from trauma is possible in all individuals, including our child clients. All children have the potential to reenact and retell their experiences through creative expression, particularly when their therapists recognize and utilize the power of art, play, stories, music, and movement to transform suffering and to help them recapture health and hope for the future.

REFERENCES

Herman, J. (1992). *Trauma and recovery*. New York: Basic Books.

Waging Peace. (2007). *Drawings of genocide*. Retrieved September 18, 2007, from *www.wagingpeace.info/?q=node/149*.

Acknowledgments

It is with great respect that I take this opportunity to acknowledge individuals in the field of trauma who have helped to make this book possible.

First, I want to thank Bruce D. Perry, whose seminal contributions to the field of child trauma are wide-reaching and inspirational to literally thousands of helping professionals. There is no one more worthy of writing a foreword to this book than Dr. Perry because of his lasting commitment to the importance of somatosensory interventions in work with children and his writings on the interface between neuroscience and human development.

I next thank the contributors for agreeing to write chapters for this text. Their expertise addresses the scope and potential of creative methods in work with children and families. I especially thank the incomparable William (Bill) Steele, founder and director of the National Institute for Trauma and Loss in Children, for his vision and influence on the field of child trauma intervention. I am indeed fortunate to have encountered Bill early enough in my work as a therapist to benefit from his wisdom and experience.

Finally, bringing together an edited book is a collaborative effort between editor, contributors, and publisher. As always, I extend a special thanks to the wonderful staff at The Guilford Press, especially my editor, Rochelle Serwator, and production editor, Anna Nelson, for facilitating yet another pleasurable editorial experience and production process.

Contents

**PART I. Creative Interventions and Children:
Basics of Practice**

Chapter 1. Creative Interventions and Childhood Trauma   3
            Cathy A. Malchiodi

Chapter 2. Effective Practice with Traumatized Children: 22
            Ethics, Evidence, and Cultural Sensitivity
            Cathy A. Malchiodi

PART II. Creative Interventions with Individuals

Chapter 3. Expressive Therapy for Severe Maltreatment   43
            and Attachment Disorders:
            A Neuroscience Framework
            P. Gussie Klorer

Chapter 4. Music and Grief Work with Children   62
            and Adolescents
            Russell E. Hilliard

Chapter 5. Grieving in the Public Eye: 81
            Art Therapy with Children Who Lost Parents
            in the World Trade Center Attacks
            Laura V. Loumeau-May

Chapter 6. Medical Art and Play Therapy   112
            with Accident Survivors
            Elizabeth Sanders Martin

Chapter 7.   Creative Approaches to Minimize the Traumatic   132
             Impact of Bullying Behavior
             Diane S. Safran and Elysa R. Safran

Chapter 8.   Trauma, Loss, and Bibliotherapy: 167
             The Healing Power of Stories
             Cathy A. Malchiodi and Deanne Ginns-Gruenberg

PART III. Creative Interventions with Families and Groups

Chapter 9.   Creative Crisis Intervention Techniques   189
             with Children and Families
             Lennis G. Echterling and Anne Stewart

Chapter 10. Working Creatively with Children   211
             and Their Families after Trauma: The Storied Life
             Ann Cattanach

Chapter 11. Vanquishing Monsters: Drama Therapy for Treating   225
             Childhood Trauma in the Group Setting
             Craig Haen

Chapter 12. A Group Art and Play Therapy Program   247
             for Children from Violent Homes
             Cathy A. Malchiodi

Chapter 13. Interventions for Parents of Traumatized Children   264
             William Steele and Cathy A. Malchiodi

PART IV. Creative Intervention as Prevention

Chapter 14. Resilience and Posttraumatic Growth   285
             in Traumatized Children
             Cathy A. Malchiodi, William Steele, and Caelan Kuban

Chapter 15. Ready . . . , Set . . . , Relax!: Relaxation Strategies   302
             with Children and Adolescents
             Roger J. Klein

             Index   321

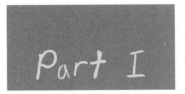

CREATIVE INTERVENTIONS
AND CHILDREN
Basics of Practice

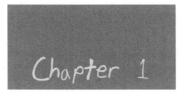

Creative Interventions
and Childhood Trauma

Cathy A. Malchiodi

Children may be in therapy for a variety of reasons related to trauma. Some children experience the death of a parent, survive a serious accident, or lose their home or possessions due to a natural disaster. Others may experience several traumatic events during their young lives or be subjected to chronically stressful situations such as abuse, neglect, or multiple foster care environments. While some children are not permanently affected by these experiences, others may suffer serious symptoms that interfere with normal emotional, cognitive, or social development.

Terr (1990) notes that "trauma does not ordinarily get better by itself. It burrows down further and further under the child's defenses and coping strategies" (p. 293). Children who are traumatized often feel helpless, confused, and ashamed and are afraid to trust others or their environment. Therapists who encounter these children must form a productive relationship with them to enable them not only to revisit painful experiences, but also to overcome intrusive memories, make meaning, and find hope. In order to reach these children effectively, therapists must use both developmentally appropriate methods

3

ations that address traumatic memories and provide emo-

nt years, recognition has been growing that trauma is an
physiological, and neurological response to overwhelming
events or experiences that creates a secondary psychological response
(Rothchild, 2000). This recognition has reframed how therapists
intervene with individuals who have symptoms of stress, and it
acknowledges that these symptoms are the body's adaptive reactions to
distressing events. There is an increasing consensus that intervention
must not only utilize evidence-based practices in psychotherapy with
children, but must also employ techniques that focus on the sensory
impact of trauma.

This chapter provides an overview of trauma from a neurobiological view and a foundation for understanding why sensory interventions such as arts therapies and expressive methods are effective and
often necessary in work with traumatized children. For therapists who
are not familiar with these modalities, a brief description of creative
arts therapies and expressive therapies is offered along with general
information on the nature of traumatic events and their impact on
children.

DEFINING TRAUMA

For the purpose of this book, "trauma" is defined as an experience that
creates a lasting, substantial psychological impact on a child. Traumatizing events may be single occurrences such as an accident or witnessing an injury to another or several experiences that become traumatic
in their totality. Extensive exposure to neglect or abuse, experience of
terrorism or war, or survival of a disaster and subsequent loss of
home, possessions, and/or family members are examples of repeated or
chronic trauma experiences. Terr's (1981, 1990) seminal work with
child survivors of the Chowchilla kidnapping incident offers some of
the first reports on the complexity of traumatic experiences and posttrauma symptoms. As a result of the Chowchilla study and subsequent
investigations, Terr identified many of the characteristics commonly
seen in traumatized children, including behaviors in art and play
activity and influences on cognitive and emotional development. She
also described two forms of traumatic events: acute or Type I trauma

(single event) and chronic or Type II trauma (multiple or cumulative events). In either type of traumatic event, children may encounter physical and/or emotional disruption and suffer bodily trauma and/or psychological effects.

Therapists who work with traumatized individuals now understand that a number of factors actually mediate how single or multiple traumas affect children and how these factors may predispose young clients to more serious problems. Posttraumatic stress disorder (PTSD) is well known to most mental health professionals; the current definition is found in the *Diagnostic and Statistical Manual of Mental Disorders* (DSM-IV-TR; American Psychiatric Association, 2000). Characteristics similar to PTSD in children were described as early as the 1930s, reflecting the currently accepted symptom cluster in assessment of PTSD (Silva, 2004). It was not until 1987 in DSM-III-R (American Psychiatric Association, 1987) that specific features of children's PTSD emerged that account for developmental differences between young clients and adults. In brief, some symptoms of PTSD in children are:

- *Hyperarousal* includes intense psychological distress and/or physiological reactivity when exposed to something that resembles an aspect of the traumatic event, difficulty concentrating, sleep problems such as difficulty falling or staying asleep, hypervigilance, and irritability or outbursts of anger.
- *Reexperiencing* includes suddenly acting or feeling as though a traumatic event is recurring in the present, intrusive thoughts about the event, and nightmares that include sensory or declarative aspects of the event.
- *Avoidance* includes attempts to avoid thoughts or feelings associated with the traumatic event, inability to recall aspects of the event, attempts to avoid activities or situations that evoke memory of a trauma, detachment from family and friends, difficulty sleeping due to nightmares associated with the event, decreased interest in previously pleasurable activities, and a foreshortened sense of the future.

These symptoms may occur in children with PTSD, but discussion continues about differences in responses in children and adults. Also, a number of factors affect how children respond to traumatic events and if children go on to exhibit emotional disorders, including PTSD. Biological aspects, temperament, resiliency, developmental stage, attachment to parents or caregivers, abilities and adaptive coping skills, and available social support are related to individual susceptibility to PTSD (Silva, 2004), acute stress reactions, and mood or behavioral disorders. Children directly exposed to a traumatic event, such as a violent crime, death, or disaster, who do not have adequate social support in the form of family, caregivers, or community or who experience multiple crises are more susceptible to trauma and may require additional, long-term treatment. These children have a higher risk of PTSD and stress-related disorders, although the prevalence rates vary depending on the research study (Silva, 2004). In brief, a number of characteristics and experiences contribute to how trauma affects children and whether or not children suffer long-lasting and disruptive symptoms.

Fortunately, only a portion of children exposed to stressful events go on to develop PTSD or serious disorders, but it is widely accepted that vulnerability and resiliency factors (see Chapter 14) impact the development of symptoms that require ongoing treatment. Most children need a minimum of intervention and usually return to normal personal and social functioning in a short time. In these cases, interventions that incorporate critical incident debriefing, prevention strategies, and brief therapies may lessen the initial distress, identify social supports, and enhance adaptive coping skills.

THE PHYSIOLOGY OF TRAUMA

It is now widely agreed that trauma reactions are both psychological and physiological experiences. In order to help children who have been traumatized, it is first important to have a working knowledge of the physiology of trauma, know how the brain is organized, and understand how the body and mind react to traumatic events. This section does not intend to provide in-depth explanations of human physiology and how trauma affects the brain; this material is widely available and is covered in numerous contemporary texts. Instead, it provides a basic overview and summarizes major concepts that pertain to trauma intervention as an introduction to creative interventions with traumatized children.

The Triune Brain

The human brain is often described as consisting of three parts: the brain stem, the limbic system, and the cortex. The brain stem is the first area to mature and is, from an evolutionary standpoint, the oldest area of the brain. It is responsible for regulating basic functions such as reflexes, the cardiovascular system, and arousal. The cerebellum is connected to the brain stem and coordinates motor, emotional, and cognitive functioning. The brain stem and cerebellum are often referred to as the "reptilian brain" because they are like the brain of reptiles (Damasio, 1999).

The limbic system includes a group of structures that form a ring around the brain stem—the hypothalamus, amygdala, and hippocampus. The limbic system is often referred to as the "emotional brain" because it is the source of urges, needs, and feelings. Its primary functions involve self-preservation, the fight or flight response, and implicit memory—learned associations that link sensations to context. The limbic system, in a sense, evaluates experiences for emotional significance and reacts to these experiences in ways that are learned by the individual over time.

The cortex and neocortex are referred to as the "thinking brain" because they are the parts of the brain where reasoning, communication, and planning occur. They contain the capacity for language and consciousness and the ability not only to think thoughts, but also to think *about* thoughts, behavior, and emotions. Despite the higher functioning of this region of the brain, the lower parts of the brain also have a significant impact on actions and responses.

Trauma reactions are believed to occur when responses of the limbic system used to mobilize oneself in the face of personal threat are not utilized in a productive way. Essentially, children who experience an event such as physical abuse, disaster, terrorism, or any other distressing experience may go into what can be considered a "survival mode." In other words, if the energy normally used for fighting or fleeing is not expended, the emotional activation is held in the nervous system and not dissipated or released (Rothchild, 2000). In the case of traumatic stress, even though the nervous system is still highly activated, children may experience a disruption or impairment in normal functioning and develop habitual responses such as explosive emotions, noncompliant behavior, psychological numbness, cognitive problems, or other reactions depending on personality factors and the type and extent of distress.

Consider 8-year-old Mark, a child who is currently in treatment at a local psychiatric facility. He has a long history of severe physical abuse, sexual abuse, and neglect and has lived in multiple foster homes. Mark has very little ability to control his impulses; in the classroom and play therapy room, he often initiates arguments with other children, steals, sets fires, and is prone to tearful outbursts when under even minimal stress. He finds it difficult to focus his attention on any one game or toy for more than a minute and reacts to fear-inducing situations with psychological numbing and withdrawal, frozen and unable to move. Mark is also developmentally delayed, behaving like a much younger child and drawing human figures at the level of a 4-year-old child (Figure 1.1).

In reviewing Mark's behavior, how the brain reacts to repetitive traumatic experiences may explain many of his current responses to others and his environment. As an individual who is profoundly or chronically distressed, Mark reacts with little self-control because he is unable to regulate his emotional responses. His behavior may be a survival response involving fighting (arguing) and sometimes freezing (psychological numbing and withdrawal), depending on the perceived

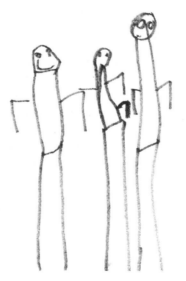

FIGURE 1.1. Human figures by Mark, age 8 years.

threats in his environment that cause fear, terror, or feelings of helplessness. He may have learning disabilities due to years of distress that have affected his cognitive and social functioning. In contrast to Mark, healthy, capable, and resilient children can use problem-solving skills, available social support, and other resources to overcome stressful events; those who have traumatic stress reactions cannot and go on to develop symptoms of PTSD or other emotional disorders.

The Mind–Body Connection

It is well accepted that the body often mirrors emotions. Different parts of the brain may become active when we look at sad faces or happy faces, imagine a happy or sad event or relationship, or hear a particular song or sound. These emotions are connected to a variety of hormonal fluctuations as well as cardiovascular and neurological effects (Sternberg, 2001). In fact, the physiology of emotions is so complex that the brain knows more than the conscious mind can reveal—that is, one can display an emotion without being conscious of what induced it (Damasio, 1999).

In the case of traumatic events, sensory experiences related to crisis, such as images, touch, sound, and smell, may become learned associations that resurface when one encounters a different, yet similar set of stimuli. For example, when Mark feels insecure around other children, he automatically reacts with uncontrollable rage, recapitulating his early relationships with an abusive sister; if he feels threatened by an adult, he becomes hypervigilant and immobilized as his body prepares for physical violence or punishment. There is general agreement that traumatic events similar to the ones Mark has experienced take a toll on the body as well as the mind. After a significant trauma, the "body remembers" (Levine, 1997; Rothchild, 2000), and, as van der Kolk (1994) notes in the title of his book, "the body keeps the score" of emotional experiences.

Memory Storage

The way in which memory is stored is also important to understanding the brain and traumatic events. In brief, there are two types of memory: explicit and implicit. Explicit or declarative memory is conscious memory and is composed of facts, concepts, and ideas; one has access to language to describe what one is thinking and feeling, and explicit memory allows processing of information, reasoning, and meaning, helping individuals define and make sense of experiences.

Implicit memory is sensory and emotional and is related to the body's learned memories. Riding a bicycle is good example of implicit memory, while narrating the chronological details of the event (getting on the bike, pedaling to the park) is an example of explicit memory. In implicit memory, there is no language. In other words, the senses are the memory—what we see, what we hear, sensations of smell, touch, and taste become the implicit containers of that experience.

Currently, there is speculation that PTSD may result when implicit memory of trauma is excluded from explicit storage (Rothchild, 2000); that is, an individual may not have access to the context in which the emotions or sensations arose. Additionally, language (a function of explicit memory) is not generally accessible to trauma survivors after a distressing event. In particular, Broca's area, a section of the brain that controls language, is affected, making it difficult to relate the trauma narrative. Positron emission tomography (PET) scans have demonstrated that trauma actually creates changes in Broca's area that lead to difficulties in identifying and verbalizing experiences, a process normally accessible via explicit memory (van Dalen, 2001). Bessel van der Kolk observes, "it is a problem with verbalization . . . the Broca's area shuts down" (Korn, 2001, p. 4) when an individual is asked to speak about a traumatic event. Because trauma is stored as somatic sensations and images, it may not be readily available for communication through language. Perhaps this inability to verbalize trauma relates to the human survival response; when an experience is extremely painful to recall, the brain protects the individual by literally making it impossible to talk about it.

CREATIVE INTERVENTIONS
AND TRAUMATIZED CHILDREN

In addition to having a working knowledge of the physiology of trauma reactions in children, it is also important to understand the variety of therapeutic approaches that use creativity, imagination, and self-expression as their core. Creative interventions have been formalized through the disciplines of art therapy, music therapy, dance/movement therapy, drama therapy or psychodrama, poetry therapy, and play therapy, including sandtray therapy. Each discipline has been applied in psychotherapy and counseling with individuals of all ages, particularly children, for more than 50 years. Art, music, dance, drama, and poetry therapies are referred to as "creative arts therapies" because of their roots in the arts and theories of creativity (National Coalition of Creative Arts Therapies Associations, 2007). These therapies and others that utilize self-expression in treatment are also called "expressive therapies" (Malchiodi, 2005). Expressive therapies are defined as the use of art, music, drama, dance/movement, poetry/creative writing, bibliotherapy, play, and sandplay within the context of psychotherapy, counseling, rehabilitation, or medicine. Additionally, expressive therapies are sometimes referred to as "integrative" when purposively used in combination in treatment.

These individual approaches are defined as follows:

• *Art therapy* is defined as the use of art media, images, and the creative process and respects client responses to the created products as reflections of development, abilities, personality, interests, concerns, and conflicts. It is a therapeutic means of reconciling emotional conflicts, fostering self-awareness, developing social skills, managing behavior, solving problems, reducing anxiety, aiding reality orientation, and increasing self-esteem (American Art Therapy Association, 2007).

• *Music therapy* is the prescribed use of music to effect positive changes in the psychological, physical, cognitive, or social functioning of individuals with health or educational problems (American Music Therapy Association, 2007).

• *Drama therapy* is the systematic and intentional use of drama/theater processes, products, and associations to achieve the therapeutic goals of symptom relief, emotional and physical integration, and personal growth. It is an active approach that helps the client tell his or her story to solve a problem, achieve catharsis, extend the depth and breadth of his or her inner experience, understand the meaning of images, and strengthen his or her ability to observe personal roles while increasing flexibility between roles (National Association for Drama Therapy, 2007).

• *Dance/movement therapy* is based on the assumption that body and mind are interrelated and is defined as the psychotherapeutic use of movement as a process that furthers the emotional, cognitive, and physical integration of the individual. Dance/movement therapy effects changes in feelings, cognition, physical functioning, and behavior (American Dance Therapy Association, 2007).

• *Poetry therapy and bibliotherapy* are terms used synonymously to describe the intentional use of poetry and other forms of literature for healing and personal growth.

• *Play therapy* is the systematic use of a theoretical model to establish an interpersonal process wherein trained play therapists use the therapeutic powers of play to help clients prevent or resolve psychosocial difficulties and achieve optimal growth and development (Landreth, 1991; Webb, 2007).

• *Sandplay therapy* is a creative form of psychotherapy that uses a sandbox and a large collection of miniatures to enable a client to explore the deeper layers of his or her psyche in a totally new format; by constructing a series of "sand pictures," a client is helped to illustrate and integrate his or her psychological condition.

• *Integrative approaches* involve two or more expressive therapies to foster awareness, encourage emotional growth, and enhance relationships with others. This approach distinguishes itself through combining modalities within a therapy session. Integrative approaches are based on a variety of orientations, including arts as therapy, arts psychotherapy, and the use of arts for traditional healing (Barba, Fuchs, & Knill, 1995; Estrella, 2005).

It is important to clarify that while some practitioners define art, dance/movement, music, or drama therapies as play therapies (Lambert et al., 2007), creative arts therapies and expressive therapies are not merely subsets of play therapy and have a long history in mental health with distinct approaches. While the arts may sometimes be a form of play, encouraging children to express themselves through a painting, music, or dance involves an understanding of the media beyond the scope of play. In brief, the arts therapies are different from play therapy because they integrate knowledge of art with principles of psychotherapy and counseling.

In addition to the disciplines and approaches mentioned above, many therapists integrate activities that enhance relaxation as part of trauma intervention. Relaxation techniques often include creative components such as music (see Chapter 4), movement, or art making. Guided imagery or visualization, meditation, yoga, and other methods of stress reduction are also used with children who have experienced traumatic events (Klein, 2001).

Art, music, and dance/movement therapies and other creative interventions such as play have sometimes been incorrectly labeled as "nonverbal" therapies. They are both verbal and nonverbal because verbal communication of thoughts and feelings is a central part of therapy in most situations. In fact, most therapists who use these methods integrate them within a psychotherapy approach, including but not limited to psychodynamic, humanistic, cognitive, developmental, systems, narrative, solution-focused, and others. For example, practitioners who describe their work with children in this book utilize specific frameworks to facilitate therapy with children based on current knowledge of best practices in trauma intervention. There are also creative interventions that specifically focus on verbal communication and self-expression as part of treatment, such as drama therapy, creative writing and poetry therapy, and bibliotherapy.

UNIQUE CHARACTERISTICS OF CREATIVE INTERVENTIONS IN WORK WITH INDIVIDUALS WITH TRAUMA

Johnson (1987) observes that creative arts therapies have a unique role in the treatment of trauma-related disorders, noting that individuals who experienced traumatic events have difficulty with verbal expression. He underscores that creative arts therapies are effective interventions with psychological trauma in children, individuals with mental illness or developmental delays, and older adults with neuro-degenerative disorders or speech problems. Johnson's observations were made almost a decade before the fields of neurobiology, psychiatry, and psychology confirmed that trauma has profound effects on the part of the brain that controls language or more fully identified the roles of explicit and implicit memory in trauma-related disorders.

For young trauma survivors with limited language or who may be unable to put ideas into speech, expression through art, music, movement, or play can be a way to convey these ideas without words and may be the primary form of communication in therapy. Creative interventions involving art, play, music, movement, or other modalities add a unique dimension to treatment because they have several specific characteristics not always found in strictly verbal therapies used in trauma intervention. These characteristics include, but are not limited to, (1) externalization, (2) sensory processing, (3) attachment, and (4) arousal reduction and affect regulation.

Externalization

In trauma intervention, externalization of trauma memories and experiences is considered central to the process of relief and recovery. All therapies, by their very nature and purpose, encourage individuals to engage in externalizing troubling thoughts, feelings, and experiences. Creative interventions encourage externalization through one or more modalities as a central part of therapy and trauma intervention. Gladding (1992) notes that using the arts in counseling may speed up the process of externalization and that expressive modalities allow people to experience themselves differently. Early studies by Terr (1990) identify specific ways that children externalize their trauma experiences through play in repetitive, abreaction, and corrective actions.

Externalization through visual means, play activity, movement, or other modalities may help shift traumatic experiences from the present to the past (Collie, Backos, Malchiodi, & Spiegel, 2006). In art therapy, for example, trauma memories can be externalized through the creative process of making or constructing an image or object. Self-expression through a painting, movement, or poem can relate past experiences, but this is only one benefit of how creative expression externalizes trauma. In fact, most therapists using creative arts or expressive therapies in trauma intervention capitalize on the ability of art, music, play, and other comparable methods of expression to contain traumatic experiences rather than encourage cathartic communication of raw emotions or mere repetition of troubling memories. Essentially, child clients are encouraged to use creative self-expression as a repository for feelings and perceptions that can be transformed during the course of treatment, resulting in emotional reparation, resolution of conflict, and a sense of well-being. When verbal communication is limited after traumatic experiences, it may be that some other form of externalization must be used in addition to verbal therapies such as cognitive-behavioral or other accepted approaches to trauma relief.

Sensory Processing

In most methods of trauma intervention, therapists encourage individuals to explore the trauma narrative—the story of what happened when the trauma occurred and feelings associated with the event—at some point during treatment. The goal is to help traumatized individuals process what is distressing; transform disturbing behaviors, thoughts, and feelings; and ultimately find relief. With children, however, expressing the trauma story with words is not always possible for developmental reasons, and, as previously mentioned, for severely traumatized clients, words may not be accessible when it comes to describing trauma memories.

Expressive therapies and creative arts therapies are defined by psychology as "action therapies" (Weiner, 1999) because they are action-oriented methods through which individuals explore issues and communicate thoughts and feelings. Art and music making, dance and drama, creative writing, and all forms of play are participatory and sensory and require individuals to invest energy in them. For example, art making, even in its simplest sense, can involve arranging, touching, gluing, stapling, painting, forming, and many other tangible experiences. All creative methods focus on encouraging clients to become active participants in the therapeutic process.

Creative interventions serve as a catalyst for individuals to explore thoughts, feelings, memories, and perceptions through visual, tactile, olfactory, and auditory experiences. Some forms of creative activity actually can enhance trauma intervention with children. Drawing, for example, facilitates children's verbal reports of emotionally laden events in several ways: reducing anxiety, helping the child feel comfortable with the therapist, increasing memory retrieval, organizing narratives, and prompting the child to tell more details than in a solely verbal interview (Gross & Haynes, 1998).

Because highly charged emotional experiences such as trauma are encoded by the limbic system as a form of sensory reality, expression and processing of sensory memories of the traumatic event are necessary to successful intervention and resolution (Rothchild, 2000). Action-oriented activities can tap the limbic system's sensory memory of the event and help bridge implicit and explicit memories of it (Malchiodi, 2003; Malchiodi, Riley, & Hass-Cohen 2001). Steele (2007) observes that trauma intervention is a matter of finding a way to access implicit memory to help children express their experiences. He cites an implicit process referred to as "iconic symbolization," a means of giving traumatic experiences a visual identity (Michaesu & Baettig, 1996). The brain creates images to contain all the elements of traumatic experience—what happened, our emotional reactions to it, the horror and terror of the experience. When memory cannot be expressed linguistically, it remains at a symbolic level, which there are no words to describe. In brief, to retrieve that memory so that it can become conscious, it must be externalized in its symbolic form. In the same vein, in order to access traumatic experiences in children, sensory interventions must be used to allow them to "make us witnesses to their experiences, to present us with their iconic representations, and to give us the opportunity to see what they are now seeing as they look at themselves" following exposure to a traumatic event (Steele, 2007, p. 3).

Sensory expression makes progressive exposure of the trauma story and expression of traumatic material tolerable, helping overcome avoidance and allowing the therapeutic process to advance relatively quickly (Collie et al., 2006). Active participation and progressive exposure through creative methods may also help reduce the emotional numbing that occurs with PTSD. It allows children actively to imagine, experiment with or reframe an event, or rehearse a desired change through self-expression; that is, it involves a tangible object, play activity, movement, or other experience that can be physically altered. The role of imagination in expressive therapies is illustrated throughout this book, but in essence it assists children in moving beyond preconceived beliefs through experimentation with new ways of communication and experiences that involve "pretend."

Attachment

Perry (2006) observes that "Experience can become biology" (p. 1). For children who have been severely traumatized, normal development during childhood can be profoundly altered by multiple traumatic events, causing attachment problems. Attachment theory (Bowlby, 1969) has been used as a theoretical base for psychotherapy for many years but has more recently become a major focus of neuroscience and renewed interest among therapists who work with trauma. Since Bowlby's initial writings, researchers have demonstrated that interactions between children and parents or caregivers determine the brain's structure for children, promoting the development of the prefrontal cortex responsible for reasoning, problem solving, flexibility, and other important functions. Siegel (1999) explains attachment as "an inborn system in the brain that evolves in ways that influence and organize motivational, emotional, and memory processes with respect to significant caregiving figures" (p. 67). Schore (1994) offers a neurological model for the importance of infant attachment throughout life. He notes that soon after birth the caregiver and the infant develop interactions that are important to the process of affect regulation. Face-to-face contact and soothing touch are examples of ways the infant learns to respond to stimulation from people and experiences.

While early childhood trauma affects relationship patterns later in life, it may be corrected, at least in part, with appropriate intervention. Research in neuroscience is demonstrating that infancy is not the only chance a person has to develop healthy attachment; there seem to be ways to reshape and repair some early experiences. Recapitulating the normal, attachment-building sensory experiences of childhood through therapeutic intervention and through strengthening the parent–child relationship may help reestablish healthy attachments. Riley (2001) cites how art and play activities are being used in early childhood attachment programs and how simple creative exercises can be used to resolve relational problems and strengthen parent–child bonds. She explains that the nonverbal dimensions of these activities tap into early relational states before words are dominant, possibly allowing the brain to establish new, more productive patterns.

Siegel (1999) and Schore (1994) believe that interactions between infant and caregiver are mediated by the right brain because, during infancy, the right cortex develops more quickly than the left. Siegel also observes that, just as the left hemisphere requires exposure to language to grow, the right hemisphere requires emotional stimulation to develop properly. He goes on to say that the output of the right brain is expressed in nonverbal ways, such as drawing a picture, using a picture, or participating in play activities to describe feelings or events. Creative interventions may be an important means of working with attachment issues as well as other emotionally related disorders or experiences. A conceptual framework for how art and play therapies can be used with children with attachment disorder is more fully explained in Chapter 3, and the importance of psychoeducation for parents and caregivers of traumatized children is presented in Chapter 13.

Arousal Reduction and Affect Regulation

The reduction of arousal or hyperarousal in young clients is a central concept in trauma intervention. For this reason, most trauma intervention begins with regulation of emotions, stress reduction, and restoration of feelings of safety. Art therapy, for example, can be used to activate the body's relaxation response. In working with children from violent homes, I observed that art activity had a soothing, hypnotic influence and that traumatized children were naturally attracted to this quality when anxious or suffering from posttraumatic stress (Malchiodi, 1990).

Benson (1996), acclaimed for his work with the relaxation reponse, observes that it is possible for everyone to remember the calm and confidence associated with health and happiness. Even when physically ill, individuals can access what Benson calls "remembered wellness," increasing the sense of well-being despite distress or illness. In trauma intervention, recalling memories of positive events that can reframe and eventually override negative ones is helpful in reducing posttraumatic stress, particularly if a sensory experience of remembered wellness is included. Simple activities such as drawing a picture of a pleasant time or hearing a soothing, familiar song, story, or rhyme appear to be effective because of the capacity of image making to recall sensory memories and details of positive moments (Malchiodi et al., 2001).

Tinnin (1994) proposes that art therapy facilitates healing in a similar way to the placebo effect because it uses mimicry, an instinctive, preverbal function of the brain that is basic to self-soothing. An example of mimicry might be a child stroking a blanket in a way that mimics a mother's soothing to activate an internal process of self-relaxation. Creative expression may stimulate a similar experience and help the client self-soothe and repair, as noted above. Music, art, and dance and movement may be helpful in tapping the body's relaxation response (Benson, 1996). Overall, expressive activities may stimulate the placebo effect through mimicking self-soothing experiences of childhood and inducing self-relaxation (Malchiodi, 2003; Tinnin, 1994). Of all creative interventions, music therapy has received the most comprehensive research on the reduction of autonomic responses such as blood pressure, heart rate, and respiration.

CONCLUSIONS

In brief, using creative interventions has enormous potential in trauma intervention, as demonstrated in this chapter and through the applications and cases described in this book. For children in general, creative activities in therapy offer many benefits: pleasure in making, doing, and inventing; play and imagination; and enhancement of self-worth through self-expression. For children who are traumatized, there are additional reasons to consider integrating creative arts therapies, play therapy, and other action-oriented approaches within intervention. For these young trauma survivors, creative expression offers a way to contain traumatic material within an object, image, story, music, or other art form; provides a sense of control over terrifying and intrusive memories; encourages active participation in therapy; reduces emotional numbness; and enhances reduction of hyperarousal and other distressing reactions. When verbal techniques fail to ameliorate trauma memory in children, art, play, music, or movement can provide the necessary means to reenact the feelings and sensations associated with traumatic experiences. In subsequent chapters, these and other advantages of creative activities as used in intervention with traumatized children are described, demonstrating in detail how these approaches facilitate emotional reparation, relief, and recovery.

REFERENCES

American Art Therapy Association. (2007). *About art therapy*. Retrieved January 22, 2007, from *www.arttherapy.org/about.html*.

American Dance Therapy Association. (2007). *What is dance therapy?* Retrieved January 23, 2007, from *www.adta.org/about/who.cfm*.

American Music Therapy Association. (2007). *Music therapy makes a difference: What is music therapy?* Retrieved January 22, 2007, from *www.musictherapy.org*.

American Psychiatric Association. (1987). *Diagnostic and statistical manual of mental disorders* (3rd ed., rev.). Washington, DC: Author.

American Psychiatric Association. (2000). *Diagnostic and statistical manual of mental disorders* (4th ed., text rev.). Washington, DC: Author.

Barba, H., Fuchs, M., & Knill, P. (1995). *Minstrels of soul*. Ontario: Palmerston Press.

Benson, H. (1996). *Timeless healing: The power and biology of belief*. New York: Scribner.

Bowlby, J. (1969). *Attachment and loss: Vol. 1. Attachment*. New York: Basic.

Collie, K., Backos, A., Malchiodi, C., & Spiegel, D. (2006). Art therapy for combat-related PTSD: Recommendations for research and practice. *Art Therapy: Journal of the American Art Therapy Association, 23*(4), 157–164.

Damasio, A. (1999). *The feeling of what happens*. New York: Harcourt.

Estrella, K. (2005). Expressive therapy: An integrated arts approach. In C. A. Malchiodi (Ed.), *Expressive therapies* (pp. 183–209). New York: Guilford Press.

Gladding, S. T. (1992). *Counseling: A comprehensive profession* (2nd ed.). New York: Macmillan.

Gross, J., & Haynes, H. (1998). Drawing facilitates children's verbal reports of emotionally laden events. *Journal of Experimental Psychology, 4,* 163–179.

Johnson, D. (1987). The role of the creative arts therapies in the diagnosis and treatment of psychological trauma. *The Arts in Psychotherapy, 14,* 7–13.

Klein, N. (2001). *Healing images for children*. Watertown, WI: Inner Coaching.

Korn, M. L. (2001). Trauma and PTSD: Aftermath of the WTC disaster—An interview with Bessel A. van der Kolk, MD. *Medscape General Medicine 3*(4), 2001 [formerly published in *Medscape Psychiatry and Mental Health eJournal* 6(5), 2001]. Available at *www.medscape.com/viewarticle/408691*.

Lambert, S. F., LeBlanc, M., Mullen, J. A., Ray, D., Baggerly, J., White, J., et al., (2007). Learning more about those who play in session: The national play therapy in counseling practices project (Phase I). *Journal of Counseling and Development, 85*(1), 42–46.

Landreth, G. (1991). *Play therapy: The art of the relationship*. Muncie, IN: Accelerated Development.

Levine, P. (1997). *Waking the tiger*. Berkeley, CA: North Atlantic.

Malchiodi, C. A. (1990). *Breaking the silence: Art therapy with children from violent homes*. New York: Brunner/Mazel.

Malchiodi, C. A. (Ed.). (2003). *Handbook of art therapy*. New York: Guilford Press.

Malchiodi, C. A. (2005). *Expressive therapies*. New York: Guilford Press.

Malchiodi, C. A., Riley, S., & Hass-Cohen, N. (2001). *Toward an integrated art therapy mind–body landscape* (Cassette Recording No. 108-1525). Denver, National Audio Video.

Michaesu, G., & Baettig, D. (1996). An integrated model of posttraumatic stress disorder. *European Journal of Psychiatry, 10*(4), 243–245.

National Association for Drama Therapy. (2007). *Frequently asked questions about drama therapy: What is drama therapy?* Retrieved January 23, 2007, from *www.nadt.org/faqs.html*.

National Coalition of Creative Arts Therapies Associations. (2007). *Definition of profession*. NCCATA fact sheet. Retrieved January 22, 2007, from *www.nccata.org/fact_sheet.htm*.

Perry, B. D. (2006, January). Death and loss: Helping children manage their grief. *Early Childhood Today, 15*(4), 1–3.

Riley, S. (2001). *Group process made visible: Group art therapy*. Philadelphia: Brunner-Routledge.

Rothchild, B. (2000). *The body remembers: The psychophysiology of trauma and trauma treatment*. New York: Norton.

Schore, A. (1994). *Affect regulation and the origin of the self*. Hillsdale, NJ: Erlbaum.

Siegel D. J. (1999) *The developing mind: Toward a neurobiology of interpersonal experience*. New York: Guilford Press.

Silva, R. (2004). *Posttraumatic stress disorders in children and adolescents*. New York: Norton.

Steele, W. (2007). When cognitive interventions fail with children of trauma: Memory, learning, and trauma intervention. Retrieved January 23, 2007, from *tlcinst.org/cognitiveinterventions.html*.

Sternberg, E. (2001). *The balance within: The science connecting health and emotions*. New York: Freeman.

Terr, L. (1981). Psychic trauma in children: Observations following the Chowchilla school-bus kidnapping. *American Journal of Psychiatry, 138*, 14–19.

Terr, L. (1990). *Too scared to cry*. New York: HarperCollins.

Tinnin, L. (1994). Transforming the placebo effect in art therapy. *American Journal of Art Therapy, 32*(3), 75–78.

van Dalen, A. (2001). Juvenile violence and addiction: Tangled roots in childhood trauma. *Journal of Social Work Practice in the Addictions, 1*, 25–40.

van der Kolk, B. (1994). *The body keeps the score*. Cambridge, MA: Harvard Medical School.

Webb, N. B. (Ed). (2007). *Play therapy with children in crisis: Individual, group, and family treatment* (3rd ed.). New York: Guilford Press.

Weiner, D. J. (1999). *Beyond talk therapy: Using movement and expressive techniques in clinical practice*. Washington, DC: American Psychological Association.

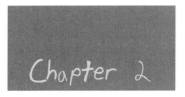

Chapter 2

Effective Practice
with Traumatized Children
Ethics, Evidence, and Cultural Sensitivity

Cathy A. Malchiodi

Creative interventions, like any therapeutic approach, require that therapists prepare to use them appropriately and effectively in practice. Creative arts therapies and expressive therapies provide the foundation for a variety of useful techniques with traumatized children, but these approaches cannot be applied without rationale, understanding of basic principles, and experience. Because so many therapists intuitively use creative approaches in their work with children, they may take for granted that a large and formalized body of knowledge on the use of these approaches already exists.

While therapists cannot possibly know every aspect of creative arts therapies and expressive therapies, there are several areas with which they should become familiar before applying these therapies in trauma work. First and foremost, using any of these interventions with traumatized children involves unique ethical issues related to each expressive modality and should include knowledge of evidence-based practice. Cultural sensitivity about play, toys, music, props, and art materials in therapy is also requisite to work with young clients, particularly those from diverse backgrounds. Finally, there are special issues in trauma intervention that are relevant to creative approaches. This chapter provides a brief overview of these ethical, cultural, evidence-based practice, and special issues, with an emphasis on aspects relevant to the use of creative arts therapies and expressive therapies with traumatized children.

ETHICAL PRACTICE
OF CREATIVE INTERVENTION

Knill, Barba, and Fuchs (2004) observe that creative approaches used in therapy have distinct characteristics that set them apart from strictly verbal techniques and from each other. For example, visual expression is conducive to more private, isolated work and introspective exploration; music often taps feeling and may lend itself to socialization when people collaborate in song or in simultaneously playing instruments; and dance/movement offers opportunities to interact and form relationships. Play incorporates many forms of creative expression and may involve a wide range of individual or interpersonal interventions. All creative arts therapies and expressive therapies utilize tactile, kinesthetic, and auditory experiences in various ways, depending on the activity. Each form of creative expression has its unique properties and roles in therapeutic work depending on its application, practitioner, client, setting, and objectives.

The differences inherent in each modality inform the ethical practice and application of creative interventions in work with traumatized children. While all mental health professionals abide by the ethical codes of their specific disciplines, creative arts therapists and play therapists have ethical standards for practice that address issues specific to the use of these methods with clients. The American Art Therapy Association (AATA), American Music Therapy Association (AMTA), American Dance Therapy Association (ADTA), National Association for Drama Therapy (NADT), National Association for Poetry Therapy (NAPT), and the Association for Play Therapy (APT) all provide helpful guidelines about the application and ethical practice of expressive modalities with clients of all ages. Familiarity with the content of these codes enhances therapists' applications of these approaches and helps them develop a clearer understanding of the purpose and characteristics of the methods they are using. While it is impossible to become an expert on all aspects of all therapies, therapists should have hands-on experience with and a working knowledge of the modalities they employ and a rationale for their use in trauma intervention.

A growing body of literature in the fields of counseling and psychology addresses some of the ethical aspects of creative expression in therapy. Special interest groups in both professional counseling and psychology discuss the use of creativity in counseling and arts in psychology; however, these groups do not have specific ethical guidelines for the use of art, play, props, or other expressive means in child therapy. In comparison, the ethical codes of professional disciplines such as play therapy and art therapy delineate issues inherent in work with children in much more detail. For example, the field of play therapy has contributed supplemental information on the issue of "touch" in therapy because of the nature of the relationship between therapists and children in the playroom (Sprunk, Mitchell, Myrow, & O'Connor, 2007). In brief, therapists must be prepared to respond not only to children's perceptions of touch, but also to touch that occurs during play interventions. Sprunk and colleagues also underscore the importance of informed consent before touch is introduced or occurs in play sessions and suggest that therapists give parents or caregivers and children examples of types of touch that might happen in play therapy and initiate discussion about physical safety and sexual boundaries. They identify special considerations in work with abused children, noting that touch is not automatically eliminated from play therapy just because a client has experienced "bad touch." In certain circumstances, children who have been physically or sexually abused may need to experience safe and positive touch in order to reestablish trust and attachment.

Art therapists stress understanding and being sensitive to specific ethical issues when it comes to introducing art expression in treatment (Malchiodi, 1998a). Art therapy involves the creation of a product that constitutes part of clients' confidential treatment record, just as written documentation, audiotapes, or videotapes of sessions would be confidential. In other words, therapists who ask child clients to make drawings, paintings, or other art must consider how they will record, store, and, in certain situations, retain original artworks produced in therapy. Digital cameras have made it possible to store photographic copies more easily, allowing children to keep their products, but, in some cases, such as those involving abuse or neglect, it is often necessary to retain the artwork.

Therapists without experience in creative approaches may use expressive modalities in a mechanical fashion and apply activities and techniques routinely rather than determining what would be best for traumatized children given their histories, presenting problems and potentials, cultural backgrounds, and goals of treatment. Because expressive therapies can include directed activities, it is easy for some therapists to fall into the habit of looking for a "recipe" for an activity or sequence of activities.

In the case of using art expression, therapists who fully understand art therapy are careful not to interpret images based on their own intuition or projections. In general, creative arts therapists, expressive therapists, and play therapists do not seek to interpret individuals' drawings, movement, poems, or play, but facilitate those individuals' discovery of personal meaning and understanding of such expressions. They use verbal techniques to help young clients explore their feelings and perceptions rather than relying solely on interpretation. As with any form of therapy, therapists listen to and respect what clients are communicating through self-expression and flexibly apply techniques that are best suited to clients' needs and treatment objectives.

EVIDENCE-BASED PRACTICE

Using creative methods in counseling or psychotherapy comes with the responsibility of learning established and emerging information on the use of these approaches with children and trauma. The term "evidence-based practice" refers to a body of scientific knowledge about specific clinical interventions or treatments (Hoagland, Burns, Kiser, Ringeisen, & Schoenwald, 2001). In brief, for an intervention or treatment to be classified as well-established, two or more studies must demonstrate that it is better than placebo, medication, or alternative treatment or that it is equal to another established intervention. Interventions or treatments are classified as "probably efficacious" if at least one study demonstrates their superiority to placebo or shows efficacy via other accepted methods. Evidence-based practice not only advances therapists' knowledge of what protocols and techniques are most effective, but also helps ensure that clients are getting the best treatment based on current knowledge.

Cognitive-behavioral therapy (CBT) is a widely accepted approach among trauma therapists with children who have experienced a traumatic event (Reinecke, Dattilio, & Freeman, 2003). Trauma-focused cognitive-behavioral therapy (TF-CBT) (Cohen, Mannarino, & Deblinger, 2006) is one of few approaches that is believed to be a well-established evidence-based practice for trauma intervention with children. TF-CBT consists of conjoint child and parent therapy and incorporates cognitive-behavioral, family, and humanistic concepts.

Creative arts therapists, play therapists, and expressive therapists often use CBT in combination with their approaches, but creative interventions themselves have not yet been extensively studied to determine if they qualify as evidence-based practices in the field of trauma intervention with children. Limited research studies that demonstrate their effectiveness with other disorders and populations exist, and there is a rapidly growing interest in producing more outcome studies of expressive therapies in general. TF-CBT lists the use of "artistic narrative" within its protocol, indicating that art and play approaches may be applied during this particular evidence-based intervention.

Gil (2006) makes an important point in reference to current evidence-based practices in trauma intervention and the use of art and play within their protocols. Like evidence-based approaches, creative arts therapies and expressive therapies both employ gradual exposure and work with affective material related to traumatic experiences. Gil (2006) notes that, unlike in models such as TF-CBT that have a specific agenda and set of instructions, in creative arts and expressive therapies, expressive activities "are initiated by children or facilitated by clinicians and employed at their pace, within the context of a therapy relationship, and with respect for children's need to utilize their defensive mechanisms in a fluid fashion" (p. 102). In other words, children are allowed to set their own pace for self-expression through play and art, depending on needs for adaptive coping, the nature of the trauma, temperament, cultural diversity, and other factors. Creative approaches may be less likely to be evaluated because they include both nondirective (spontaneous or authentic self-expression) and directive (specific activities) approaches. Nevertheless, therapists who use these methods should regularly review the available literature on evidence-based practice (see Resources at the end of this chapter).

"Best practices" in creative arts therapies have been identified in an effort to establish which methods show promise and demonstrate reliable outcomes when compared to other treatments. Best practices are different from evidence-based practices in that they are derived from clinical data from practitioners about particular applications or commonly used protocols within a discipline. Evidence-based practices are the result of research studies that include both experimental and control groups and, often, multiple trials. Because creative approaches stimulate sensory parts of the brain and its memories, creative arts therapists and play therapists are providing emerging data that indicates that best practices, in part, are found in the use of creative approaches as methods of nonverbal processing. Collie, Backos, Malchiodi, and Spiegel (2006) reviewed art therapy interventions for posttraumatic stress disorder (PTSD) to determine best practices and found that art therapy techniques emphasized the provision of psychological safety through specific techniques, stress reduction, and opportunities for nonverbal expression and processing of trauma narratives through art. They emphasize the importance of contemporary knowledge of how trauma affects individuals, current definitions of PTSD symptoms, and advanced training in the use of art therapy with stress-related disorders as part of overall best practices.

CULTURALLY SENSITIVE
CREATIVE INTERVENTION

Sue and Sue (2002) define "cultural competence" as the recognition of individuals' cultures and the development of skills, knowledge, and procedures in order to provide effective services to those individuals. In trauma intervention with children, cultural competence includes knowledge of how culture may affect trauma in young clients, based on a variety of factors including, but not limited to: ethnicity; degree of acculturation; location (rural or urban); regionalization (e.g., northern or southern United States); family, extended family, and peers; socioeconomic status (SES); gender; development; and religious or spiritual affiliation. The National Child Traumatic Stress Network (NCTSN) (2006) cites "cultural identity"—the culture with which someone identifies and looks to for accepted standards of behavior—as a factor in the treatment of childhood trauma. The NCTSN (2005) underscores that children and adolescents from minority backgrounds are at "increased risk for trauma exposure" (p. 1). Disasters also pose risks for children of ethnic minorities and in developing countries because of socioeconomic and political conditions, increasing the likelihood of more severe symptoms. In brief, many aspects come together to determine children's worldviews and preferences for participation and disclosure in therapy.

In brief, therapists using culturally sensitive creative methods in trauma treatment consider how children appraise their experiences and cope with events, including biological, psychological, social, and cultural perspectives. They also consider developmental aspects and children's capacity and preference for creative expression as intervention. Finally, therapists evaluate child clients for risk and resilience (see Chapter 14 for more information) in choosing activities and goals and base their choices on cultural aspects.

Diversity and worldview influence how children perceive toys, props, and play, depending on cultural background or experiences. Gil and Drewes (2005) provide one of the few comprehensive overviews of how culture specifically affects children's play within therapy, including a chapter on art therapy. They note that there are some obvious ways that therapists who use play activities, toys, and props can enhance intervention with attention to diversity issues. They underscore that therapists serious about using play in treatment should maintain an organized collection of toys and props that are developmentally, gender, and culturally diverse. For example, toy animals differ among cultures, so it is important to provide figures that are typical to many different cultures and that have distinctive cultural meanings. Similarly, books, dolls, games, and props should take diversity issues into consideration. Kao (2005) notes that the most traditional and preferred toys in Asian cultures actually fall into five distinct categories: social, intellectual, seasonal, physical, and gambling.

Therapists should have on hand art materials that support and nurture creativity with children of various cultures, such as crayons, felt-tip markers, and clay in a range of tones that approximate different skin colors. Photo collage materials should reflect a variety of crosscultural images, including ethnicity, families, lifestyles, and beliefs. Craft materials such as fabric, yarn, beads, or other objects may be helpful in stimulating some children whose experiences with art evolved around fabric decoration, jewelry making, or traditional needle arts.

Generally, children's self-expression is influenced by what they are exposed to in their communities, particularly by the media (Malchiodi, 1998a, 2005). Television, movies, video games, computers, and print material are an extremely important element of culture that has a powerful and often direct impact on children's view of themselves (Villani, 2001). Exposure to media is one of the strongest sources of images and stories, and children adopt those images and stories that have had a significant impact on them. One of the most memorable examples in recent years involves the events of September 11, 2001; any child who saw the repeated footage of the planes hitting the World Trade Center buildings reenacted that image in drawings and play activities for weeks, months, and, in the case of those most severely affected through traumatic loss, years (Malchiodi, 2002). In addition to significant events, television, movies, and the Internet are powerful influences on children's adoption of clothing and fashion as well as language, behaviors, and worldviews. These influences are recognizable in children's drawings that reference cartoon characters, popular film or music stars, or movie, television, or video game plots; older children and adolescents may include cultural conventions from peer groups such as graffiti, gang symbols, or tattoo art (Riley, 1999).

In providing culturally sensitive creative intervention, therapists must be flexible in how they initiate creative expression as therapy with children. Art, music, movement, and play provide a means of communication that bypasses language to some extent, and in situations where verbal communication is difficult, the use of creative approaches may be preferable; however, this does not automatically mean any method or activity is culturally appropriate in all cases. In fact, creative approaches have not been sufficiently examined within a cultural framework. Mental health professionals who use these approaches with children must continually appraise how culture may impact clinical applications of creative arts therapies and expressive therapies with traumatized clients.

Many cultures expect individuals to contain and regulate their feelings, implying that sharing emotions or personal experiences is a sign of immaturity. For example, for some children, a nondirective approach ("draw anything you want to" or "improvise a movement from your imagination") may be threatening, perceived as intrusive, or counterproductive to developing trust and establishing a safe, comfortable environment for creative expression. Children may prefer the security of copying images or the familiarity of learning dance steps, practicing a song, or hearing a story to creating something original, particularly if their cultural identity dictates the former as the preferred way to experience art, music, or dance. This should be accepted and understood as part of who the child is because it may recall positive memories of success or high self-esteem in children.

Therapists must also be especially sensitive to the preferences, values, and worldviews of parents, caregivers, and family of child clients when employing creative approaches. For example, parents of school-age children may question the use of play, toys, art, or props, questioning or misunderstanding free expression as a technique to help ameliorate traumatic symptoms. Adult family members may not fully comprehend why play or art is being used as a primary method, may see the use of these modalities as frivolous or unproven, or simply be uncomfortable with creative interventions because of personal or cultural reasons. Families often want to know that their children will get some immediate benefits or may even see the therapist as ineffective if there is not immediate change in their children or solutions to their children's emotional distress. Because children's parents or caregivers are usually involved in the treatment of their children's trauma symptoms, culturally sensitive therapists help them understand the creative interventions that will be used. Therapists should be sure to ask parents or caregivers what indicators of change they expect to see in their children, respecting their opinions and views about the content and desired outcome of intervention. In brief, all children and their families want to be treated with respect, to know that their concerns and preferences are heard, and to feel their opinions are important, valued, and accepted when their children participate in any therapy, including creative approaches.

POSTTRAUMATIC PLAY

Rosa was 7 years old when she, her mother, and a younger brother arrived at a shelter for battered women and their children. Rosa's mother, Tasha, had been only 15 years old when she gave birth to Rosa, and Rosa's biological father abandoned them at that time. For the next 7 years, Rosa lived in public housing in a large midwestern city in an environment regrettably dominated by drug abuse, neighborhood violence, and poverty. In addition, Tasha and Rosa were often physically abused by various boyfriends Tasha brought into the home; reports made to child protective services indicated that Rosa was sexually abused on several occasions, but the details and types of abuse remained unclear. Social services and law enforcement documented numerous incidents of domestic violence to Rosa and her mother, and in each case Rosa became both a child witness and a victim of physical brutality.

When Rosa was 5 years old, her mother could no longer afford to pay rent, and they became homeless. Rosa's life was chaotic and nomadic during her first years in elementary school, limiting her attendance at school to only a few months each year. Tasha gave birth to a son whose biological father also abandoned the family, adding to the stress of continued poverty, homelessness, domestic violence, and abandonment. During this time, Rosa became increasingly anxious, withdrawn, and preoccupied. Fortunately, Tasha realized that she could no longer manage her family's situation by herself, called a domestic violence help line, and was taken to a local shelter.

While Rosa received some limited intervention from school counselors, she did not obtain the type of regular treatment needed to ameliorate the effects of the multiple traumatic events she had experienced. She now exhibited many of the classic signs of PTSD, including avoidance, hyperarousal, and recurrent memories of multiple abuses to herself and her mother. She could no longer sleep through the night, had frequent nightmares, and developed phobias of school because she feared separation from her mother. The birth of her brother exacerbated the stress she experienced, and she became increasingly aggressive when her mother directed her attention to her sibling and away from Rosa.

Like many children who have encountered multiple traumas, Rosa presented a repetitive narrative in her art and play during early therapy sessions. Over the course of several meetings, Rosa related the following story in drawings and spontaneous narrative:

> "A little girl is being hurt by a man who hits her with a baseball bat and sometimes his hands. He hurts the mother, too. The mother and the little girl try to run. He keeps hurting them with the bat. He hits the little girl really hard and hurts her face. There is blood on the mother. They get into the bathroom and close the door [Figure 2.1]. The little girl is real afraid that the man will get in. The little girl's face is hurt and there is blood [Figure 2.2]. The mother takes the little girl to the hospital and she gets a bandage put on. She is still real afraid."

I am __9__ years old and in the __3__ grade.

I was __9__ years old when __I was hurt__.

This is a picture of me:

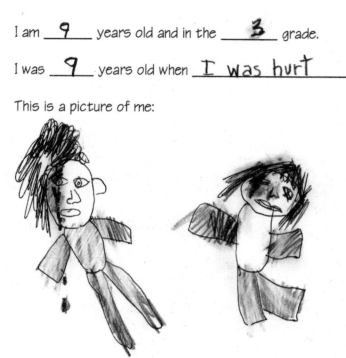

FIGURE 2.1. Rosa's drawing of "what happened" to a "little girl" and her mother during domestic violence.

Rosa spontaneously related an important personal story about "what happened" through her artwork, but she is not getting relief from telling her story through art and play. Like many children who are affected by significant traumatic experiences, Rosa often reexperiences these events through repetitive and intrusive thoughts. She also reenacts the traumatic events through art expression or play (Scheeringa, Zeanah, Drell, & Larrieu, 1995); in Rosa's case, the story is specific to events she experienced, but for other children these themes can be nonspecific and symbolically related to traumatic events. For example, children who survived Hurricane Katrina in the Gulf Coast region of the United States created miniature towns inundated by rising floodwaters in sandplay with toy figures, while others constructed sandtrays with monster themes or battle scenes.

The term "posttraumatic play" is used to describe both the recurrent memories and the reenactment common to children who are distressed by single-incident or chronic traumas. Terr (1979, 1990) first used the term to describe the play activity of children who have experienced traumatic events but not resolution of the emotions associated with those events. In contrast to normal play, which leads to pleasure, satisfying expression, problem solving, and learning, posttraumatic play is often anxiety-ridden and constricted, repetitive, rigid, and without resolution. For example, a child may consistently attempt to destroy a toy house, repeatedly saying, "House goes boom," to describe the devastation experienced during a tornado. For the child engaged in this type of play, mastery over the event is not possible, and emo-

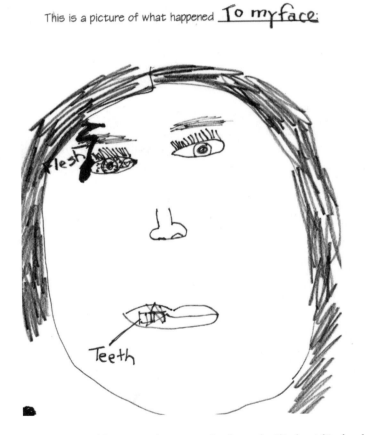

FIGURE 2.2. Rosa's self-portrait depicting the face of a "little girl" after being hurt.

tional relief from play is unavailable. During the first several weeks of treatment, Rosa unproductively repeated the story of a particularly brutal incident of domestic violence involving physical abuse and terror without receiving needed relief from her fears and anxiety. It also conveyed her hopelessness and lack of belief in rescue and resolution of her situation; in Rosa's initial art expressions, no one is able to save her mother and her from "hurt" and "blood." At this stage of intervention, it is important for Rosa to communicate what happened and her feelings about it, but her art expression is stagnant, stuck, and unproductive in finding solutions to her trauma experiences, without hope of support from caregivers or other adults.

Gil (2006) provides an excellent summary (see Table 2.1) of the differences between "stagnant posttraumatic play" and what she defines as "dynamic posttraumatic play." According to Gil, dynamic posttraumatic play addresses and resolves traumatic material, as opposed to the stagnant version that may leave the child retrauma-

TABLE 2.1. Differences between Dynamic and Stagnant Posttraumatic Play

Dynamic posttraumatic play	Stagnant posttraumatic play
• Affect becomes available.	• Affect remains constricted.
• Physical fluidity becomes evident.	• Physical constriction remains.
• Interactions with play become varied.	• Interactions with play remain limited.
• Interactions with clinician become varied.	• Interactions with clinician remain limited.
• Play changes, or new elements are added.	• Play stays precisely the same.
• Play occurs in different locations.	• Play is conducted in same spot.
• Play includes new objects.	• Play is limited to specific objects.
• Themes differ or expand.	• Themes remain constant.
• Outcomes differ, and healthier, more adaptive responses emerge.	• Outcomes remain fixed and nonadaptive.
• Rigidity of play loosens over time.	• Play remains rigid.
• After-play behavior indicates release or fatigue.	• After-play behavior indicates constriction/tension.
• Out-of-session symptoms may remain unchanged or peak at first, but then decrease.	• Out-of-season symptoms are unchanged or increase.

Note. From Gil (2006, p. 160). Copyright 2006 by The Guilford Press. Reprinted by permission.

tized or feeling hopeless and helpless. In brief, children who engage in dynamic posttraumatic play are less rigid, interact more freely with the therapist, take a more active role on their own behalf, and are generally more emotionally relieved by the experience. The differences between the two types of play are subtle but discernible with careful observation over time. These differences are important to all therapists who observe traumatized children's play, art, or other expressive work because, as Gil notes, the lack of positive resolution is a signal that a child needs appropriate clinical intervention.

Because play encompasses a number of forms of self-expression, including movement, dramatic enactment, and storytelling, therapists should have a solid understanding of what differentiates posttraumatic play from healthy play activity. Art expressions, too, may be rigid and repetitive and contain unresolved narratives about trauma. In all cases, the challenge is how to help children find corrective, self-soothing, and productive experiences through creative approaches. Creative activity in and of itself does not necessarily lead to positive resolution, no matter how carefully selected. Therapists should be prepared to make both appropriate creative and verbal interventions to assist children in this process; the goal is to facilitate play and other expression that helps children explore feelings and experiences but does not reinforce traumatic memories. This process includes actively helping children transform these memories, providing creative activities to enhance relaxation, teaching children self-soothing, and assisting children in finding solutions and reframing traumatic stories.

SENSORY-BASED METHODS

As discussed in Chapter 1, creative approaches are sensory-based methods because they use tactile, auditory, visual, and kinesthetic experiences for the purpose of nonverbal processing. These experiences can assist individuals in expressing sensory aspects of traumatic experiences, help reduce hyperarousal through stress reduction, and may be useful in bridging declarative and nondeclarative memories. In using these approaches, therapists face the challenge of employing art, play, music, movement, stories, and dramatic enactment in treatment both to ease trauma-related symptoms and to facilitate the expression and resolution of trauma narratives.

In order to be effective, therapists should have a clear understanding of why and how creative approaches support sensory work with children. For example, creative arts therapies can be useful in helping children recognize body reactions to stress and trauma-related memories. Asking a child to indicate through color, shapes, and lines on a body outline "where you feel the fear/worry/anger/sadness in your body" begins the process of identifying how the child reacts to an intrusive memory or distressing event. Similarly, a child could be asked to use sound or a musical instrument to communicate a feeling or express it through movement. Therapists serve as facilitators of self-expression and, more important, as entities who encourage children to use creative methods to transform fear, worry, anger, and sadness, helping them identify their own healing responses through sensory experiences. Because this sensory work with children is both directive and nondirective, therapists should be ready to face the challenge of trauma intervention with both flexibility and sensitivity to application of media.

Because trauma-related symptoms may include intrusive memories, anxiety, and hyperarousal, which can be psychologically paralyzing for some individuals, helping young clients take small steps toward expression of feelings and experiences is a necessary skill. Rothchild (2000) refers to this as "titration," a process of helping individuals release distressing emotions, memories, and thoughts in small amounts. Rothchild compares titration to shaking up a bottle of soda and then carefully unscrewing the top to slowly release the contents. If done correctly, only a small fizz is heard and no liquid escapes the bottle; however, if the top is removed too quickly, the contents of the bottle will explode. Rothchild's metaphor effectively demonstrates that therapists must consistently provide interventions that help their clients safely release troubling feelings and memories at an appropriate pace.

In using creative approaches, titration involves an understanding of materials, props, toys, stories, music, and movement and how to modulate their use, depending on children's needs and degree of symptoms. In particular, it is important to know that a material, prop, or method can be productive (leading to self-soothing, affect regulation, or corrective experiences) or nonproductive (leading to distress). For example, large paper and watery paint can provide an experience of free play and expression but may not be appropriate for some traumatized children who need structure, safety, and consistency. In using music or sound, it is important to understand how rhythm, affect, and content may influence the pace of a session, promote relaxation, or stimulate positive emotions. Similarly, toys and props should be selected for specific purpose, based on knowledge of how children who have been traumatized may react. If therapists have not had experience with and preparation in the creative methods they plan to use, they may not be able to appropriately and gradually assist children in finding relief and recovery.

Expressive methods can and do stimulate the flow of traumatic memories, either in the form of trauma narratives (stories about the event) or implicit experiences (sensory memories of the event) because of the tactile, kinesthetic, auditory, olfactory, or visual aspects inherent to creative activities. For example, in an art therapy group of four children from the same family, the youngest child, age 6 years, attempted to clean his brush in a plastic water jar and accidentally knocked it over, spilling water everywhere. At that moment, he froze, intensely watching the therapist for a reaction. In the same moment, two of the children jumped from their seats and ran to the door. The fourth child hid beneath the table, becoming silent and watchful. The children reacted to the sights and sounds of the water spilling just as they would if someone accidentally spilled milk at their dining table at home. The spilled water jar triggered implicit memories of fear, anxiety, and responses including hypervigilance, escape routines, and other physical strategies for survival (such as hiding under the table or running for the door). In this family, each child had developed automatic reactions for survival when threatened by the possibility of retaliation from an adult who was verbally and physically abusive.

Creative expression can also become a way to rehearse positive experiences of safety, stability, attachment, and self-esteem. Many children, if given a safe environment and opportunity, will intuitively use creative expression for pleasure and to self-soothe. Some children may find relief through cuddly toys (tactile); some through brightly colored tissue paper, glitter, and paints (visual); and others may respond positively to dance or movement (kinesthetic) or making or listening to music (auditory). In other situations, therapists may use directive approaches to help children have positive experiences through self-expression. For example, an activity such as creating a safe place for an animal (Malchiodi, 1998b), in which children select or are given small plastic or soft toy animals and are encouraged to use a box or other materials to make a place where the animal feels safe and has all its needs met. Through imaginative caretaking of the toy animal and constructing a safe place for it, issues of protection and nurturance can be explored and practiced in a tangible, sensory way with help and prompting from the therapist if needed.

Finally, the sensory nature of creative approaches can evoke self-soothing experiences common to childhood—rhythmic movements and sounds, tactile and visual pleasure, and imagination and fantasy. Imagination and fantasy are the first adaptive coping strategies children have available to them, especially during preschool years. By using imagination, children can formulate a more appealing narrative for what has happened or divert themselves from it momentarily. Art making, play, drama, music, stories, and movement allow children to escape their fears, worries, and sadness, if only during the time they are engrossed in an activity. The experience of losing oneself in a pleasurable activity can induce feelings of relaxation and self-satisfaction and reinforce positive sensations, but, as described in the previous section on posttraumatic play, becoming engrossed in an activity in a nonproductive, rigid way that leads to feeling worse afterwards is not helpful to children over time. In providing activities to traumatized children, therapists are consistently challenged to observe their young clients' responses to expressive interventions and to reevaluate whether these interventions and are providing the sensory experiences necessary for emotional restoration, resolution, and eventual recovery.

CONCLUSIONS

Therapists with an understanding of ethical, evidence-based, and culturally sensitive creative approaches are in a unique position to do effective and rewarding work with traumatized children. Therapists who use creative approaches also must continually learn how to recognize posttraumatic play, art, and other similar expressions and to capitalize on sensory aspects of creative arts and expressive therapies in treatment. Learning these concepts is an ongoing process that forms the foundation of successful and effective creative intervention and advances the range of therapeutic skills that professionals can offer their child clients.

REFERENCES

Cohen, J., Mannarino, A., & Deblinger, E. (2006). *Treating trauma and traumatic grief in children and adolescents*. New York: Guilford Press.

Collie, K., Backos, A., Malchiodi, C., & Spiegel, D. (2006). Art therapy for combat-related PTSD: Recommendations for research and practice. *Art Therapy: Journal of the American Art Therapy Association, 23*(4), 157–164.

Gil, E. (2006). *Helping abused and traumatized children: Integrating directive and nondirective approaches*. New York: Guilford Press.

Gil, E., & Drewes, A. (Eds.). (2005). *Cultural issues in play therapy*. New York: Guilford Press.

Hoagland, K., Burns, B., Kiser, L., Ringeisen, H., & Schoenwald, S. (2001). Evidence-based practice in child and adolescent mental health services. *Psychiatric Services, 52*(9), 1179–1189.

Kao, S. C. (2005). In E. Gil & A. Drewes (Eds.), *Cultural issues in play therapy* (pp. 180–194). New York: Guilford Press.

Knill, P., Barba, H., & Fuchs, M. (2004). *Minstrels of the soul*. Toronto: EGS Press.

Malchiodi, C. (1998a). *Understanding children's drawings*. New York: Guilford Press.

Malchiodi, C. (1998b). *The art therapy sourcebook*. New York: McGraw-Hill.

Malchiodi, C. (2002). Editorial. *Trauma and Loss: Research and Interventions, 2*(1), 4.

Malchiodi, C. (2005). The impact of culture on art therapy with children. In E. Gil & A. Drewes (Eds.), *Cultural issues in play therapy* (pp. 96–111). New York: Guilford Press.

National Child Traumatic Stress Network. (2005). *Culture and trauma brief: Promoting culturally competent trauma-informed practice*. Durham, NC: National Child Traumatic Stress Initiative.

National Child Traumatic Stress Network. (2006). *Culture and trauma brief: NCTSN resources on culture and trauma*. Durham, NC: National Child Traumatic Stress Initiative.

Reinecke, M., Dattilio, F., & Freeman, A. (Eds.). (2003). *Cognitive therapy with children and adolescents: A casebook for clinical practice* (2nd ed.). New York: Guilford Press.

Riley, S. (1999). *Contemporary art therapy with adolescents*. London: Jessica Kingsley.

Rothchild, B. (2000). *The body remembers*. New York: Norton.

Scheeringa, M., Zeanah, C., Drell, M., & Larrieu, J. (1995). Two approaches to the diagnosis of posttraumatic stress disorder in infancy and early childhood. *American Academy of Child and Adolescent Psychiatry, 34*(2), 191–200.

Sprunk, T. P., Mitchell, J., Myrow, D., & O'Connor, K. (2007). *Paper on touch: Clinical, professional, and ethical issues.* Retrieved February 16, 2007, from *www.a4pt.org/download.cfm?ID=9971.*

Sue, D. W., & Sue, D. (2002). *Counseling the culturally diverse: Theory and practice* (4th ed.). New York: Wiley.

Terr, L. (1979). Children of Chowchilla. *Psychoanalytic Study of the Child, 34,* 547–623.

Terr, L. (1990). Childhood trauma—An outline and overview. *American Journal of Psychiatry, 148,* 10–20.

Villani, S. (2001). The impact of media on children and adolescents: A 10-year review of research. *Journal of the American Academy of Child and Adolescent Psychiatry, 40*(4), 392–400.

RESOURCES ON EVIDENCE-BASED PRACTICES

California Evidence-Based Clearinghouse for Child Welfare
www.cachildwelfareclearinghouse.org

Campbell Collaboration
www.campbellcollaboration.org/index.html.

Cochrane Collaboration
www.cochrane.org/index0.htm

National Registry of Evidence-Based Programs and Practices
modelprograms.samhsa.gov/template.cfm?page=nreppover

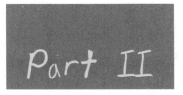

CREATIVE INTERVENTIONS
WITH INDIVIDUALS

Chapter 3

Expressive Therapy for Severe Maltreatment and Attachment Disorders
A Neuroscience Framework

P. Gussie Klorer

Recent developments in neuroscience provide important information for therapists working with maltreated children. Severe maltreatment and lack of significant attachment figures in the crucial early years lead to adverse brain development (Bremner, 2001; Chugani et al., 2002; De Bellis, 2001; De Bellis et al., 1999; Perry, 1997; Rutter & O'Connor, 2004). It appears evident that traumatic memories are stored in the right hemisphere, making verbal declarative memory of the trauma more difficult (Glaser, 2000; Rauch et al., 1996; Schiffer, 2000; Schiffer, Teicher, & Papanicolaou, 1995). This research lays the groundwork for understanding why nonverbal, expressive therapies can be more effective than verbal therapies in work with severely maltreated children exhibiting attachment difficulties. This chapter explores current research in neuroscience and provides a rationale for expressive therapy as a treatment intervention for this population.

DEFINITION OF TERMS

Defining severe maltreatment is not an easy task. When child abuse is reported, there has been an indicator that a child is being or has been abused in the eyes of the person reporting it. In order for abuse to be substantiated, there must be physical evidence, reliable witnesses, and/ or disclosure by the child. If the report is substantiated and the child is referred for treatment, the treatment focus may need to go much deeper than the initial sign of abuse that brought the child to the attention of authorities. For example, Erin's black eye, which initiated an investigation, will heal, but it is nothing compared to the emotional effects of Erin not being fed and being forced to sleep on the floor of a closet amid urine-soaked clothes, waiting for someone to free her from imprisonment. Erin will not readily talk about this. Children rarely talk about experiencing severe maltreatment, especially when it is inflicted upon them by the person on whom they rely to meet their basic needs. Much more often, we see children protecting the abusive parent and longing to return home if placed with a foster family. Erin is not talking and cries for her mother. When a child is not talking, ascertaining when he or she has been severely maltreated is difficult.

A special issue of *Child Maltreatment* defined severely maltreated children as those who display behaviors suggesting severe disturbance, even if their reported maltreatment does not seem severe, because the extent of what these children have experienced may be unknown. It also includes those children who have experienced forms of maltreatment that are likely to result in severe disturbance, even if that disturbance is not evident behaviorally, because research shows that consequences may emerge later (Haugaard, 2004). Severe maltreatment can be characterized as chronic, involves considerable pain, is physically invasive, or causes the child to fear death or permanent injury (Haugaard, 2004; Saywitz, Mannarino, Berliner, & Cohen, 2000).

Defining attachment difficulties is also hard. According to the American Psychiatric Association's (2000) *Diagnostic and Statistical Manual of Mental Disorders* (DSM-IV-TR), the diagnosis of reactive attachment disorder includes evidence of pathogenic care and persistent disregard of the child's basic physical or emotional needs, as well as criteria of disturbed and developmentally inappropriate social relatedness, beginning before 5 years of age. The inhibited type is described as a failure to initiate or respond appropriately in social interactions, and the disinhibited type is characterized by a failure or inability to discriminate in social interactions (American Psychiatric Association, 2000). As with defining severe maltreatment, evidence of pathogenic care prior to age 5 may be difficult to obtain because often the child's history is unknown (Hanson, 2002; Hanson & Spratt, 2000).

For the sake of this chapter, attachment difficulties will include the entire range of attachment problems, not just the diagnosis of reactive attachment disorder, because children are so often misdiagnosed and the diagnosis can and does change throughout the course of treatment. Behavior patterns of poorly attached children include a lack of joy, humor, reciprocal enjoyment, eye contact, empathy, guilt/remorse, appropriate communication, appropriate physical boundaries, and demonstration of indiscriminate relationships (Hughes, 1998).

NORMAL BRAIN DEVELOPMENT

Before looking at what happens to the brain in situations of long-term exposure to trauma, it is useful to see what happens in normal brain development. The human brain during the early years of life is dependent upon both genetic information and proper external stimulation. During the first 2 years, the basic circuits of the brain are being established (Balbernie, 2001; De Bellis, 2001; Schore, 2002). "Neuroplasticity" is the brain's ability to change its structure in response to environmental stimuli. When a baby is born, about 100 billion neurons are present in its brain, although they are not all functioning yet. Those that are not used become disabled, and those that become part of neuropathways thrive. A "synapse" is the electrical impulse that crosses between connecting neurons, creating neuropathways. When a neuropathway of synapses is stimulated, then all the synapses become engaged and store a chemical pattern, which, if repeated, becomes strong enough to be a permanent circuit (Balbernie, 2001). The child's brain develops in a "use-dependent" fashion, meaning that the more any neural system is activated, the more likely it is to become permanent (Perry, Pollard, Blakley, Baker, & Vigilante, 1995). There are crucial windows of opportunity for development of certain parts of the brain that, if not activated, will wither. Other areas may be amenable to rewiring later, after the crucial period has passed. Balbernie (2001) writes: "The regions of the cortex that play an operational part in hearing and sight can be permanently compromised if some biological, or even social, condition has deprived them of normal input early on in life. The neural circuits for language and emotion retain (reducing) plasticity for most of childhood" (p. 241). For example, when an infant is spoken to, the neural system responsible for speech and language is activated, which helps the child develop the capacity for language. By contrast, when a child is in an environment where he or she is not spoken to, he or she will develop language more slowly and may have communication delays because those parts of the brain were not stimulated at a crucial developmental stage (Perry, 2001).

The relationship between external stimulation and the development of the brain is increasingly recognized as reciprocal, as both animal and human studies show. For example, when a kitten's eye was artificially closed at birth, the kitten did not develop sight in that eye. When researchers subsequently looked at the kitten's brain to study the area that governs sight, it was found to be underdeveloped (Baer & Rittenhouse, 1999; Wiesel & Hubel, 1963, 1965).

Schore (2001) postulates that the emotional communications of the attachment between the primary caregiver and the infant directly impact the experience-dependent maturation of the infant's developing brain. The neuropathways that are reinforced in the baby's brain are selected by the quality and content of the emotional surroundings within the caregiving/attachment relationship (Balbernie, 2001). The mother–child bond is crucial to both psychological and physiological development. Schore (2001, 2002) describes the neurobiology of a secure attachment: In order to enter into the bond of communication, the mother must be psychobiologically attuned to the infant. Each partner in this dyad learns the emotional rhythm of the other. In moments of affect synchrony, the pair is in affective resonance and is like a single biological unit. After moments of stress for the child, the mother invokes a reattunement, which helps regulate the child's negative state. When the child is living in a secure environment, the maternal interactions act as an external organizer of the child's biobehavioral regulation (Schore, 2002). This stimulation helps the developing brain reach its potential.

Research shows that the right hemisphere of the brain is dominant in human infants until the age of 3. This is confirmed by positron emission tomography (PET) scans showing developmental changes in cerebral blood flow measured at rest. These changes appear to follow the emergence of functions localized initially on the right hemisphere (visuospatial) and later on the left hemisphere (language abilities) (Chiron et al., 1997). This research supports Schore's (2001) notion that the right hemisphere stores an internal working model of the initial attachment relationship that assists the child in developing strategies of affect regulation for coping and survival. Mahler (1979) talked about the child in rapproachement learning to tolerate the stress of the mother's absence through experimenting with leaving. The securely attached child learns to self-regulate the stress associated with separations and the fear that previously required the mother's physical presence and external regulation. This learning happens as a result of practicing, as Mahler noted, but new research shows that it is also a result of neurophysiological development. The early relationship helps stimulate the connections in the brain that form the neuropathways for growth.

BRAIN DEVELOPMENT IN POORLY ATTACHED OR TRAUMATIZED CHILDREN

Neuropsychiatrists today are providing solid scientific evidence of theories developed 30 years ago by Bowlby (1969) and Mahler (Mahler, Pine, & Bergman, 1975) regarding attachment theory and object relations. According to Schore (2002), traumatic attachment histories affect the development of frontolimbic regions of the brain, especially the right cortical areas that are prospectively involved in affect-regulating functions. Evidence shows that early relational trauma is expressed in right-brain hemispheric deficits in the processing of social–emotional and bodily information. If the optimal conditions for brain development include a secure attachment figure who provides external stimulation and emotional connections, what happens when a child is raised in an environment where this figure is lacking? Unfortunately, there have been opportunities to examine this question through studies of Romanian orphans.

In the 1980s a number of Romanian orphans who were brought to the United States and the United Kingdom and adopted began exhibiting serious behavioral, cognitive, and attachment problems. One report states that more than 100,000 children throughout Romania were warehoused in situations with minimal food, heat, or clothing, with few caregivers for many children (Kaler & Freeman, 1994). The staff did not provide stimulation or personal attention for the children, even during activities that would normally involve contact, such as feeding. Instead of being held, children were propped up in their beds with their bottles (Beckett et al., 2002). Loving adoptive families who believed that a change in the child's environment was all that was needed were frequently surprised to find that both the behaviors and the remedies were much more complex. Behaviors associated with institutional experience and duration were noted in a study of 144 of these children and fell into three basic categories: inattention/overactivity, attachment difficulties, and quasi-autistic behavior. Specific behaviors included patterns of rocking, difficulties with chewing and swallowing, self-injury, and unusual sensory interests (Beckett et al., 2002).

A longitudinal study of Romanian orphans adopted at ages ranging from infancy to 3½ years and then followed up on at the ages of 4 and 6 revealed a close association between duration of deprivation and severity of attachment disorder behaviors, which were correlated with attention and conduct problems and cognitive level (O'Connor, Rutter, & English and Romanian Adoptees Study Team, 2000). There was no evidence of a decrease in attachment disorder behavior over a 2-year period. The researchers found that these problems were not related to nutritional deprivation. Half of the total group of Romanian adoptees had a weight below the third percentile at the time of adoption, but weight was normal or nearly normal by the age of 6 for most. Head circumference was a different matter. Even for those without severe malnutrition at the time of adoption, head circumference at age 6 was still about 1½ standard deviations below the general population mean. With respect to cognitive impairment, this study found that subnutrition and a small head circumference both point to the likelihood of abnormal brain development, as brain growth largely determines head size (Rutter & O'Connor, 2004).

The authors provide several hypotheses, among them that an institutional environment such as the Romanian orphanages falls outside the range of what is necessary for normal brain development with respect to the neural systems underlying social relationships (Rutter & O'Connor, 2004). They further point out that when numerous caregivers come and go and cannot be relied upon for relationships and interaction, it may be adaptive for children to seek interactions in a nonselective way.

Chugani and colleagues (2002) applied functional neuroimaging with PET in a group of adopted Romanian children. The 10 children, all over the age of 6, had been placed in the orphanages at approximately 4–6 weeks of age and resided there for a mean of 38 months before being adopted by U.S. families. The neuropsychological assessment showed the adoptees as having mild neurocognitive impairment, impulsivity, and attention and social deficits. Distinct abnormalities were found in various areas of the brain connected with emotion (Davies, 2002), and deficits in language processing, memory, and executive functioning were found, suggesting that the stress of early global deprivation is involved in long-term cognitive and behavioral deficits (Chugani et al., 2002).

Perry (1997) discovered that a lack of sensorimotor and cognitive experiences in a child's early years leads to underdevelopment of the cortex. The cortical and subcortical areas of the brain are smaller in individuals who have suffered "global environmental neglect," or children who were rarely touched, spoken to, or allowed to play with toys. Perry did brain-imaging studies and found "cortical atrophy" in 7 of 12 of the children studied. He discovered that these areas of the cortex were underused, resulting in profound underdevelopment of those areas of the brain that assist in inhibiting, modulating, and regulating the functioning of the lower parts of the central nervous system.

Perry's work is supported by others who have found that the overwhelming stress of child maltreatment is associated with adverse brain development. Using magnetic resonance imaging (MRI) technology, brain development in medically healthy clinically referred children with chronic posttraumatic stress disorder (PTSD) was compared with nontraumatized healthy controls who were case matched for age, handedness, sex, height, weight, and race (De Bellis, 2001; De Bellis et al., 1999). This group of maltreated children had smaller MRI-based brain structural measures of intracranial volume than did the nonabused controls. PTSD cluster symptoms of intrusive thoughts, avoidance, hyperarousal, or dissociation correlated negatively with intracranial volume. The study suggests neurobiological consequences of trauma. The earlier in childhood the abuse occurs, the more severe the effects on intracranial volume. Additionally, a negative correlation of intracranial volume with abuse duration suggests that childhood maltreatment may have a cumulative effect on brain development.

Bremner's work focuses on how changes in brain structures and systems mediating memory may offer reasons for delayed recall of child abuse in patients with abuse-related PTSD (Bremner, 2001). Through his study of both Vietnam War veterans and abuse victims, he found that patients with PTSD show changes in structure and function in brain regions mediating memory, including the hippocampus and medial prefrontal cortex, as well as brain chemical systems involved in stress response and retrieval of memories. In order to test the hypothesis that traumatic stress results in hippocampal damage in abuse victims, he used MRI to quantify hippocampal volume in survivors of child abuse with a diagnosis of PTSD, as compared to healthy subjects. Patients with abuse-related PTSD had left hippocampal volume 12% below the control group. Bremner (2001) hypothesizes that atrophy and dysfunction of the hippocampus following exposure to abuse leads to distortion and fragmentation of memories. These patients' difficulty talking about the abuse may be at least partially a function of changes in their brain structures.

Early trauma affects the child throughout his or her life. Studies of Vietnam War veterans with PTSD support the notion that child abuse may predispose soldiers to combat-related PTSD (Bremner, Southwick, Johnson, Yehuda, & Charney, 1993). A later study found that insecure attachment style classification was an even stronger predictor of PTSD in prisoners of war than was trauma severity (Dieperink, Leskela, Thuras, & Engdahl, 2001).

Does the smaller hippocampal volume seen in individuals with PTSD represent a preexisting condition that makes the brain more vulnerable to stress, or does early childhood trauma in fact cause smaller hippocampal volume? A study of twins explored this issue, with inconclusive results (Gilbertson et al., 2002). Hippocampal volumes of combat-exposed Vietnam War veterans (some with and some without PTSD) and their twins with no combat exposure were compared. Smaller hippocampal volume was found in trauma-exposed veterans with severe PTSD but also in their twin brothers. What was impossible to decipher was whether this finding represented heredity or shared environment. Although a preexisting familial vulnerability seemed likely, there was a nonsignificant trend for this group to share higher rates of childhood abuse. It appears that most studies do not infer a causal relationship between posttraumatic stress and hippocampal volume (Marko & Merckelbach, 2004). More studies in this area are needed.

HEMISPHERIC ASPECTS OF HOW TRAUMA IS STORED IN THE BRAIN

Sudies of the brain help us understand how traumatic memories are stored. Schiffer and colleagues (1995) measured hemispheric activity of the brain in subjects with a history of trauma while they thought about a neutral, work-related memory and then about an unpleasant early memory. The responses were compared with a control group (no known trauma) in which subjects recalled a neutral work-related situation. The trauma group showed significant left-dominant asymmetry during the neutral memory, which shifted markedly to the right during the unpleasant memory. This research implies that traumatic memories may be stored in the right cerebral hemisphere, which would make verbal declarative memory of the trauma more difficult.

Further work by Schiffer (2000) suggests that the two hemispheres of the brain can have distinct personalities, memories, and perspectives. His review of the split-brain studies and his own experiments with lateral visual stimulation in patients with trauma histories suggests that the "immature side maintains a perspective very similar and consistent with that which a child in troubled circumstances might be expected to experience" (p. 98). In a sense, Schiffer is suggesting that the traumatized child maintains those feelings and that identity in one side of the brain while the other side matures. Finding access to that troubled side may be instrumental in healing.

Other studies show that exposure to violence or trauma affects the developing brain by altering neurodevelopmental processes. Rauch and colleagues used PET scanning to study patients suffering from PTSD. When presented with vivid accounts of their own traumatic experiences, these individuals showed autonomic arousal and concomitant heightened activity in the right amygdala and associated areas of the temporal and frontal cortex, as well as in the right visual cortex. At the same time, the area concerned with language in the left hemisphere was "turned off." This evidence suggests that the tendency of patients with PTSD to reexperience emotions as physical states rather than as declarative verbal memories has a neurobiological explanation (Glaser, 2000; Rauch et al., 1996).

According to Munns (2000), the right hemisphere controls sensorimotor perception and integration, processes social–emotional input, and is dominant in the first 3 years of life. Memories of trauma and poor attachment experiences in the early years are processed in the right side of the brain. Munns states, "This suggests that since these experiences are processed and stored in a part of the brain that is preverbal or nonverbal, it makes sense to pay more attention to non-verbal methods of treatment (Schore, 1998) such as Theraplay, sand-play therapy, dance and movement therapy, touch therapy, eye move-ment therapy, nondirective play therapy, and others" (2000, p. 13).

CLINICAL IMPLICATIONS

Unfortunately, one does not have to go to a Romanian orphanage or look to Vietnam War veterans to study the effects of long-term trau-ma. The trauma histories of some children in the foster care system in the United States are akin to torture. Unlike the Romanian orphans, who were abandoned and neglected, these are children who were mal-treated by those who were supposed to be significant attachment fig-ures: parents, grandparents, guardians. Not only is there is a lack of attunement to the attachment figure, but the very person on whom the child must rely for safety is the person the child most fears. Although some children with histories such as these have a compul-sion to tell their story, more often they do not. Those for whom the abuse has gone on for a long time often *cannot*.

How can we understand and treat these clients more effectively with new developments in neuropsychiatry? What does this research tell us clinically? After 25 years working with severely maltreated chil-dren, I have come to believe that nonverbal expressive therapy approaches are highly effective interventions in working with this population because they do not rely on the client's use of the left brain and language for processing. Neuroscientists are helping us understand why this is so after many years of dutifully writing treatment goals and objectives that included talking about the abuse as a measure of prog-ress, only to discover that this treatment goal was rarely, if ever, met with children who had long-term exposure to severe maltreatment at an early age. According to Schiffer and colleagues (1995):

> Previous reports have suggested that early abuse may be associated with enduring neurobiological effects . . . early trauma may lead to a lack of integration of left–right hemisphere function, and we further speculate that traumatic memories may be preferentially stored in the right hemi-sphere. This hypothesis of deficient hemispheric integration and prefer-

ential right-sided storage of traumatic memories provides an interesting theoretical explanation for the fact that memory recollection following trauma can be both deficient (constricted or amnestic) and intrusive. (p. 174)

In children with histories of severe maltreatment and attachment difficulties, one has to wonder whether the child even has full access to the memories of trauma. The safety of the child is paramount, so pressing for disclosure in order to help substantiate an abuse allegation and provide a safety plan may be crucial in the early stages. Once the child is protected from further abuse, pressing him or her to talk may be counterproductive and countertherapeutic. This does not mean that the child should not be given an opportunity to approach and work through traumatic issues, but it makes sense to help the child use right-brain functions, where the trauma memories are stored, to express and work through issues of severe maltreatment in a way that supports the child's cognitive, developmental, and emotional levels.

CASE EXAMPLES

Two vignettes illustrate this point. Seven-year-old Peter was removed from his mother's home because of inappropriate discipline that included her spraying her children with mace and locking them in dog cages for many hours at a time. The children were also witnesses to and participants in multiple layers of incestuous behavior. Peter vehemently denied any abuse throughout several years of therapy. His art, however, revealed a different perception of the world and his home life. In his first art therapy session Peter was told that he could draw anything he wanted. "Anything?" he asked incredulously. After repeated assurances, he asked, "Can I draw the vampire that kills my mom?" Peter's medium of choice was sculpture, as he responded to the tactile nature of found objects and materials and manipulated them into structures that defined a world much different from the one he projected consciously. One day, Peter created a holiday living room scene, a diorama made from a cardboard box. He carefully added a braided rug, which he made from yarn, drew little pictures to hang on the walls, and created a Christmas tree in the corner of the room, festively decorated. He then added a chain to the tree, which was attached to the walls of the room, "so nobody can just come in and steal the tree." To the outside of the house he added scores of tooth-picks, protruding from the exterior walls in a way that appeared both aggressive and defensive. This, too, appeared to be a way to protect the tree inside the house. For a child such as Peter, articulating the pain of living in his own home was impossible, and many Christmasses had been "stolen" from him; this metaphor appeared to be a way that he could deal with the memories in his brain, both those he was willing to talk about and those that he could not.

The second case, Tammy, is an example of a child able to work through an incredibly complex array of maltreatment and attach-ment issues without ever having to talk about them. Unfortunately, Tammy's social history is not unlike that of many of the children in state custody. Tammy entered the foster care system and therapy at age 4, when she was removed from her mother's care due to severe abuse and neglect. During her subsequent 3 years of therapy, Tammy was placed in three different foster homes, one residential treatment cen-ter, and four day care centers and had a succession of three social workers. The only consistent person in her life was her therapist. Her various foster mothers complained that she sexually acted out, was physically aggressive with other children, and could not bond. Her diagnoses at age 4 were adjustment disorder with depressed mood and reactive attachment disorder (American Psychiatric Association, 2000).

Throughout her therapy, Tammy was never able to talk about the abuse she endured while in her mother's care. In fact, like many chil-dren in foster care, Tammy cried often because she wanted to see her mother. Talking about the bad things her mother did would have been a betrayal. Tammy was abused over a long period of time, and much of the abuse likely occurred at preverbal levels of development. Hence, the memories may not have had words associated with them, but rather were stored in nonverbal parts of the brain as physical and emo-tional sensations.

Tammy's therapy went through many stages over the course of 3 years (for a more detailed account of Tammy's story, refer to *Expressive Therapy with Troubled Children* [Klorer, 2000]). After about 2 years of therapy, Tammy's mother's rights were terminated due to her lack of followthrough on court orders, frequent incarcerations, drug use, and apparent lack of interest in even visiting her daughter. Tammy was moved into a preadoptive foster home, where her ambivalence about attachment was played out with her foster family as it played out in all of her relationships. When her foster parents disappointed her or set a limit for her, she cried inconsolably for her mother. The word "no" meant dissolution of all love in her eyes, and she would become distraught, tearful, and withdrawn when she heard it. Tammy wanted a family, yet she struggled with attaching to this family because she still longed for her mother. She was adamant that she did not want to be adopted because she was sure her mother was going to stop using drugs and come get her.

Two pieces of art stand out as significant of the intensity of the work she was doing expressively surrounding her attachment issues. One day Tammy announced that she wanted to make a sculpture of "a sister" in art therapy. Tammy had no sister in her biological or in her preadoptive family. The idea came up several times, and each time she would gather materials to reserve for this project, but she did not actually began assembling it until about 4 months after the idea emerged. When she was finally ready to begin the project, she pulled out the Styrofoam, cardboard boxes, doll hair, and other items she had reserved, and over the course of several weeks she constructed a life-sized doll. The therapist had no idea of the importance of this doll until Tammy's foster mother called to tell her what transpired once she brought the doll home. Tammy named her sister Tina, and Tina took on the roles that Tammy could not for fear of betraying her mother. Tina asked to sleep with the foster parents. Tina watched the foster mother work on the computer and cook dinner. Tina told the foster mother that she loved her.

Tammy could not betray her own mother by loving her foster parents, although she did love them. She was able to work toward some resolution of this dilemma through her art making. She created a self who could be affectionate without betraying her mother, a self who could express feelings that were too difficult for her to consciously acknowledge, a self who could say and do the things that she could not. Tammy was able to practice with Tina, try on a different role, and see what it felt like to be a full member of a family.

As Tammy became more comfortable with the possibility of adoption, she needed art again to help her resolve what to do with her feelings for her mother. One day she came into therapy and asked for a coffee can. She assembled a pair of scissors, glue, and white, pink, and blue paper. Tammy began cutting tiny pieces of white paper, about $\frac{1}{16}$ inch square, and dropping them into the can with much concentration and purpose. When asked what she was making, she announced,

"Ashes," as if that were the most natural thing in the world. "You know how when people die, they have something with ashes? That's what I want to make . . . . I'm making my mom's ashes." She then instructed the therapist to continue cutting tiny pieces of paper to fill the can, while she took on the more important job of decorating the can with pink and blue hearts and stars.

Tammy's mother had not died, but this was Tammy's way of conceptualizing the process of letting go that was necessary in order for her to move on with her own life. Through this art piece, Tammy symbolically mourned the loss of her mother. Several months later, Tammy was adopted, terminated therapy, and at last report continues to do very well.

DISCUSSION

How does this work? How is it that Tammy and Peter were able to approach their feelings in art but could not articulate them? Could this ability relate to the functions of the brain, to where trauma memories are stored and how they are stored? Could it be that Tammy and Peter had access to the feelings in the emotional centers of their brains, the right-brain functions, and therefore could express those feelings through art when they were impossible to put into words? Tammy was able to do the work necessary to move on in her emotional life without ever having to confront her issues directly. Art therapists see this over and over again; clients can express feelings through art before they can put into words what they are feeling. Ulman, a founder of art therapy, referred to art as "the meeting ground of the world inside and the world outside" (Ulman, 1975, p. 7). Perhaps it is also the means of integrating the inside and outside worlds. Along with art, the other nonverbal expressive therapies, such as movement, music, poetry, and drama, have the potential to lead people to long-forgotten emotions and feelings.

For true transformation to happen in expressive work with a severely maltreated child, it appears that expression has the most potential for therapy when it comes from the child and is not imposed by the therapist. Directives aimed at certain issues are not nearly as effective as what the client brings in terms of metaphor. The therapist cannot choreograph the work or be too directive in this kind of approach. Rather, the therapist provides the resources and creative environment so that the child can find his or her own curative path.

Today, a number of art therapy clinicians are looking to neuroscience for answers in their trauma work (Chapman, 2002; Gantt, Tinnin, & Tabone, 2002; Klorer & Chapman, 2004; Klorer & Malchiodi, 2003; Malchiodi, Kaplan, & Riley, 2002). Recent trends in conference presentations of the American Art Therapy Association suggest that practitioners of both eye movement desensitization and reprocessing (EMDR) and art therapy are seeing parallels between their processes (Chapman, 2003; Gruber, 2003; McNamee, 2003). Others are finding that the bridge between neuroscience and art therapy is becoming more pronounced (Henley, Kaplan, & Shore, 2003; Kaplan, 2000, 2004; Lusebrink, 2004; McNamee, 2004; Stewart, 2004). Two promising collaborations between art therapy and neuroscience are looking at electroencephalograph (EEG) recordings to understand what happens in the brain during and after art making (Belkofer & Konopka, 2003; Kruk, 2004). More such collaborations are needed. It is a marriage that supports the attachment theories so long believed to be true, and it will enhance therapeutic work with severely maltreated children.

ACKNOWLEDGMENT

This chapter is adapted from Klorer (2005). Copyright 2005 by American Art Therapy Association. Adapted by permission.

REFERENCES

American Psychiatric Association. (2000). *Diagnostic and statistical manual of mental disorders* (4th ed., text rev.). Washington, DC: Author.

Baer, M. F., & Rittenhouse, M. (1999). Molecular basis for induction of ocular dominance plasticity. *Journal of Neurobiology, 41,* 83–91.

Balbernie, R. (2001). Circuits and circumstances: The neurobiological consequences of early relationship experiences and how they shape later behavior. *Journal of Child Psychotherapy, 27*(3), 237–255.

Beckett, C., Bredenkamp, D., Castle, J., Groothues, C., O'Connor, T., Rutter, M., et al. (2002). Behavior patterns associated with institutional deprivation: A study of children adopted from Romania. *Journal of Developmental and Behavioral Pediatrics, 23*(5), 297–303.

Belkofer, C., & Konopka, L. (2003, November). *A new kind of wonder: EEG and art therapy research*. Paper presented at the American Art Therapy Association's 34th Annual Conference, Chicago, IL.

Bowlby, J. (1969). *Attachment* (2nd ed., Vol. 1). New York: Basic Books.

Bremner, J. D. (2001). A biological model for delayed recall of childhood abuse. *Journal of Aggression, Maltreatment and Trauma, 4*(2), 165–183.

Bremner, J. D., Southwick, S. M., Johnson, D. R., Yehuda, R., & Charney, D. S. (1993). Childhood physical abuse and combat-related posttraumatic stress disorder in Vietnam veterans. *American Journal of Psychiatry, 150*(2), 235–239.

Chapman, L. (2002, November). *A neuro-developmental approach to treating posttraumatic stress disorder and symptoms*. Paper presented at the American Art Therapy Association's 33rd Annual Conference, Washington, DC.

Chapman, L. (2003, November). *Neuro-developmental art therapy: Treating acute and chronic posttraumatic stress disorder and symptoms*. Paper presented at the American Art Therapy Association's 34th Annual Conference, Chicago, IL.

Chiron, C., Jambaque, I., Nabbout, R., Lounes, R., Syrota, A., & Dulac, O. (1997). The right brain hemisphere is dominant in human infants. *Brain, 120*(Part 6), 1057–1065.

Chugani, H. T., Behen, M. E., Muzik, O., Juhasz, C., Nagy, F., & Chugani, D. C. (2002). Local brain functional activity following early deprivation: A study of postinstitutionalized Romanian orphans. *Neuroimage, 14*(6), 1290–1301.

Davies, M. (2002). A few thoughts about the mind, the brain, and a child with early deprivation. *Journal of Analytical Psychology, 47*(3), 421–435.

De Bellis, M. (2001). Developmental traumatology: The psychobiological development of maltreated children and its implications for research, treatment, and policy. *Development and Psychopathology, 13,* 539–564.

De Bellis, M., Keshavan, M., Clark, D., Dasey, B., Giedd, J., Boring, A., et al. (1999). Developmental traumatology. Part II: Brain development. *Biological Psychiatry, 45,* 1271–1284.

Dieperink, M., Leskela, J., Thuras, P., & Engdahl, B. (2001). Attachment style classification and posttraumatic stress disorder in former prisoners of war. *American Journal of Orthopsychiatry, 71*(3), 374–378.

Gantt, L., Tinnin, L., & Tabone, C. (2002, November). *Time-limited trauma therapy using art therapy*. Paper presented at the American Art Therapy Association's 33rd Annual Conference, Washington, DC.

Gilbertson, M., Shenton, M., Ciszewski, A., Kasai, K., Lasko, N., Orr, S., et al. (2002). Smaller hippocampal volume predicts pathologic vulnerability to psychological trauma. *Nature Neuroscience, 5*(11), 1242–1247.

Glaser, D. (2000). Child abuse and neglect and the brain—A review. *Journal of Child Psychology and Psychiatry, 41*(1), 99–116.

Gruber, L. (2003, November). *Alleviating trauma: Art therapy and eye movement desensitization and reprocessing (EMDR).* Paper presented at the American Art Therapy Association's 34th Annual Conference, Chicago, IL.

Hanson, R. (2002). Reactive attachment disorder: What do we really know about this diagnosis? *APSAC Advisor, 14*(3), 10–12.

Hanson, R., & Spratt, E. (2000). Reactive attachment disorder: What we know about the disorder and implications for treatment. *Child Maltreatment, 5*(2), 137–145.

Haugaard, J. (2004). Recognizing and treating uncommon behavioral and emotional disorders in children and adolescents who have been severely maltreated: Introduction. *Child Maltreatment, 9*(2), 123–130.

Henley, D., Kaplan, F., & Shore, A. (2003, November). *Art therapy: When is it science? When is it arts and humanities?* Paper presented at the American Art Therapy Association's 34th Annual Conference, Chicago, IL.

Hughes, D. (1998). *Building the bonds of attachment.* Northvale, NJ: Aronson.

Kaler, S., & Freeman, B. (1994). Analysis of environmental deprivation: Cognitive and social development in Romanian orphans. *Journal of Child Psychology and Psychiatry, 35,* 769–781.

Kaplan, F. (2000). *Art, science and art therapy: Repainting the picture.* London: Jessica Kingsley.

Kaplan, F. (2004). Inner space. *Art Therapy: Journal of the American Art Therapy Association, 21*(3), 122–123.

Klorer, P. G. (2000). *Expressive therapy with troubled children.* Northvale, NJ: Aronson.

Klorer, P. G. (2005). Expressive therapy with severely maltreated children: Neuroscience contributions. *Art Therapy: Journal of the American Art Therapy Association, 22*(4), 213–220.

Klorer, P. G., & Chapman, L. (2004, November). *Cumulative trauma and art therapy: Neurodevelopmental advances in theory and practice.* Paper presented at the American Art Therapy Association's 35th Annual Conference, San Diego, CA.

Klorer, P. G., & Malchiodi, C. (2003, November). *Acute vs. long-term trauma: Therapeutic interventions.* Paper presented at the American Art Therapy Association's 34th Annual Conference, Chicago, IL.

Kruk, K. (2004, November). *EEG and art therapy: Brain activity during artmaking.* Paper presented at the American Art Therapy Association's 35th Annual Conference, San Diego, CA.

Lusebrink, V. (2004). Art therapy and the brain: An attempt to understand the underlying processes of art expression in therapy. *Art Therapy: Journal of the American Art Therapy Association, 21*(3), 125–135.

Mahler, M. (1979). *The selected papers of Margaret S. Mahler: Vol. II. Separation–individuation*. New York: Aronson.

Mahler, M., Pine, R., & Bergman, A. (1975). *The psychological birth of the human infant: Symbiosis and individuation*. New York: Basic Books.

Malchiodi, C., Kaplan, F., & Riley, S. (2002, November). *A neuroscience approach to art therapy*. Paper presented at the American Art Therapy Association's 33rd Annual Conference, Washington, DC.

Marko, J., & Merckelbach, H. (2004). Traumatic stress, brain changes, and memory deficits: A critical note. *The Journal of Nervous and Mental Disease, 192*(8), 548–553.

McNamee, C. (2003, November). *Bilateral art: A creative response to advances in neuroscience*. Paper presented at the American Art Therapy Association's 34th Annual Conference, Chicago, IL.

McNamee, C. (2004). Using both sides of the brain: Experiences that integrate art and talk therapy through scribble drawings. *Art Therapy: Journal of the American Art Therapy Association, 21*(3), 136–142.

Munns, E. (2000). *Theraplay: Innovations in attachment-enhancing play therapy*. Northvale, NJ: Aronson.

O'Connor, T., Rutter, M., & English and Romanian Adoptees Study Team. (2000). Attachment disorder behavior following early severe deprivation: Extension and longitudinal follow-up. *Child and Adolescent Psychiatry, 39*(6), 703–712.

Perry, B. (1997). Incubated in terror: Neurodevelopmental factors in the "cycle of violence." In J. Osofsky (Ed.), *Children in a violent society* (pp. 124–148). New York: Guilford Press.

Perry, B. (2001). *Violence and childhood: How persisting fear can alter the developing child's brain*. Available at *www.ChildTrauma.org*.

Perry, B., Pollard, R., Blakley, T., Baker, W., & Vigilante, D. (1995). Childhood trauma, the neurobiology of adaptation, and "use-dependent" development of the brain: How "states" become "traits." *Infant Mental Health Journal, 16*(4), 271–291.

Rauch, S., van der Kolk, B., Fisler, R., Alpert, N., Orr, S., Savage, C., et al. (1996). A symptom provocation study of postraumatic stress disorder using positron emission tomography and script-driven imagery. *Archives of General Psychiatry, 53*, 380–387.

Rutter, M., & O'Connor, T. (2004). Are there biological programming effects for psychological development? Findings from a study of Romanian orphans. *Developmental Psychology, 40*(1), 81–94.

Saywitz, K., Mannarino, A. P., Berliner, L., & Cohen, J. A. (2000). Treatment of sexually abused children and adolescents. *American Psychologist, 55*, 1040–1050.

Schiffer, F. (2000). Can the different cerebral hemispheres have distinct personalities?: Evidence and its implications for theory and treatment of

PTSD and other disorders. *Journal of Trauma and Dissociation*, *1*(2), 83–104.

Schiffer, F., Teicher, M., & Papanicolaou, A. (1995). Evoked potential evidence for right brain activity during the recall of traumatic memories. *Journal of Neuropsychiatry and Clinical Neurosciences*, *7*, 169–175.

Schore, A. (1998, November). *Early trauma and the development of the right side of the brain*. Paper presented at the C. M. Hincks Institute Conference on "Traumatized Parents and Infants: The Long Shadow of Early Childhood Trauma," Toronto, Ontario.

Schore, A. (2001). The effects of a secure attachment relationship on right brain development, affect regulation, and infant mental health. *Infant Mental Health Journal*, *22*, 7–66.

Schore, A. (2002). Dysregulation of the right brain: a fundamental mechanism of traumatic attachment and the psychopathogenesis of posttraumatic stress disorder. *Australian and New Zealand Journal of Psychiatry*, *36*, 9–30.

Stewart, E. G. (2004). Art therapy and neuroscience blend: Working with patients who have dementia. *Art Therapy: Journal of the American Art Therapy Association*, *21*(3), 148–155.

Ulman, E. (1975). Therapy is not enough: The contribution of art to a general hospital psychiatry. In E. Ulman & P. Dachinger (Eds.), *Art Therapy in Theory and Practice* (pp. 14–32). New York: Schocken Books.

Wiesel, T. N., & Hubel, D. H. (1963). Effects of visual deprivation on the morphology and physiology of cells in the cat's lateral geniculate body. *Journal of Neurophysiology*, *26*, 978–993.

Wiesel, T. N., & Hubel, D. H. (1965). Comparison of the effects of unilateral and bilateral eye closure on cortical unit responses in kittens. *Journal of Neurophysiology*, *28*, 1060–1072.

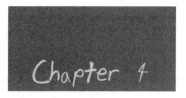

Chapter 4

Music and Grief Work
with Children and Adolescents

Russell E. Hilliard

Music has been a source of healing for centuries, and humankind has utilized this powerful medium to develop a sense of connectedness and to express emotions and thoughts. Quite often, words fail to convey the depth and breadth of one's emotions, and the elements of music (melody, harmony, and rhythm) can serve us when verbal expression is too limiting. Grief is one of the most complex emotional experiences because the grieving person often experiences myriad emotions, such as sorrow, anger, guilt, anxiety, fear, denial, disappointment, and relief, among others. Grieving adults often struggle through their bereavement, and the experience can be even more complicated for children and adolescents due to their developing understanding of the cycle of life and death (Doka, 2003). Music is a creative tool that can provide a form of emotional expression and assist children in understanding basic death education concepts (Hilliard, 2001).

Music therapy is an established allied health profession, and the American Music Therapy Association (AMTA) defines music therapy as "the clinical and evidence-based use of music interventions to accomplish individualized goals within a therapeutic relationship by a credentialed professional who has completed an approved music therapy program" (American Music Therapy Association, n.d.). While music therapy is conducted by a credentialed music therapist, music therapists are supportive of other professionals using music within their practice with proper education and experience. While this use of music is not "music therapy" per se, counselors, social workers, psychologists, and other health care professionals may find that music can support their discipline-specific interventions.

Very little is available in the literature regarding counselors' use of music interventions for grieving children and adolescents, but it does reflect the use of music interventions for the terminally ill provided by counselors. In his descriptive article, Brown (1992) claims to have been a health care troubadour providing music to the terminally ill for more than 12 years. He states, "though an associate member of the National Association for Music Therapy, I am by no means a professional therapist" (p. 13) and "my own working definition of music as therapy is the applied use of music in the context of a nurturing relationship to bring about change" (p. 15). Through case vignettes, the author illustrates how his singing and guitar playing brought about change with his clients. He suggests listening to audiotapes as a means for facilitating communication and getting people to open up. He encourages performance as a means for expression and socialization, imagery with music to increase relaxation, and song writing to communicate feelings and experiences. Although he identifies the highly specialized training of professional therapists, Brown encourages all caring professionals to use music with their patients and clients.

Lochner and Stevenson (1988) explain how they used music with the terminally ill in their professionally trained roles as counselors. Although they admit they are not therapists, the authors make no clear distinction between professionally trained therapists and counselors using music in therapy. They report on music composed by Lochner and how it was used in therapy. Music often opened communication between therapist and client. In one case, the music allowed a 20-year-old man with cancer to begin sharing his feelings about his impending death after listening to Lochner's song "I Love You, My Friend." In another case, Lochner wrote a song that he felt reflected his patient's feelings about the separation from her family she would soon experience. The patient was a 40-year-old woman with ovarian cancer and had processed her feelings in a verbal therapy session, but she wanted to communicate them to her family. Lochner wrote a song titled "Stay by My Side" and sang it to the family with the patient's permission. Family members clung to one another and cried as they realized what the patient was feeling. The music provided a way to increase awareness within the family and build a sense of higher cohesion. The authors conclude with a suggested music list for counselors to use when working with the terminally or tragically ill.

Music is an important form of creativity for children and adolescents; as such, it has been used therapeutically for a variety of clinical needs. In a study of 19 bereaved children, music therapy significantly reduced grief symptoms and taught participants a variety of healthy coping skills (Hilliard, 2001). It has been used as an alternative form of treatment to traditional verbal therapy for children and adolescents who experienced grief and trauma following the tragedies of September 11, 2001 (Gaffney, 2002). In pediatric health care settings, music therapy has been utilized to provide diversion during routine medical procedures, to supply emotional support, and to address the developmental needs of hospitalized children and adolescents (Robb, 2003). Music therapy has played a vital role in children's hospices to help terminally ill children and their families cope with their feelings of anticipatory grief (Hilliard, 2003; Pavlicevic, 2005). Through case vignettes and sample session plans, this chapter will describe the use of music therapy and music-based interventions in grief work with children and adolescents.

MUSIC AND GRIEF WORK

The session format and plans described in this chapter embrace a cognitive-behavioral music therapy model. Cognitive-behavioral music therapy has been used with a variety of client populations and has been demonstrated to be a highly effective and efficient treatment modality (Standley, Johnson, Robb, Brownell, & Kim, 2004). Within this philosophy, "undesirable behaviors and symptoms are modified, beliefs that interfere with healing are re-evaluated, and traumatic reminders are reframed to become normal parts of a child's life, not harbingers of yet another traumatic event" (Gaffney, 2002, p. 58). Cognitive-behavioral music therapy in child and adolescent grief work emphasizes "behavior modification, the identification and expression of emotions, the intellectual understanding of grief, and challenges cognitive distortions while assisting with cognitive reframing and reshaping" (Hilliard, 2001, p. 296).

An essential component of treatment is recognition of the developmental stage of the client. The child's developmental stage plays an important role in understanding and coping with losses. For young children (ages 4–5 years), the idea that the deceased may return is common as the permanence of death is not yet clearly understood. Children in this age group engage in magical thinking, think of death as punishment for bad behavior, and may have a fear of separation. The elementary-school-age child (ages 6–11 years) may feel guilt or regret when a loved one dies, especially if the child disagreed with the deceased. Children in this age group may still engage in magical thinking, are likely to personify death (e.g., see it as a monster), can understand facts, and may have a high degree of death anxiety. Adolescents (ages 12–20 years) may internalize their grief or use unhealthy forms of coping such as experimenting with drugs and alcohol, embrace an adult concept of death, or defy death by engaging in reckless behavior (Doka, 2003). It is essential to utilize music interventions appropriate for the developmental stage of the client.

In addition to the developmental stage of the client, the therapist assesses the client's strengths and problem areas, communication style, learning style, cultural and religious/spiritual background, history with music, and preferred musical styles and genres. In many cases, therapists utilize standardized music therapy assessments, especially in pediatric health care and special education settings (Chase, 2004; DeLoach-Walworth, 2005). Meta-analyses of the medical music therapy literature indicate that the most effective type of music intervention is live music. Recorded music conditions, however, show a more positive effect than do no-music conditions. The type of music shown to have the most positive effect is patient-preferred music. Based on these data, the best types of music interventions are those that utilize patient-preferred live music (Dileo & Bradt, 2005; Standley, 2000; Standley & Whipple, 2003). Therefore, learning the type of music preferred by the grieving child or adolescent is an important component of the music therapy assessment.

Following the music therapy assessment, the therapist begins the process of treatment planning and the formation of session plans. Much of the work described here was conducted in child and adolescent bereavement support groups under the auspices of a hospice's bereavement center. The format of the sessions remained fairly consistent, regardless of the age of the clients. Each session began with an opening experience designed to help clients motivate themselves to engage in the group and reduce any feelings of defensiveness or emotional guardedness. These opening group experiences included drumming, singing, or music and movement. Following the opening experience, the therapist facilitated a brief discussion with an emotional check-in for each client, and clients shared how they were feeling at that moment. The central part of the group was the theme of the day. These themes varied depending on the type of group and age of the clients but included "the memorial service," "coping with anger (or sorrow)," and "remembering." Because clients often shared intense emotions during the theme-based aspect of the group, the therapist facilitated a closing experience designed to elevate mood and encourage creative musical play. These closing experiences included musical improvisation and the playing of musical games such as name that tune or musicopoly (a music version of Monopoly).

The music and grief work described here has been utilized in bereavement centers associated with hospice programs. Music therapy has been provided for children in a variety of settings: family sessions, individual sessions, time-limited school-based bereavement groups, child and adolescent grief camps, and open bereavement groups at a bereavement center. Family therapy sessions utilizing music therapy have been facilitated prior to the death of the loved one to help children cope with the anticipated death as well as following the death to help children with the mourning process. These sessions are typically facilitated in the home environment and include various family members, such as siblings. Music provides opportunities for the family to engage in intergenerational therapy activities where each person's developmental stage is respected. Individual music therapy sessions for grief and loss can be facilitated as needed either in the home or at the bereavement center. These sessions are particularly useful for the child or adolescent who may be nervous or unsure about attending a group setting. Engaging in individual therapy initially may open the door for group participation later. Additionally, individual therapy is essential for clients experiencing complicated mourning or multiple clinical needs.

Time-limited school-based groups are useful in helping maintain continuity and lead a curriculum focused on grief and loss. Children and adolescents attend groups at their schools during the school day for 1-hour sessions once weekly for 8 weeks. The structure of these groups contrasts with the open-group format often facilitated at a bereavement center. In the open groups, clients participate as needed, there is an ebb and flow of clients attending, and the sessions are planned by topic or theme rather than following a systematic curriculum. Child and adolescent grief camps that utilize music have been offered in hospices throughout the country. Clients rotate through many small groups, and music therapy is often offered in these groups. Music is also used in large groups such as memorial services or the closing ceremonies for grief camps.

MUSIC TECHNIQUES

A variety of music therapy techniques are used in grief work. While most of these techniques employ live music, recorded music may be substituted whenever live music is not possible. The music techniques presented here are easily modified to be appropriate for youngsters of all ages. Drumming is a popular technique for children and adolescents alike. The important thing to remember when drumming with teenagers is that it is essential to use age-appropriate rhythm instruments. Rhythm instruments such as djembes and bongos can be purchased for a fair price from most local or online music retailers. Paddle drums, hand drums, and tambourines as well as other popular rhythm instruments can be enjoyed by children of all ages. Younger children like drums with bright colors or cartoon characters. There are a variety of ways to facilitate a group drumming experience (Stevens, 2003; Wajler, 2002), such as engaging in call and response where the facilitator plays a short rhythm and the group participants play it back. This call and response is passed around the group until each member has had an opportunity to play an original rhythm and hear it played back. A short discussion about the experience may follow, with the therapist helping the clients see that the experience resembles a conversation, with times for listening and times for responding.

In addition to call-and-response drumming, the facilitator can encourage improvisation by holding a steady beat while group members play any rhythm, style, and dynamic they wish. By keeping a steady beat, the facilitator grounds the improvisation. One can also divide the group in half and alternate the grounding steady beat with the improvisation, half the group keeping the steady beat at all times. Exploring dynamics (loud/soft) and tempo (fast/slow) and adding movements (marching, playing up high or down low) can also add to the drumming experience. Drumming the rhythm of a group member's name can be a fun welcoming musical experience, and playing multiple members' names can create a rich polyrhythmic experience. For example, the group can learn to drum Nancy Middleton's name by practicing playing and saying the name in rhythm (i.e., Nan-cy Middle-ton). Once the group can play and say the name together, they can fade out saying the name and just drum. Selecting multiple names to play in small groups creates a richer rhythmic experience. These drumming experiences are useful to open and close the group process. They can create a sense of group cohesion, motivate clients who may have depressive symptoms, provide an outlet for hyperactive clients, and foster a sense of working together.

Rhythmic improvisation can be used for the identification and expression of emotions as well. Group members can play what they are feeling, and other group members can guess the emotion. To facilitate this process, it is sometimes necessary to place a variety of instruments on a table or on the floor in the back of the room and have the group members face away from the instruments or close their eyes as the client playing selects the instrument and plays. This encourages the group members to listen respectfully, decreases off-task behavior, and assists the self-conscious client to play expressively and creatively. Free play can also be used with instruments, the therapist simply responding to the music as it is made by the clients. In both cases, clients are able to identify and express their emotions, one of the goals of grief work.

Singing well-known songs can assist in developing group cohesion as clients get to know one another through their musical preferences. Songs chosen can also reflect an emotional state when clients choose a song that reflects how they feel when they think of the person who died. To remember the deceased, the clients may also be asked to bring a recording of his or her favorite song to be played in the group. Clients can sing along with a recording of the song, but therapists primarily use live music with guitar or piano accompaniment. Using song lyric sheets helps prompt the clients to sing along with the recording or accompaniment.

Combining music and art techniques is useful in fostering creativity among children. There are a variety of ways that therapists facilitate this type of activity, such as by having clients create a grief collage to music. The therapist brings a recording of short segments of different types of music, and, as the music plays, clients draw freely on a large piece of paper. Each time the music changes, the clients move one seat to the right and begin drawing around the drawing of the client previously seated there. After each musical segment, a short discussion about the clients' drawings follows. The end result is a collage of art based on the clients' grief experiences. This activity can also be facilitated with live music with the therapist playing or improvising a variety of musical styles or selections.

Another music and art activity that is well liked by grieving children and adolescents is to create CD covers. The therapist asks the clients to create a series of song titles that reflects their grief experiences. Examples of instruction include "Write a song title about how you felt when you first found out your loved one died," ". . . . about how you viewed your relationship with your loved one," " . . . about how you felt at the memorial service (if you attended it)," " . . . about how you feel now when you think about your loved one," etc. Clients are instructed to write the song titles on a piece of paper and then decorate it as though it were the cover to a musical recording. During discussion of the song titles, it is useful to have instruments at hand to ask clients to give a demonstration of how the songs might sound. This type of activity can encourage verbal expression of emotions and help clients engage more easily in verbal counseling.

Music bibliotherapy combines music techniques with story reading and has been used in the field of music therapy to promote academic successes (Register, 2001, 2004) and for counseling after traumatic experiences (Altilio, 2002). While this technique is primarily used with younger children who enjoy being read stories, it can be used with adolescents as well. Adolescents are encouraged to write their own grief story or poem, and music is added to the story or poem. For young children, music is added to an existing children's book about grief and loss. There is a variety of such books available, and sample titles include *Lifetimes: A Beautiful Way to Explain Death to Children* (Mellonie, 1983), *The Tenth Good Thing about Barney* (Viorst & Blegvad, 1971), and *The Memory String* (Bunting & Rand, 2000). *Grateful: A Song of Giving Thanks* (Bucchino & Hakkarainen, 2006) is useful to help children cope with grief and the holidays because it deals with being grateful in spite of a loss, and it includes a CD recording of Art Garfunkel's original song for the book.

Therapists who use music bibliotherapy often compose original songs to accompany the story reading. During breaks in the reading of the book, the therapist and the clients sing the song, and this singing reinforces the lesson being taught by the book. Therapists may choose a highly rhythmic chant in lieu of an original song composition for a similar effect. The therapist also identifies main characters or actions that are repeated throughout the story. These characters or actions are then assigned a musical instrument (e.g., Barney = maracas; purred = shakers). Each time the character's name or the action is heard during the reading of the story, the client who has that character or action plays the assigned instrument. This technique helps increase on-task behavior and attention to the story. Books about grief and loss provide opportunities for discussion of the group members' experiences and help normalize the grief process. The musical elements assist in the understanding of the lessons learned, provide opportunities for active engagement, and encourage listening skills.

Writing lyrics has been used successfully with children and adolescents in an effort to address a variety of emotional needs (Hilliard, 2001; Keen, 2004). Song or rap lyric writing can be a useful tool in helping children and adolescents express their grief, contract to use healthy coping skills, and remember the person who died. Young children often need structure in helping to elicit lyrics. The therapist can ask questions about their grief process in a systematic way to develop each line of the song. Questions may include "How did you feel at the memorial service?"; "What are some of the things you remember about the person who died?"; and "How do you express your anger (or sorrow or any other emotion)?" Answers to these questions form the lyrics of the song or rap. Writing a rap is often easy to facilitate because clients readily provide the rhythmic structure. The task of the therapist is to fit the lyrics into the rhythmic structure provided by the clients. Sometimes this requires a rewording of the lyrics or a collapsing of ideas into shorter lines. By providing a selection of musical elements such as various keys, tempos, dynamics, and styles, the therapist helps clients compose their own music to fit their song lyrics. Another popular song-writing activity is for the therapist to provide a musical structure in the style of the blues and encourage clients to improvise singing over it.

Analyzing song lyrics can help facilitate an understanding of death, provide a sense of normalcy, educate clients about grief, and help them identify and express emotions. Therapists often lead a sing-along with guitar or piano accompaniment and then lead a discussion analyzing the song's lyrics. Recorded music can also be used, and there are several children's songs that deal with emotional content such as feeling sad, lonely, or angry and that work well in children's bereavement groups. Peter Alsop has written several songs helping children cope with death, dying, grief, and loss. His videotape *When Kids Say Goodbye* (Alsop, 1996) and audio recording *Songs on Loss and Grief* (Alsop, 1995) contain songs with lyrics to help children understand their grief emotions and also provide basic death education concepts (e.g., the difference between sleep and death). Playing either of these provides opportunities for discussion and counseling of the children's needs. Adolescents are often encouraged to bring their own recordings that express their grief emotions and reactions to the group, but it is sometimes necessary for the therapist to require that the clients bring edited versions of the recordings to prevent others from becoming offended by the sometimes graphic language. It is useful to have lyric sheets to accompany the songs, and the therapist can point out lines for discussion and opportunities for counseling.

Orff–Schulwerk is an approach to music education created by Carl Orff that embodies the concept that children learn by doing. In this approach, children experience the music through playing, singing, and moving as they learn about various musical concepts. It has been adopted by therapists because the musical elements in Orff–Schulwerk lend themselves to many therapy goals. A variety of instruments are used in Orff–Schulwerk that may include xylophones, metalophones, glockenspiels, recorders, drums, and other rhythm instruments (Colwell, Achey, Gillmeister, & Woolrich, 2004). A curriculum for grieving children based on the Orff–Schulwerk approach has been developed (Hilliard, 2007) and empirically tested. In this curriculum, children engage in song writing, improvisation, singing, playing instruments, and moving with music. All of the music is based on issues related to bereavement, and children are able to achieve therapeutic goals through their participation in musical dialogue.

SESSION PLANS

The following session plan is an example of a music-based bereavement group for young children ages 3–6 years. It is the third session in an 8-session format. Either live or recorded music can be utilized in the plan, and it is designed for a group of five to eight with a duration of approximately 45 minutes.

Session Theme: Distinguishing sleep from death

Purpose

Young children can become confused about the differences between sleep and death, especially if parents or guardians explained the death of the loved one by making statements like "Grandma is at rest; it's like she's asleep." Sometimes children are unable to distinguish between death and sleep, and they may experience fear or anxiety when they see their living loved ones asleep or when it is time for them to go to bed. The purpose of this session is to help children understand the differences between sleep and death.

Goals

1. Reduce fear/anxiety regarding sleeping situations.
2. Differentiate between sleep and death.
3. Understand basic death education concepts.
4. Learn effective coping skills.

Materials Needed

- A variety of rhythm instruments
- "While I'm Sleepin'" song sheet (music from the *Stayin' Over Songbook*) or recording of the song by Peter Alsop (from *Songs on Loss and Grief*)
- Guitar or piano for therapist accompaniment or player for recorded music

Procedure

1. Opening experience: Facilitate rhythm and movement experience by passing out rhythm instruments (egg-shaped shakers are good for this age group) and encourage children to shake their instruments while standing in place. Next, have each child take turns adding a movement to the shaking of the rhythm instruments for other children to mirror. Continue this until everyone has a chance to lead. If the children are still quite active, add a popular children's song to the shaker rhythm such as "Shake My Sillies Out" or "She'll Be Comin' 'Round the Mountain." Begin to slow the music and shaking rhythm and lead the children in sitting on the floor as they play slower and

softer. When they are seated in a circle, stop the music. Instruct the children to toss the instruments in the circle for you to collect. This will help reduce off-task behavior.

2. Play the song "While I'm Sleepin'" by Peter Alsop. Lead a sing-along of the chorus: "While I'm sleepin', I'm alive. My heart's beatin', deep inside. I keep breathin', soft and slow. How I do it? Well, I don't know." Each verse of the song provides examples of how being asleep is different from being dead and normalizes the fear, anxiety, and confusion about this issue.

3. Lead a short discussion of the song lyrics by asking concrete questions such as "What's the difference between being asleep and being dead?" or "Does a person's heart beat when he or she is asleep? How about when he or she is dead?" Have each child identify a difference between sleep and death. A nice way to end the discussion is to ask, "If you had to explain how being asleep is different than being dead, what would you say?"

4. Pass out the rhythm instruments again and play a variety of rhythms. Call and response is useful, and adding movement as needed will help reduce off-task behavior. Begin to slow and soften the music again to get the children in a seated position. Collect the instruments.

5. Pass around the most interesting instrument (e.g., rainstick or ocean drum). Explain that the instrument is the talking instrument and that when you say, "stop," whoever is holding the instrument gets to talk. Ask questions of each child such as "How was it that your special someone died?" or "Who told you about the death?"

6. For a closing exercise, engage the children in singing, rhythmic improvisation, and movement. This will allow the children to elevate their mood and end the group feeling uplifted.

The following session plan is taken from a music-based bereavement group for adolescents. Using an open format, the group meets twice monthly at the bereavement center, and music sessions are planned for each meeting. This session plan is an example of a typical music-based experience with this type of group.

Session Theme: The grief rap

Purpose

Adolescents can struggle with the recognition that grief changes over time and that most grieving people begin to feel better as they process their experiences. It can be useful for clients to see how their grief has changed over time. This activity is designed to help them recognize these changes and honor their own processes.

Goals

1. Identify and express emotions.
2. Recall memories of the deceased.
3. Engage in peer support.
4. Learn effective coping skills.

Materials Needed

- A variety of rhythm instruments
- Client-preferred live or recorded music
- Guitar or piano for therapist accompaniment or player for recorded music
- Grief worksheets and pencils
- Large piece of paper or dry-erase board and markers

Procedure

1. Opening experience: With clients sitting in a circle, play client-preferred music (either live or recorded). Distribute two medium-sized soft, foam balls and have clients toss the balls to each other while the music plays. Stop the music periodically at random and have the two clients holding the balls share how their time has been since the previous group and how they are feeling in their grief process now. Continue the activity until everyone has had an opportunity to share.

2. With music playing quietly in the background, distribute pencils and a prepared worksheet for each client to complete that contains the following questions:

What is something your loved one taught you for which you are grateful?
Where were you when you found out your loved one died?
How did you feel when you first found out about the death?
How did you deal with or express that feeling?
When you think of your loved one now, how do you feel?
What is one of the best memories you have of your loved one?

3. Lead a short discussion of the responses to the questions on the worksheet as clients feel comfortable.

4. Following the discussion, the responses provided on the worksheet will be used to write a rap. Using a drum, play a basic rhythm and ask the clients to provide the first line to the rap by choosing one of the responses they wrote on the worksheet. Most rap writing is easily completed by the adolescents, but sometimes they need prompting or suggestions. This guidance can be necessary if the clients get off task or become inappropriate with their lyrics.

5. Write the rap on a large piece of paper or dry-erase board. At the end of the group, the rap will be written on a smaller piece of paper to be photocopied for each client.

6. For a closing exercise, pass around a bongo drum and ask the clients to identify at least one person they trust and with whom they can share their grief emotions until the next group.

CASE VIGNETTES

Jackie, a 4-year-old European American female, was referred to the children's bereavement program after her father died in a tragic accident. On a Saturday afternoon, she was playing in her next-door neighbor's yard when her father arrived home with a new piece of lawn equipment. While he was unloading the equipment from the trailer, he lost control of it and was crushed to death. Jackie witnessed her father's sudden death and experienced an intense state of shock. She had been seeing a child psychologist for individual sessions who referred her to the bereavement group to give her opportunities to engage with other grieving children.

During the music therapy assessment, Jackie's mother reported that Jackie had problems sleeping at night, displayed an intense level of dependence, became increasingly inattentive in her preschool, and complained of somatic concerns such as head- and stomachaches. Jackie participated in live music experiences with the therapist during the assessment visit, was creative and engaging, and initiated free musical play with rhythm instruments. When asked about her father, she became withdrawn, looked downward, displayed a sad affect, and would not talk about him. Therapeutic goals for Jackie included increasing her awareness of basic death education concepts (e.g., the finality of death), identifying and expressing emotions, decreasing problems with sleeping and overdependency on her mother, developing coping skills, and remembering times with her father.

Initially, Jackie was quiet, withdrawn, and timid but quite polite and respectful of her peers and the therapist. It took her several weeks before she felt comfortable enough to initiate expression of her own thoughts and feelings, and then she became quite expressive and participatory in the sessions. She was musically motivated, and even before she talked about her experiences, she was readily able to engage in musical dialogue. She enjoyed choosing instruments to play during the rhythmic improvisation and Orff-based musical experiences. While playing, she smiled, giggled, and was able to share with her peers. These experiences seemed important for her as they helped her develop therapeutic rapport with other children in the group and the therapist.

Over time, Jackie began to share her grief experiences. Following a musical improvisation, Jackie identified feeling sad about her father's death. One of the other children asked her how he died, and, without hesitation, she told the group what had happened to him. This was the first time she had acknowledged the actual event. She said, "I thought it was a bad dream, but he's not coming home." Immediately afterward, she began playing a melancholic improvised melody on the xylophone that was in front of her. Jackie displayed an awareness of her father's death, and she was able to recognize that he was not going to return. The music helped her cope with her grief emotions after verbally sharing with the group, and it seemed as though her engagement in the musical dialogue helped her feel comfortable enough to share her thoughts and feelings verbally with the group.

In subsequent music therapy sessions, Jackie became increasingly expressive and talked openly about her father's death, memories of him, her family's spiritual beliefs, and her reactions to her mother's grief (she became nervous when she witnessed her mother crying). She often initiated musical experiences by making requests or leading musical improvisation experiences. Jackie's mother reported that Jackie's symptoms (sadness, sleep disturbance, overdependency, somatic concerns) continued to improve, although she remained unable to sleep through the entire night. With a curious affect, her mother reported that Jackie enjoyed coming to group and would often ask, "Is this group night?" This is a common reaction among group participants, who apparently feel supported and affirmed in the group and are able to make friends with one another; even though the topic of the group can be emotionally heavy, the music experiences seem to offer a sense of lightness and provide opportunities for mood elevation and even joy.

Tyrone, a 13-year-old African American male, was participating in music therapy sessions prior to his mother's death. His mother, diagnosed with HIV-AIDS, received home care hospice services, and, as part of the interdisciplinary team, the therapist visited the patient and family prior to the patient's death. Tyrone was present for and participated in several of his mother's music therapy sessions. At times, the therapist and Tyrone met together without his mother, and these sessions were important in helping Tyrone deal with her impending death. Tyrone wanted to learn how to play the guitar, and the therapist taught him several basic chord progressions. Tyrone's music therapy treatment was part of the overall interdisciplinary care plan for his mother. Goals for Tyrone included: engaging in meaningful experiences with his mother, identifying and expressing emotions, and learning healthy coping skills.

His mother's symptoms became difficult to manage at home, and she was admitted to the hospice's freestanding inpatient unit. When Tyrone's mother died, he went to the therapist's office in the inpatient unit and informed the therapist of her death. Tyrone's affect was flat, his eyes were vacant, and he was not crying; he appeared to be numb. He picked up the guitar in the corner and began playing a D chord repeatedly while improvising a song about his mother. While vocalizing and playing, he became tearful, and these tears quickly led to intense sobbing. With his eyes closed, he sobbed as he sang and played in an apparently cathartic experience. As his sobs lessened, he stopped vocalizing and eventually stopped playing the guitar. After the music and cathartic expression, he appeared tired and was able to begin talking about his mother's life and death.

Tyrone continued participating in individual music therapy sessions and eventually agreed to attend an adolescent bereavement group. In the group, he openly engaged with his peers and continued to prefer expressing his emotions nonverbally through his participation in live musical dialogue. Music helped Tyrone engage in meaningful experiences with his mother prior to her death, and he often shared memories of these experiences with his peers in the bereavement group. He also used the music experiences as a means to express his emotions and typically resisted verbally discussing his emotions. In his time outside of the therapy sessions, Tyrone used music to alter his mood and help him cope with his grief. He rarely left his home without his MP3 player, and he often brought his favorite recordings to the group to share with his peers.

CONCLUSIONS

Music therapy has been used effectively in helping children and adolescents cope with traumatic experiences and subsequent feelings of grief and loss. Research documenting music therapy's effects on mood and behavior of grieving children supports that music therapy is a viable treatment option for significantly reducing the symptoms associated with bereavement (Hilliard, 2001). It has also been used to help children and adolescents cope with the aftermath of the September 11, 2001, tragedies (Altilio, 2002). Although music therapy is most effectively conducted by a board-certified therapist, other mental health professionals may find that the use of music in their practice can support their therapeutic interventions. By using recorded music in lieu of live music, counselors may explore new and creative ways to help children and adolescents in the counseling process. A variety of musical techniques used by therapists can lend themselves to verbal therapy sessions. Such techniques include lyrical analyses and using background music combined with art activities. When counselors and therapists work together, clients benefit from the expertise provided by both disciplines. Sharing information is essential for children and adolescents to have better access to treatment in a world they understand—the world of creativity and play.

REFERENCES

Alsop, P. (1995). *Songs on loss and grief.* Minneapolis: Moose School.
Alsop, P. (1996). *When kids say goodbye: Helping kids with sad feelings.* Minneapolis: Moose School.
Altilio, T. (2002). Helping children, helping ourselves: An overview of children's literature. In J. Loewy & A. Hara (Eds.), *Caring for the caregiver: The use of music and music therapy in grief and trauma* (pp. 138–147). Silver Spring, MD: American Music Therapy Association.
American Music Therapy Association. (n.d.). Retrieved November 11, 2005, from *musictherapy.org/*.

Brown, J. (1992, March/April). When words fail, music speaks. *American Journal of Hospice and Palliative Care*, 13–17.

Bucchino, J., & Hakkarainen, A. (2006). *Grateful: A song of giving thanks*. New York: HarperCollins.

Bunting, E., & Rand, T. (2000). *The memory string*. London: Clarion Books.

Chase, K. M. (2004). Music therapy assessment for children with developmental disabilities: A survey study. *Journal of Music Therapy, 41*(1), 28–54.

Colwell, C. M., Achey, C., Gillmeister, G., & Woolrich, J. (2004). The Orff approach to music therapy. In A. Darrow (Ed.), *Introduction to approaches in music therapy* (pp. 103–124). Silver Spring, MD: American Music Therapy Association.

DeLoach-Walworth, D. (2005). Procedural support for music therapy in the healthcare setting: A cost-effectiveness analysis. *Journal of Pediatric Nursing, 20*(4), 276–284.

Dileo, C., & Bradt, J. (2005). *Medical music therapy: A meta-analysis and agenda for future research*. Cherry Hill, NJ: Jeffrey Books.

Doka, K. (2003). *Living with grief children, adolescents, and loss*. Washington, DC: Hospice Foundation of America.

Gaffney, D. (2002). Seasons of grief: Helping children grow through loss. In J. Loewy & A. Hara (Eds.), *Caring for the caregiver: The use of music and music therapy in grief and trauma* (pp. 54–62). Silver Spring, MD: American Music Therapy Association.

Hilliard, R. E. (2001). The effects of music therapy-based bereavement groups on mood and behavior of grieving children: A pilot study. *Journal of Music Therapy, 38*(4), 291–306.

Hilliard, R. E. (2003). Music therapy in pediatric palliative care: A complementary approach. *Journal of Palliative Care, 19*(2), 127–132.

Hilliard, R. E. (2007). The effects of Orff-based music therapy and social work groups on grieving children. *Journal of Music Therapy, 44*(2), 123–138.

Keen, A. W. (2004). Using music as a therapy tool to motivate troubled adolescents. *Social Work in Health Care, 39*(3–4) 361–373.

Lochner, S. W., & Stevenson, R. G. (1988). Music as a bridge to wholeness. *Death Studies, 12*, 173–180.

Mellonie, B. (1983). *Lifetimes: A beautiful way to explain death to children*. London: Banton.

Pavlicevic, M. (2005). *Music therapy in children's hospices*. London: Jessica Kingsley Publishers.

Register, D. (2001). The effects of an early intervention music curriculum on prereading/writing. *Journal of Music Therapy, 38*(3), 239–248.

Register, D. (2004). The effects of live music groups versus an educational children's television program on the emergent literacy of young children. *Journal of Music Therapy, 41*(1), 2–27.

Robb, S. L. (2003). *Music therapy in pediatric healthcare: Research and evidence-based practice*. Silver Spring, MD: American Music Therapy Association.

Standley, J. M. (2000). Music research in medical treatment. In D. Smith (Ed.), *Effectiveness of music therapy procedures: Documentation of research and clinical practice* (3rd ed., pp. 1–64). Silver Spring, MD: American Music Therapy Association.

Standley, J., Johnson, C. M., Robb, S. L., Brownell, M. D., & Kim, S. (2004). Behavioral approach to music therapy. In A. Darrow (Ed.), *Introduction to approaches in music therapy* (pp. 103–124). Silver Spring, MD: American Music Therapy Association.

Standley, J., & Whipple, J. (2003). Music therapy in pediatric palliative care: A meta-analysis. In S. Robb (Ed.), *Music therapy in pediatric healthcare: Research and evidence-based practice* (pp. 1–18). Silver Spring, MD: American Music Therapy Association.

Stevens, C. (2003). *The art and heart of drum circles*. Milwaukee, WI: Hal Leonard Corporation.

Viorst, J., & Blegvad, E. (1971). *The tenth good thing about Barney*. New York: Atheneum.

Wajler, Z. (2002). *World beat fun: Multicultural and contemporary rhythms for K–8 classrooms*. Miami: Warner Brothers Publications.

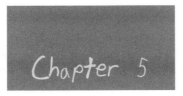

Grieving in the Public Eye

Art Therapy with Children Who Lost Parents in the World Trade Center Attacks

Laura V. Loumeau-May

Mass terrorism has an impact on children that exceeds the loss of life and property. More than 3,000 children and teenagers lost parents on September 11, 2001, in the worst terrorist attack in U.S. history. Even those children who did not lose a parent were affected. Thousands witnessed the terror firsthand from their homes and schools, while millions more saw the destruction of New York City's World Trade Center towers on television. This chapter discusses the use of art therapy in recovery from traumatic grief academically and through case studies. Interventions with children whose parents died in these attacks demonstrate the role of creativity in healing. Names have been changed to protect children's identities.

MASS TERRORISM

The trauma of mass terrorism is inflicted upon a large group such as a community or nation. Populations affected by terrorist activity identify themselves as being part of a targeted group. Terrorism is purposeful and intersocietal rather than interpersonal as in familial abuse or random violence. The goals exceed physical and economic destruction; they are psychological, with the aim of demoralizing the targeted population. Mass terrorism differs from other trauma in scope, cause, and intent.

Within the category of terrorism, mass terrorism is substantially different from typical terrorist acts consisting of repeated incidents on a small scale. People living in communities where isolated car, subway, and suicide bombings occur intermittently experience a state of constant hypervigilance (McGeehan, 2005). Although multiple deaths may result from these acts, they are generally limited in scale and the targets arbitrary. No one knows when or where the next incident will occur. People live with the awareness that they are in constant danger of losing their lives or homes (Abu Sway, Nashashibi, Salah, & Shweiki, 2005). According to Kalmanowitz and Lloyd (2005), "When violence is ongoing, pervasive and unremitting, it may form an integral part of each individual's internal world, identity, values, beliefs and history and not only affect a part of their present, but also inform whom each person will become. It will invariably inform the community itself" (p. 15). Furthermore, political violence affects the cultural memory of a society when the artifacts or symbolic structures of a community that represent its identity are destroyed. This is true of the World Trade Center's Twin Towers, which were symbols of Western economic might, free trade, and power.

Mass terrorism is characterized by the scale of human and property loss. Targets are often large, symbolic public sites thought to be invulnerable, which creates widespread panic. The ripple effects of terrorism impact the society and create a massive diversion of resources to control and repair damage (Doka, 2003). Political and social institutions can be temporarily immobilized; the worldview of those affected can change focus, and their values are perceived as endangered. On September 11, 2001, the United States experienced mass terrorism and trauma. People throughout the nation perceived serious threat to themselves, their country, and its institutions. Identification with the victims was powerful. The people who died could have been anyone; the majority of victims were simply going about their everyday business. The sacrifice of the rescue personnel who perished trying to save them augmented the pathos of their situation (Doka, 2003). The perception of the country being under attack lasted long after the final plane went down in Pennsylvania that morning. Trauma-induced fear spread to the nation as a whole. Repercussions remain today, as exemplified by the Department of Homeland Security's suspension of habeas corpus and the right to privacy, and the war on terrorism spreading from Afghanistan to Iraq.

Creative expression plays an important role in healing in the aftermath of a public tragedy involving terrorism (Bertman, 2003). Although art has been described as insubstantial to address the immensity of human suffering from such experiences as the Holocaust, Bertman argues that it is relevant and healing; art helps a society to cope. It is an outlet for grief and provides comfort. Art expression helps to resist and protest what has occurred. Art consoles and gives voice to the philosophical, political, and spiritual questions.

Public and private art making started to help the process of recovery from 9/11. Almost immediately after the tragedy, a number of ad hoc altars, walls plastered with pictures and tokens of love and memory, and firehouses and an armory filled with gifts of children's artwork appeared around New York (Santino, 2006). Art was created and displayed publicly in lower Manhattan. Drawings and paintings from children all over the tri-state area (Goodman & Fahnestock, 2002) attested to the healing role of creative expression in exorcising the pain, communicating hope, and narrating this unacceptable experience. Art therapists throughout the nation (Henley et al., 2001) addressed the trauma with workshops to help the public process the anguish. Music concerts and compositions provided lyrical response to the tragedy. Websites sprung up across the United States and around the world to reach out and share creative responses to the suffering. Public ceremonies addressed the need for healing, not only for the loved ones of the victims, but also for the collective soul of the society (Benke, 2003). Dealing with the attack preempted other concerns, even for individuals not directly affected (Testa & McCarthy, 2004).

BEREAVED FAMILIES AND THE 9/11 ATTACKS

There are traumatic aspects of grief, especially among children, and there are aspects of grief present in the recovery from trauma. The two experiences overlap but are not identical. Families of victims of the September 11, 2001, terrorist attacks not only had to recover from trauma, but also to undergo the process of grieving.

My clients were children who all lost a parent in the New York City attacks, one mother and the rest fathers. The surviving parents all remembered where they were and what they were doing when they heard the news. Some received a phone call from a friend or relative telling them to turn on the television. Others actually received calls from their husbands who were trapped in the towers and were able to talk to them before they died. A few returned home to find goodbye messages on their answering machines. Some parents were working. One parent, a nurse, was at work in Manhattan. She hoped her proximity and work would improve her husband's chances; unfortunately, no wounded were brought to her hospital.

The surviving parents wanted to determine their missing spouse's status. Telephone lines quickly became jammed and only intermittently accessible. Entry to and exit from Manhattan was closed. Some of the mothers rushed to schools to fetch their children. School officials varied in how they told their students. Some informed the children and held group discussions, while others left it for parents to handle. In schools where no news was officially announced, rumors and misinformation spread. Students saw their peers being called out of the classroom and taken home. The remaining children sensed the dire atmosphere and their teachers' moods. Some children of the victims remained in school for the full day, either knowing or not knowing what had happened.

Many of the home-based mothers cannot remember what their non-school-age children may have witnessed in those first hours. They do not recall the things they said on the phone in their children's presence or how soon they thought to turn off the television; their primary focus was on the fate of their husbands.

Despite the growing evidence to the contrary, many families refused to give up hope that their loved ones could be found alive. Many spent hours and days on the phone and in the city searching. This focus drained the families. Even when the inevitability of death was acknowledged, it could not be tolerated emotionally. It could not be spoken: their loved one was just missing, not dead. To give up hope was felt to be a betrayal. The emotional atmosphere of these homes was chaotic and tense. One parent was suddenly missing, while the other parent was in shock. One child later said of this time, "It was as if I lost both parents."

Open acknowledgment of death came reluctantly, days later, when Mayor Rudy Giuliani announced that only recovery and not rescue efforts were possible (Hartley, 2004). Many surviving families only conceded later when they were visited by an officer informing them that their loved ones' remains had been recovered or identified through DNA. Some families never received that visit. The absence of identifiable bodies compounded the trauma and complicated bereavement. Families held memorial services once they had acknowledged the death, but the absence of physical remains compromised closure spiritually, culturally, emotionally, cognitively, and legally. The traditional practice of viewing, touching, and burying the dead body of a loved one was not possible. A more insidious challenge ensued in the months following as the children's increased knowledge of death gradually made them aware of the significance of the absence of a body.

Media coverage of the events and repercussions of September 11 (or 9/11) was unprecedented. Among the most common symptoms of posttraumatic stress disorder (PTSD) are recurrent memories of the traumatizing event. Grieving families were reexposed to the images of the planes hitting the Twin Towers—the murder of their loved ones— every day. No television or radio could be turned on and no newsstand passed without seeing images of the destruction and discussion of the attacks. Parents tried to escape the constant coverage and the omnipresent replays by turning off their televisions and stopping news deliveries (Rathkey, 2004). While child witnesses throughout the United States drew pictures of the horrific images they had seen in order to process the trauma, children who had lost a parent tried to avoid these images. In my work with children of the victims, no bereaved child consciously drew the now famous image of a plane flying into a tower until 8 months later. Grieving children were focusing on their parents.

TREATING GRIEF AND TRAUMA IN CHILDREN

Traumatic factors complicate bereavement (Rando, 2003), and this was true for the families of 9/11 victims. The sudden, violent, and intentional nature of the events and the constant media coverage of the attacks, combined with nationwide hysteria, intensified the trauma that, in some cases, overtook the grief itself. Before a person can fully mourn the death of a loved one, he or she must feel safe (see Figure 5.1).

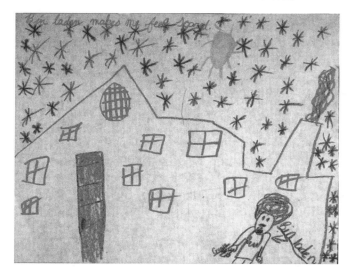

FIGURE 5.1. Addressing issues of fear and safety is essential in the treatment of traumatic grief. Hypervigilance was experienced by U.S. citizens following 9/11, especially by those most directly affected. Early drawings by children of 9/11 victims revealed the fear that they would be attacked again in their homes. In this picture, Bin Laden approaches a child's home with a gun.

Eth and Pynoos (1985) identify several factors common to traumatic grief in children, including (1) visual horror seen or imagined that interferes with remembering pleasant interactions with the deceased parent, (2) guilt that inspires a child to create rescue or revenge fantasies, (3) ego constriction that can result in blocked emotions as well as long-term cognitive deficits, (4) stigma, and (5) reunion fantasies in which the violent death is often reversed or undone. Therapists should address these issues early in treatment because normal mourning may be delayed if insufficient attention is given to relief of trauma-related anxiety. Rando (1996) also recommends treating trauma that overwhelms the ego before addressing bereavement issues.

Rankin and Taucher (2003) outline a systematic task-oriented approach in using art therapy with victims of trauma. Their approach features (1) safety planning, (2) self-management, (3) telling the trauma story, (4) grieving traumatic losses, (5) self-concept and worldview revision, and (6) self- and relational development. Early art directives use collage and writing to focus on recognition and regulation of psychic as well as actual danger with the development of a safety plan. Self-management techniques, including bodywork, visualization, and art, help clients become calm, regulate intense emotions, and ground themselves during flashbacks. Clients decide whether and when to tell the trauma story. Narrative techniques help them accept reality while reducing the negative effects of recall. Art directives aim to integrate sensations, emotions, and cognitions at the time of the trauma while recreating chronology. Self-soothing artwork follows completion of the narrative.

Once the overwhelming anxiety of the trauma is managed, grief work can begin. Treatment objectives in acknowledging and accepting losses include aspects of Rando's (1993) "6-R" tasks of bereavement: (1) recognize the loss, (2) react to the separation, (3) recollect and reexperience the deceased and the relationship, (4) relinquish old attachments to the deceased and the assumptive world, (5) readjust by adapting to the new world or life without the deceased without forgetting the old world, and (6) reinvest emotionally and psychologically. Rankin and Taucher (2003) emphasize recognizing ways in which losses affect current life and exploring barriers to grief and anger. They recommend breaking a loss into small pieces and grieving for each piece in turn. Integration of the experience into a revised self-concept and worldview is important in order for clients to perceive a hopeful continuum in their lives. Finally, returning to a sense of normality, reframing what has happened, and cultivating the ability to reinvest in new relationships and interests are vital for both bereavement and trauma recovery.

THE JOURNEYS PROGRAM AND 9/11

Of the 2,801 people who died at the World Trade Center, 694—almost one-fourth—resided in New Jersey. The Journeys Program of Valley Home Care began in 1990 and is one of the few northern New Jersey resources for grieving children. It provides individual and group art therapy to children and teenagers facing actual or anticipated loss of a loved one. Over the years, it has grown from a 3-day-a-week program to a 5-day-a-week program and has guided children through bereavement for normal as well as traumatic death. Following the attacks, the program anticipated an unprecedented need for bereavement services for the children of victims, but although many of the victims lived in local communities, there were no immediate referrals. Families were still looking for their loved ones and not ready to admit that death had occurred.

A few families started to attend the Journeys Program by the end of September 2001. Hand in Hand, a Saturday afternoon workshop with therapeutic follow-up, was offered to victims' families with children. Although Journeys programming normally provides weekday services for children only, to meet the needs of the large number of people affected by the attacks it expanded to include Saturdays and to serve the widowed parents of the children. An 8-week program ran on alternate Saturdays for 4 months. Three age-coordinated art therapy groups facilitated by myself, Juliana Mansfield, and Pamela Ullmann were provided concurrently with a parent group that was facilitated by a social worker. After the completion of this 8-week group, children were offered customary weekly programming. Many joined weekly 9/11 groups already in progress and continued for 3 to 4 more years. The Journeys Program provided therapy for a total of 31 families who suffered losses on September 11, 2001.

Over the course of 4 years, the involvement of Journeys with 9/11 victims' families changed. In the first academic year, six separate age-appropriate groups were established and well attended. By the end of June 2005, three teenage boys remained in the program and were placed in inclusive traumatic loss groups to complete their bereavement work. Unlike other Journeys families, 9/11 clients took a break during the summer months. With the return of school each fall came the anniversary of the attacks, with painful reminders and renewed media interest. During the second and third years, Journeys organized anniversary memorials for 9/11 families. In 2002, 10 families attended the first memorial, which aimed to help them bond through the creation of one joint memorial piece. The next year, only five families participated; by the third anniversary, in 2004, one mother said, "I want to take my kids away. This year I want it to be just our family's grief." Although many initially believed that they would require years of therapy, most children and families developed inner resources and strengths to cope with pain and reorganize their lives.

Initial Goals: Coming to Terms with the Trauma

Children who entered the program in the first months following the attacks presented a need to release and share fearful images and a need to avoid overwhelming emotions. During the first 8 months of treatment, therapy provided psychological stability and structure to increase opportunities for feelings of safety and mastery. This goal was accomplished by creating an open atmosphere that encouraged catharsis. Art materials as well as directives simultaneously provided the structure to contain and the stimulation to express.

Children expressed diverse reactions to their parents' deaths. Some were experiencing trauma and anxiety, others were confused and angry, and many just missed their parents. Working individually with the first children who entered the program allowed specific focus on each child. Later, as the 9/11 population grew, group work was possible and, in fact, necessary due to the large number of participants. Group work provided peer support for the children, reinforcement of safety, management of anxiety, and life adjustment. While switching between directive and nondirective art tasks, specific therapeutic goals were achieved while empowering the children. Allowing them some choice of activities or materials and voice for their primary concerns decreased the helplessness induced by the traumatic deaths.

Because children were traumatized as well as bereaved, it was essential first to provide a psychologically safe holding environment. Once this environment was established, trauma-related goals (Rando, 1996) included teaching them (1) ways to self-soothe and self-regulate, (2) to understand and express emotions, (3) to identify and develop healthy defenses, (4) to achieve mastery to counteract helplessness, (5) to recall and narrate trauma witnessed or imagined, and (6) to manage anxiety related to memory or present fears.

A number of techniques were used, including but not limited to: guided imagery, music, and group quilts to provide containment and comfort; painting, clay work, expressive movement, multimedia collage, and scratchboard to release energy and emotions; storyboard, puppetry, and sandplay to encourage literal and symbolic narrative; and "before and after" drawings to ascertain how each child perceived events and how his or her coping skills improved after treatment.

Creating "safety boxes" was one of the early projects designed to facilitate a sense of safety, expression of emotions, and understanding of traumatic events. This directive is a variation on "comfort boxes" described by Cohen, Barnes, and Rankin (1995). Children were given an array of photographs and other materials and asked to collage images of safety, comfort, and protection on the outside of boxes. On the inside, they were asked to represent their fears, anger, sadness, and other experiences of vulnerability. Verbal processing focused on fears and how the children could obtain comfort or protection. The box directives aimed at a contained expression of feeling that would not overwhelm the children emotionally and could help them focus on the acquisition of self-help skills.

Kalmanowitz and Lloyd (2005) discuss the importance of remembering and forgetting in the amelioration of trauma. Remembering and being able to tell the traumatic experience is validating and healing, but remembering can also overwhelm the psyche. Even for a skilled therapist, it is not always possible to modulate when and how memories emerge. It is important to respect defenses and recognize the vulnerability of clients before encouraging them to narrate traumatic events too quickly. In initial individual sessions children of 9/11 victims were provided with freedom to choose art or play materials as well as topics. These children alternated between dealing directly with or responsively to what they remembered and engaging in "fun" projects to calm, soothe, and distract them.

Vulnerability and fragmentation were nowhere more evident than in the early images produced by this first group of children. Even when offered an abundance of materials, many produced impoverished and skeletal images of transparent houses and floating objects. They did not fill the paper with the brilliant colors and images characteristic of young children. Nine-year-old Sharon and her younger siblings had had private art lessons prior to their Journeys sessions and demonstrated their skill and experience by how they handled the materials. Yet the cheerful images of their family produced by the younger sisters that featured bright suns and hearts were fragmented—faces without bodies, words and sentences filling the gaps between images, disembodied tears and stereotyped gravestones labeled "RIP" to indicate death. They were guarded and hesitant to fully explore their feelings. Much later, in a group session, Holly, one of the girls, painted a tower with herself next to it, depicted as large as the tower. She added the words "But it was real." Holly needed to remind herself of the truth of what had happened; numbness from the trauma and disbelief still guarded her against the full impact of her loss.

Coping and resilience are cultivated by the creative and physical properties of the art-making process and are enhanced by catharsis, expression, and exploration within the structure of the media and a supportive therapeutic relationship (Kalmanowitz & Lloyd, 2005). Through development of imagery and symbolism, meaning is given to experience, sometimes highly personal and sometimes numinous and spiritual. The ability to create requires trust and flexibility. The act of creation itself counters the powerlessness caused by traumatic loss. When Sharon entered the Journeys room for her first individual session, she excitedly noticed mask projects drying on the shelves. The masks piqued her interest, and she asked to make one, cheerfully stating that she wanted to make a portrait of her father. He was a redhead, she said as she selected and mixed the right shades of hair color, eye color, and skin tone before painting. Very carefully, she painted a fairly realistic portrait, then sat looking at the portrait for a few moments before starting slowly, as if in a trance, to pour the remaining red, pink, orange, and brown paint over the face, even getting more brown paint out of the bottle.

At first the shining red and orange blobs covering the face glistened like fire. The subsequent brown paint she poured over half of the face lumped on like mud, making it appear partially buried in dirt. Her initially loving portrait had become a ghastly, deformed human face (Figure 5.2). When she finished, Sharon remained sitting quietly, looking at the mask. After a few minutes, I asked her if she would like to talk about it. She shook her head no. Together in silence, we contemplated the mask lying on the table. An interpretation or discussion would have been a violation of her privacy and the power of the image she had created. Through the process of responding to the media with her unconscious, Sharon had allowed this fearful image to emerge. She had externalized it and could tolerate looking at it; she could assimilate its meaning without turning away. The image and the process of

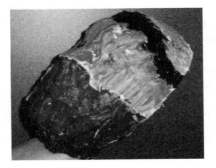

FIGURE 5.2. Eth and Pynoos (1985) indicate that imagined visual horror can interfere with pleasant memories of the deceased parent.

making it transcended verbal description. Later, while cleaning up, Sharon said that next week she would like to make a different mask, a beautiful one, as a gift to a new friend whose family had helped hers after the attacks.

Telling the trauma narrative, an essential step in recovery, was challenging during the first several months after the attacks. Consistent with PTSD reactions, children attempted to avoid recalling the events and were not helped by the media saturation of replays. To assist them in speaking through metaphor, children were encouraged to use narrative in sandtray, dollhouse and puppet play, and storyboard drawings. They were given a choice of sharing dreams or personal or created stories. This offered them control; many, including Sharon, provided symbolic versions of the trauma. In her storyboard, Sharon created the tale of a "little blue man" who built his house on the shore; it was swept out to sea by a gigantic tidal wave and destroyed. In the story, 2 years later, the little blue man, alone on an island and situated between two palm trees, was still yelling, "Help!" as loud as he could (Figure 5.3). The blue in this story may be a verbal metaphor for sadness, death from lack of oxygen, or vaporizing. The tale was of an isolated person overwhelmed by a catastrophic event. The tidal wave may have symboliized the suddenness of the attack that killed her father as well as the experience of being overcome by a deluge of tears.

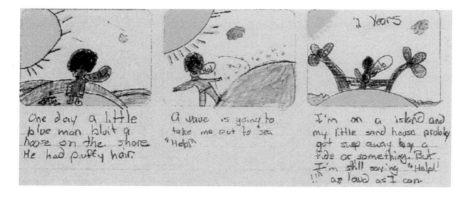

FIGURE 5.3. The use of storyboard and other narrative techniques offers traumatized children control over disclosure. They may use metaphor or symbolism, as Sharon did, to retell their experience in a manageable, less direct way.

The home may have represented both a building and home life. The number two may have represented both the towers and the anticipated duration of grief. The little blue man had large puffy hair that resembled a turban, which may have been a subconscious association to Bin Ladin; the blue man could also be a combination of aspects of both the victim and the perpetrator of the trauma. Through the rich metaphor of her story, Sharon was able to discuss her psychic process without direct confrontation.

The creation of "inside/outside" masks addressed the use of outward defenses as well as the vulnerable feelings inside. Mask projects were started in January, 4 months after the attacks. Families had "survived" the first holidays without their loved ones. Once the excitement associated with the holidays had passed, the reality of the loss and deeper sadness became pervasive. Children were grieving more openly but were also looking for normalcy in their lives. They did not always want to be seen by their classmates as children of the victims. They wanted to be treated like everyone else while they dealt with their own emotions. Over the course of three or four sessions, the mask project addressed both coping strategies and feelings. Children began by studying masks from around the world and discussing their symbolism of transformation, disguise, or "becoming a new character." Then they created masks that represented habitual ways they hid feelings or protected themselves. Once the masks were completed, they were asked to paint inside the masks the feelings they usually hid. Discussion about their masks helped them understand the importance of having defenses, as well as of honoring, acknowledging, and expressing their feelings at the right times.

Some children continued to block their feelings. A different approach was taken to help these children release them. One project in the Saturday preteen group involved a multimedia experience that utilized Wallace's (1990) tissue paper collage technique while listening to New Age music and Pablo Neruda's (1970) poem "Loneliness." In addition to tissue paper, phrases from the poem were provided to be included in the collage. My goal in this complex directive was to use the tearing of the tissue paper, augmented by discordant music and Neruda's lament, to tap into and provide release for the emotions of those who were still guarded, apprehensive, and superficial in their engagement. Ambiguous music intermingled with the soothing process of brushing glue over tissue paper, and seeing brilliant colors emerge, provided an opportunity for both the expression of pain and containment. Bob, who had joined the program with his brother Alan, stated that his image was of the fire trucks rushing to the scene of the attack (Figure 5.4). In the image, what could be a tall bearded figure in shadow dissolves into the image of two sagging towers with large chunks of debris flying everywhere; one piece may even recall a plane. Bob selected many of the poetry phrases and glued them onto his collage: "on that day," "not happening," "so sudden," "not knowing," and "I have no idea." He used the effect of the tissue paper colors bleeding when brushed with the watered glue as a way of depicting yellow-orange flames emanating from the burning buildings. The collage itself is a visual catharsis of shock, pain, destruction, and confusion.

In another group session, participants were offered the medium of scratchboard. The sharp instruments needed to scratch out an image harnessed controlled aggression to depict aspects of the attack or death that made them angry. Bob's brother Alan methodically divided his scratchboard into quadrants and carefully depicted four separate views of the attack as if he were a film director. He cut from scene to scene to show aspects of what happened: a high aerial view of the towers, including the Hudson River; a view from above of the North Tower

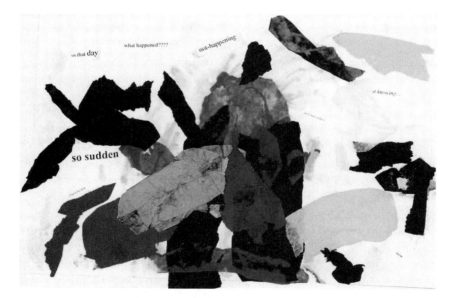

FIGURE 5.4. A multimedia approach that combined tissue paper collage with New Age music and poetry helped participants release blocked feelings.

getting hit by a plane and its antenna falling off; a view looking straight down over the South Tower with debris and smoke coming out of it; and, last, an image of a news helicopter flying over the destroyed towers. Like a director, he distanced himself from the event, looking down, trying to see the big picture. He maintained control of his emotions even as he aggressively etched these images. He became observer and narrator, trying to make sense of what had happened. Alan highlighted the ever-present aspect of media that took away privacy and ownership from his deeply personal loss. He felt that he and his family were made more vulnerable to unwanted attention from strangers.

Toward the end of June 2002, the children made "before and after" drawings to help them understand how their responses to the trauma and deaths had changed. They were instructed to divide a piece of paper in half and draw on one side what they remembered as the most difficult part of 9/11 itself and on the other side what the most difficult thing was now. Several drew the familiar image of the attack itself as the memory and changes in the family as the current challenge. Holly drew herself in her classroom on September 11 hearing from her teacher about the attacks and thinking of her father. On the other side, she drew a picture of herself playing softball, saying her father would be proud of how well she was doing now. In the "after" drawing, a large cloud passing behind her figure is shaped like an enormous plane silhouetted against the blue sky. Similar images of penetration or rupture reminiscent of the attack continued to appear in many children's artwork throughout their time in the program. These images reflected the lingering unconscious presence of the frightening experience even as they regained a conscious sense of security and worked through their grief.

The power of memory is important in both trauma and loss. In the bereavement process it is a symbolic way to hold onto the deceased. It attests to the endurance of love and relationship; it is not merely the physical presence of the loved one that constitutes the connection, but what the lost person has been to the bereaved and all that has transpired between them. Grief work is a dance between holding on and letting go. Native American wisdom reminds us: "A person is alive as long as someone can tell their story." Young children, because of their developmental stage, will forget much. Sharon's youngest sister, Mary, was poignantly aware of this: "I'm scared . . . because sometimes I think . . . when I grow up I won't remember him" she said of their father (Payson, 2002). In the earliest stages of trauma, images of their parents' violent death interfered with children's ability to remember their parents as whole and healthy, as illustrated by Sharon's mask. In subsequent months, as they addressed aspects of their trauma and began to feel safe, many children started to have pleasant dreams in which they spent time with their late fathers or mother. Toward the end of the first year, the children created portraits from photographs. Through time spent looking intently at the faces of their parents and the act of recreating their images, they started to recreate memories.

Bereavement Goals: Experiencing the Reality of Death

After the camaraderie of public grief and the nakedness of public exposure disappeared, families of the victims were left with the existential loneliness of their own grief and a private hole as bottomless as Ground Zero. One of the characteristics of early grief and of trauma is numbness, a feeling that the loss is only a terrible dream. When that passes, the reality of the loss can be devastating. In the second and third years of therapy the weight of reality settled on many of the children.

In the second year, two exclusive younger 9/11 groups resumed, and three older boys who had lost fathers opted to join a nonexclusive group of adolescents. These boys attended a weekend camp for survivors of 9/11 several times a year, which satisfied their need to be with peers who had experienced the same loss. They decided to join a weekly non–9/11 Journeys bereavement group in order to be in a larger ongoing group with kids their age.

In the second year, a few children had not yet dealt directly with the traumatic aspects of their parents' death, and some of the younger children were just becoming fully cognizant of what had actually happened. Many were beginning to explore specific questions about the attack and death. Traumatic images that had been successfully repressed by the 5-to-7-year-olds in the first year now emerged. Families had developed new routines and started to grieve on a deeper level. Many of the children—younger and older—wanted to hold on to positive memories to ward off the frightful ones. Goals of the second year included examining changes, providing continued structured review of the deaths, fuller acceptance of uncomfortable emotions, memory work, and life review.

A warm-up technique I often use with bereavement groups as a way of addressing the cognition of death includes having participants look at, touch, and examine natural objects such as driftwood, sharks' teeth, bone, amber, petrified wood, birds' nests, carbuncles, and worm-wood. This is followed by a discussion of the life cycle. Children get very excited about sharing their knowledge of nature, life, and death with each other. They sometimes speculate about the emotional reactions of animals to the death of their kin. At the end of the second year, these objects were presented to the now 6-to-8-year-old group. Interest stimulated a lively discussion that stopped short when one child, citing the movie *Jurassic Park* (Kennedy & Molen, 1993), excitedly proclaimed that the amber might have some DNA in it. Anna, whose mother had died in the towers, asked, "What is DNA?"

Following the answer, Anna told the group that her father had to take her mother's hairbrush and toothbrush into Manhattan to give her mother's DNA. She asked, "Why?" but then answered herself. Searchers had later found a part of her mother that they had identified through DNA testing. Others in the group started talking about whether their fathers had been found or not. The children wanted to know why only parts had been found and started to share what they remembered: the planes, the fire, the collapse, and how everyone was trapped inside. "That is why so many people were hurt so badly," I told them.

Animatedly, the children, who had avoided the topic up until now, interrupted each other to tell what they knew and what they thought. Suddenly, they needed a way to share the awful facts they had heard and to find out if the others harbored similar scary thoughts and unpleasant memories. As Sharon had done with her mask a year and a half earlier, each child now filled in the blanks of his or her knowledge with imagination. In the drawings they later produced, they replayed the impact of the terrorist attack—not merely what they had seen on television, but what they imagined their parents to have experienced during the attacks. A dreaded question emerged next: "Miss Laura, why did they jump?" Before I could formulate a response, other children chimed in with their own explanations, some plausible and realistic, others not. Some used macabre humor to deflect the truth: "Maybe they wanted to go for a swim," or "They wanted to get out of the building fast!" They giggled nervously. All knew what had happened to the towers, but they could not know what had happened to their parents. They wondered if their parents had jumped, how they had died, or what they had been thinking and feeling at the end. Their jokes and clamorous answers yielded to an uneasiness that silenced further discussion.

The children were offered oil pastels and paper and I told them, "It's very hard to think about what we all are talking about. You all are thinking so much about what happened that day. There are many things none of us will ever know. If you want, draw a picture of what you think happened. If you don't want to do that, you can draw a picture of something that makes you feel good." All drew the outlines of the towers; several showed staircases with flames rising up through the center of the building and tiny stick figures of people trapped inside. Marian, who had joined the group in March with her two siblings, selected black paper, outlined a tower with red pastel—hardly visible against the black—and drew a skeletal image of her father screaming to get out as others jumped or fell (Figure 5.5). She drew a large heart next to the building to show her love for him. All of the children said they had thought about these images before but tried not to. They did

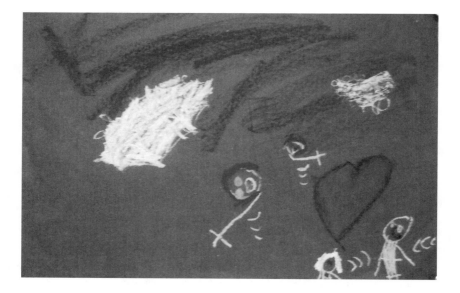

FIGURE 5.5. In the second year, the younger children were beginning to more fully realize what had actually happened on September 11, 2001, and a few had not yet dealt with the traumatic aspects of their parents' death. Frightening images that had been repressed by some 5-to-7-year-olds in the first year now emerged.

not like talking about it at home because it was too scary and it upset their remaining parent. Steele (2002) suggests that adults are so fearful of their children being overwhelmed by trauma that they encourage them to avoid thinking about it. Traumatized children need to tell their story and have their internal experiences witnessed. It took more than a year for these children, who had been 5 to 7 years old at the time of the attacks, to externalize their images and have the courage to ask unanswerable questions. In addition to facing the trauma, this group had started to tackle two important aspects of bereavement—the cognitive understanding of death and empathy for the plight of their parents.

Many children of the victims revealed that the defining moment of the loss for them was not the attack itself but the arrival at their homes of policemen to inform them that the body of their father or mother had been identified (Freeman, 2005). For example, the shock that Bob had so vividly portrayed in his collage during the first year contrasted with the loneliness he depicted 2 years later in a drawing of when he found out about the death. Bob drew himself sitting alone on the edge of his bed in his room (Figure 5.6). In the picture, the large bed, on which he braces his arms, makes him look small. The emptiness of the room is broken only by the two open windows behind him, a calendar on the wall, and the light fixture on the ceiling. Bob described looking out his window and seeing the police car pull up to his house; he remained in his room because he knew why the officers were there. Like others whose loved ones' bodies were found, Bob admitted that up until the point when the police came, he had held out hope that maybe his father was trapped and surviving on water and food found in the rubble. It was not until he saw the police car that he admitted to himself that his father was dead. The reality of the loss swept over him as he sat alone in his room; he did not need to hear the words.

Bob had a highly developed capacity for empathy and spent time worrying about what the end had been like for his father. When doing a heart-box collage, he illustrated both the inside and outside with all the positive and negative feelings he experienced in relation to his father's life and death. On the interior, he filled the bottom of the box with several images of intense suffering or trauma: a man in a gas mask, a string of seaweed underwater, a dog dragging the lifeless body of a large fish, a cartoon rendering of a sweaty man struggling to climb a rope, an animal trapped behind barbed wire, someone searching

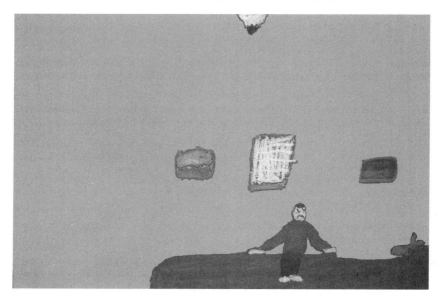

FIGURE 5.6. In the second year of therapy, Bob depicted the loneliness he felt when his father's body was found and he was forced to give up the hope that his father had somehow survived. Bob drew himself sitting alone on the edge of his bed in his room, bracing himself against the emptiness overwhelming him.

through stones and rubble, and the word "suffer?" On the underside of the bottom, he showed two dinosaurs in a life-and-death struggle and a human skull. For Bob, thinking of the ways his father might have suffered and not knowing if he had or not distressed him even more than his own loss. In the same group exercise, his brother Alan used the collage process to depict the experience of confusion and loneliness he had felt as well as to show the ways in which his father would be proud of him now—how he was coping and living a good and worthy life (Figure 5.7).

Donald, Marian's brother, who was 10 at the time of the attacks, denied his grief but enjoyed participating in group. He tended to focus exclusively on positive memories of his father and on how well he felt he was coping. In June of 2003, when the school year ended and many children would break for summer, "journey" drawings were assigned. Journey drawings, adapted from a technique by McElligott and Webb (1989) that was originally developed for addictive populations, pro-

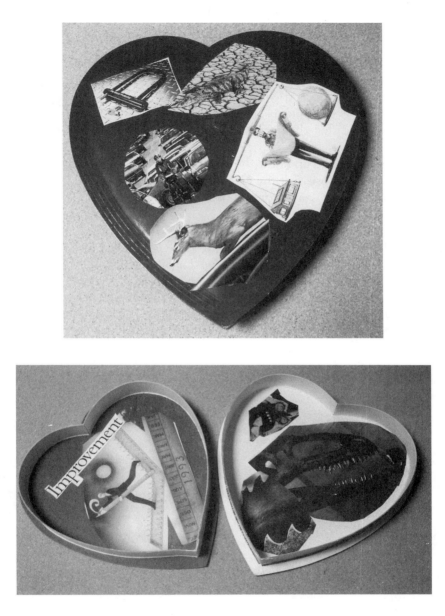

FIGURE 5.7. Heart-box collage is a technique I developed. It combines the resistance of selecting superficial symbols such as hearts for love with the control offered by finding and using photographic images created by others. Participants are asked to cover the inside and outside of a heart-shaped box with pictures that represent the gamut of their emotions—positive and negative—about their late loved ones. The act of juxtaposing often startling images with the heart shape brings a visual and emotional depth to the final product.

vide a way to have participants look at the current stage of their grief and their anticipated recovery. Group participants were asked to envision themselves on a trip to a chosen destination after completing therapy and to imagine an obstacle en route barring their way. They were then told that they could have any means possible to overcome this obstacle and complete the journey. The task was to draw the obstacle envisioned and how they overcame it. Donald's trip involved driving to New York over the George Washington Bridge (Figure 5.8). The bridge had broken apart and he and his family could not proceed, so they got off the bridge and found a way to get to New York by land. In his drawing, the aerial view of a road with a jagged hole ahead looks more like a stark white skyscraper with blue sky streaming through a hole in its structure than a bridge. The danger posed by such an obstacle, his unrealistic solution, and the lingering unconscious image of the attack indicated that Donald was not coping as well as he thought he was.

People who have experienced trauma or bereavement are prone to sleep disturbances. In December 2003, Donald's mother expressed concern about a dream he had shared with her. An individual session

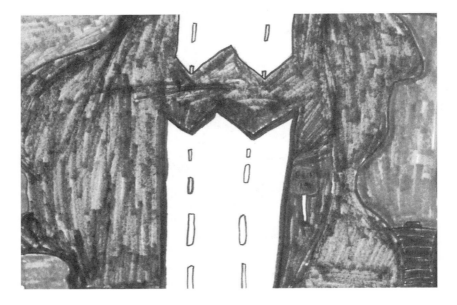

FIGURE 5.8. Journey drawings provide a metaphor for current grief and anticipated recovery.

was scheduled to allow him to process this dream. In his dream, Donald and his father were in one of the towers as it was attacked. Both managed to get out safely, but his father went back in to save someone, as he had done in the 1993 terrorist attack on the World Trade Center. Donald was safe outside as the building collapsed with his father inside. Donald told the story with much hesitation and difficulty. I asked him to paint it. The painting resembled those from Marian's group a year earlier (Figure 5.9). In his painting, the black skyline is silhouetted against a purple sky. The interior of one tower is dominated by a fiery red crisscrossing stairwell. On the burning stairs are three small yellow figures that look like flickering flames against the red and black. Outside, the top of the page is filled with yellow. Donald had painted himself back in the building. He spoke of his father's bravery and was reassured that it takes courage to enter a burning building, even in one's imagination; he had allowed himself to experience what he felt his father had. Out of love for his father, he had faced the imagined horror of being trapped inside the building. Not

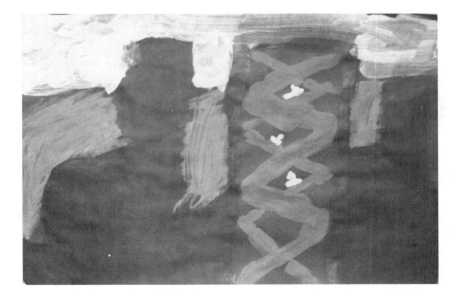

FIGURE 5.9. In his imagination, Donald had recreated the horror of his father's death and tried to replay it and change the ending but without success. By processing his dream through imagery, Donald was able to face the trauma.

only survivor's guilt, but also his longing to be reunited with his father took him back into that building. Even in his imagination, he could not change what had happened. He could not effect a rescue as his father had years earlier. The sense of helplessness, of not being able to change reality, was palpable. Donald had faced the trauma and begun a deeper and more conscious exploration of his grief.

In the third year, the adolescents explored the impact of their parents' deaths on their lives through "before and after" drawings. In one drawing, Alan used his father's vegetable garden as a metaphor for the change that had occurred in his family (Figure 5.10). Both he and his brother Bob told how their father liked to grow traditional Chinese vegetables with the boys to keep their culture alive. They also talked about his pride, hard work, and the many other skills he had taught and the experiences he had shared with them. On one side of his drawing, Alan depicted his family busily working in the garden together, each of them intent on his or her task. On the other side, his father's garden had gone to waste because everyone was either too sad or too busy with family obligations to tend to it and because his father

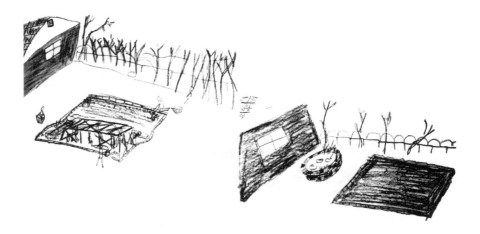

FIGURE 5.10. "Before and after" drawings help clients measure real changes in their lives as well as psychological changes caused by trauma and loss.

was not there to guide them. A solitary plant to memorialize their father wilts in the barren plot while nearby is a fancy raised brick flower bed that his mother paid someone else to install. No one is outside enjoying it.

Alan repeated this garden theme later in a "window in time" painting. Group participants were instructed to paint a view through a window showing a scene in the past, present, or future. This time Alan painted a solitary, unused lawnmower seen from inside the house through the windows of two closed doors. He again told the group that he and his brother used to help their father with all the chores; now they pay someone else "too much money" to do something they can do themselves. Donald approached this task differently; he painted himself and his father sitting together quietly talking at the kitchen table of their old house, separated by the window panes through which they were viewed. Looking at this image seems like spying on an intimate conversation. Group members thought the colors of the kitchen cupboards made the whole picture look like a football field; the sharing of sports interests was a frequent theme in Donald's artwork. Donald was acknowledging the separation more completely by placing his relationship with his father in the past.

Final Goals: Preserving the Connection

By 2003, many children were no longer actively grieving but had come to identify themselves as members of an exclusive group who shared experiences that no one else could understand. They wanted to normalize their lives. They were not interested in continuing to focus on the events and trauma of 9/11 but wanted to maintain a bond with each other. Memories were fading, and perspectives were changing. Art directives and projects now concentrated on revised life perspectives, review of the previous relationship with their deceased parents, and memorializing their parents.

Toward the end of the third year, the spring of 2004, controversial plans to replace the towers were being formulated and made public. Some children and teenagers were in favor of the plans. Donald hoped to work there as his father had. Some opposed it. Anna said, "Our parents died there; it is sacred ground." This debate provided an appropriate beginning point for participants' culminating memorial projects (Figure 5.11).

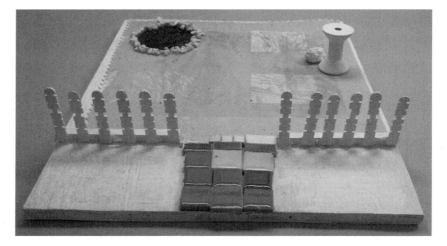

FIGURE 5.11. In her memorial project, Anna designed a meditation garden in which she would feel close to her mother.

By the fourth year following the attacks, only the three oldest boys remained in the program, continuing for 10 monthly group sessions. Life and grief reviews indicated that they had reinvested and found new focus in their lives. Letting go of active mourning as a way to maintain attachment to their fathers provided a final challenge. Self-portraits in which they represented incorporated aspects of their parents helped reveal internalized strengths.

Donald was in the Journeys Program for 4 years and grew from 10 to 14 years old in that time. The death of his father left him in a home with two younger sisters and a mother. He was the only male in the household without the father who had been his anchor. Donald attempted to be the man of the house, accepting responsibility for his younger sisters while maintaining a fierce loyalty to his father. He resisted the efforts of his uncles to become confidants and support figures as his father had been. Much of Donald's early artwork had been nostalgic and idealized. It took a brave leap for him to let go of his façade of strength and allow himself to feel the full pain and sorrow of separation, which he eventually had done. He had to fully experience the separation before he could reconnect with his father on a deeper level.

In his last year in the Journeys Program, Donald came in for individual sessions twice a month and attended his group meeting once a month. His favorite project was a combined self-portrait based on a group directive I devised (Figure 5.12). The group was requested to remember a scene from *The Lion King* (1994) where Rafiki tells Simba to look into his own reflection to find his father who "lives in" him. Group participants then created self-portraits that mirrored how their fathers lived in them. Donald divided his portrait in half. He drew his father's face on one side and his own on the other. He surrounded the portrait with a series of stripes symbolizing the various sports teams they both enjoyed (Freeman, 2005).

In individual therapy, he noted that he had changed physically; he had grown taller and could now fit into his father's clothes that his mother had saved. He also noted with pride that everyone told him how much he looked like his father. He was proud to have been accepted into the same high school his father had attended. Previously, when exploring ways in which he missed his father's guidance, he had despaired that he would not be able to perform in school as

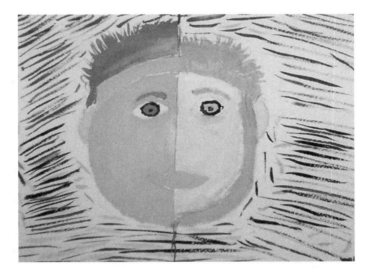

FIGURE 5.12. In this image, Donald's and his father's identities mingle and separate. Donald realized his father lived in him through their deep relationship, through all his father had taught him, and through the man he was becoming as he matured.

well without his father's help. In a drawing, he depicted how he had difficulty concentrating and how his father always managed to make studying fun. At first, he struggled on his own and was afraid of failure. Over time, however, he recognized that he had developed his own strengths and, after initial setbacks of bereavement that affected his concentration, was now able to understand, concentrate, and achieve good grades on his own. He even thought he might have inherited his father's abilities, especially in math. Now he realized on a deeper level that his father resided in him not just in the memories he tried to preserve, in their shared name, or in their similar physiques, but on a deep level through the way they had connected, what he had learned from his father, and whom he was growing up to be. This growth occurred as a result of what his father had taught him and the strength he had developed in coping with his father's death.

CONCLUSIONS: IMPLICATIONS FOR THE TREATMENT OF TRAUMATIC GRIEF

In discussing their work with traumatized families, Abu Sway and colleagues (2005) say, "the special therapeutic techniques developed to help in the healing of trauma . . . are very helpful but lack the ability to empower the individual . . . the power of the arts as a means of self-expression is that it brings out the deep-rooted pain in the self without posing a threat to it. The arts can provide a safe transitional space to allow the self to experiment until it attains integrity and control" (p. 159). This chapter demonstrates the use of art for treating trauma and grief in work with children who lost a parent in the mass terrorist attacks against the United States in 2001. Art therapy provided a safe vehicle through which full self-expression was possible. The use of drawing and other art modalities actively engaged children in their own healing (Steele & Raider, 2001).

Establishing safety and instilling the inner strength to modify overwhelming emotions and memories produced by trauma was necessary before grief work could begin. Short-term trauma-related goals used in the Journeys Program include safety, self-regulation, the use of metaphor, and attention to the adaptive use of defenses. The reintroduction of positive images of the deceased enhances the transition between trauma and bereavement work. Long-term goals of bereavement work include helping children deal with recognizing and adjusting to external and internal life changes, evaluating self-growth, experiencing the fullness of grief, internalizing aspects of deceased parents, and creating memorials to them.

Finally, the role of the therapist as a supportive witness who provides unconditional acceptance is vital to intervention. In grief and trauma work, therapists must be fully present and able to tolerate children's pain, help decrease their isolation, and provide structure and containment. With the power of creativity and guidance through the recovery process, children experiencing combined trauma and grief can develop innate courage and resilience, complete the tasks of bereavement, and reinvest in their lives (Rando, 1993).

REFERENCES

Abu Sway, R., Nashashibi, R., Salah, R., & Shweiki, R. (2005). Expressive arts therapy—healing the traumatized: The Palestinian experience. In D. Kalmanowitz & B. Lloyd (Eds.), Art therapy and political violence (pp. 154–171). London: Routledge.

Benke, D. (2003). A healing ritual at Yankee Stadium. In M. Lattanzi-Licht & K. Doka (Eds.), Living with grief: Coping with public tragedy (pp. 191–201). Washington, DC: Hospice Foundation of America.

Bertman, S. (2003). Public tragedy and the arts. In M. Lattanzi-Licht & K. Doka (Eds.), Living with grief: Coping with public tragedy (pp. 203–217). Washington, DC: Hospice Foundation of America.

Cohen, B., Barnes, M., & Rankin, A. (1995). Managing traumatic stress through art: Drawing from the center. Baltimore, MD: The Sidran Press.

Doka, K. (2003). What makes a tragedy public? In M. Lattanzi-Licht & K. Doka (Eds.), Living with grief: Coping with public tragedy (pp. 3–13). Washington, DC: Hospice Foundation of America.

Eth, S., & Pynoos, R. (1985). Post-traumatic stress in children. Washington, DC: American Psychiatric Press.

Freeman, V. (2005, October) Between trauma and transformation: The alchemy of art therapy. Alternative Medicine, 43–48.

Goodman, R., & Fahnestock, H. (2002). The day our world changed: Children's art of 9/11. New York: New York University Child Study Center and the Museum of the City of New York, Harry N. Abrams.

Hartley, B. (2004). Bereavement groups soon after traumatic death. In N. Webb (Ed.), Mass trauma and violence: Helping children and families cope (pp. 167–190). New York: Guilford Press.

Henley, D., Rosner David I., Greenstone, L., Goodman, R., Spring, D., Stoll, B., et al. (2001). Art therapists in their own words. *Art Therapy: Journal of the American Art Therapy Association, 18*(4), 179–189.

Kalmanowitz, D., & Lloyd, B. (2005). Art therapy and political violence. In D. Kalmanowitz & B. Lloyd (Eds.), *Art therapy and political violence* (pp. 14–34). London: Routledge.

Kennedy, K., & Molen, G. (Producers), Crichton, M. (Writer), & Spielberg, S. (Director). (1993). *Jurassic park* [Film]. Los Angeles: Universal Pictures.

McArthur, S., & Schumacher, T. (Executive Producers), Mecchi, I., Roberts, J., & Woolverton, L. (Writers), & Allers, R., & Minkoff, R. (Directors). (1994). *The lion king* [Film]. Burbank, CA: Walt Disney.

McElligott, D., & Webb, K. (1989, November). *Clinical art therapy with addicted populations: Application of the systemic model.* Preconference course presented at the meeting of the American Art Therapy Association, San Francisco, CA.

McGeehan, I. (2005). Creativity from chaos: An art therapist's account of art work produced in the aftermath of a bombing in her community, Omagh, Northern Ireland. In D. Kalmanowitz & B. Lloyd (Eds.), *Art therapy and political violence* (pp. 126–141). London: Routledge.

Neruda, P. (1970). *Selected poems.* New York: Delta Publishing Company.

Payson, J. (Executive Producer). (2002, March 7). Tender hearts: Art helps children of 9/11 express emotions and heal. *Primetime Thursday* [Television series]. New York: American Broadcasting System.

Rando, T. (1993). *Treatment of complicated mourning.* Champaign, IL: Research Press.

Rando, T. (1996). Complications in mourning traumatic death. In K. Doka (Ed.), *Living with grief after sudden loss* (pp. 139–159). Washington, DC: Hospice Foundation of America.

Rando, T. (2003). Public tragedy and complicated mourning. In M. Lattanzi-Licht & K. Doka (Eds.), *Living with grief: Coping with public tragedy* (pp. 263–274). Washington, DC: Hospice Foundation of America.

Rankin, A., & Taucher, C. (2003). A task-oriented approach to art therapy in trauma treatment. *Art Therapy: Journal of the American Art Therapy Association, 20*(3), 138–147.

Rathkey, J. (2004). *What children need when they grieve.* New York: Three Rivers Press.

Santino, J. (2006). *Spontaneous shrines and public memorialization of death.* New York: Palgrave Macmillan.

Steele, W. (2002). Using drawing in short-term trauma resolution. In C. Malchiodi (Ed.), *Handbook of art therapy* (pp. 139–151). New York: Guilford Press.

Steele, W., & Raider, M. (2001). *Structured sensory intervention for traumatized children, adolescents and parents strategies to alleviate trauma.* Lewiston, NY: Edward Mellen Press.

Testa, N., & McCarthy, J. (2004). The use of murals in preadolescent inpatient groups: An art therapy approach to cumulative trauma. *Art Therapy: Journal of the American Art Therapy Association, 21*(1), 38–41.

Wallace, E. (1990). *A queen's quest pilgrimage for individuation.* Santa Fe, NM: Moon Bear Press.

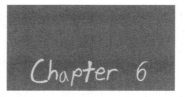

Chapter 6

Medical Art and Play Therapy with Accident Survivors

Elizabeth Sanders Martin

Accidents are the leading cause of injury in children between the ages of 1 and 17 years. Schreier, Ladakakos, Morabito, Chapman, and Knudson (2005) reported that more than 8 million children a year in the United States sustain some form of physical injury, with more than 200,000 requiring hospitalization. Accidents may involve one person or many people; some may die in an accident or shortly thereafter. These accidents can completely change patients' lives in an instant. Survivors may sustain traumatic brain injuries, spinal cord injuries, amputations, broken bones, and/or burns. Each of these injuries may leave a lasting traumatic memory on patients, families, friends, and even the medical personnel who come in contact with them.

Perry and Azad (1999) report that 30% of children exposed to traumatic events develop posttraumatic stress disorder (PTSD). Meiser-Stedman, Yule, Smith, Glucksman, and Dalgleish (2005) observe in their research that patients who developed acute stress disorder following a traumatic injury were more likely to be diagnosed with PTSD. This chapter will focus on art and play therapy interventions in the hospital setting for pediatric patients with traumatic brain injury, spinal cord injury, and burns, with an emphasis on addressing traumatic stress in child and adolescent survivors.

MEDICAL SETTINGS AND TRAUMATIZED CHILDREN

Working in a medical setting presents a unique challenge to trauma specialists. In contrast to other types of settings where intervention is provided, hospitals can be a source of both hope and distress to the patient and family (Councill, 2006). Receiving treatment for injuries offers hope for relief from suffering, but the sights, smells, sounds, and other aspects of the hospital environment may leave patients and their families feeling as though they have traveled to a foreign land (Spinetta & Spinetta, 1981). Therapists may work with pediatric patients in hospital rooms where medical personnel are regularly present to give medications or take vital signs or in waiting rooms where play areas are provided for patients and their siblings. Hospital environments, in contrast to private offices or playrooms, sometimes demand attention to infection or medical needs and often are chaotic, filled with health care providers, family, and visitors.

A serious physical accident such as a burn, spinal cord injury, or brain injury is often experienced by both patient and family as not only a surprise, but also as an event that robs them of the functional illusion that bad things happen to other people, not to good people (Kushner, 1981). Patients in hospitals lose a sense of control due to the injury and the necessary regime of medications, procedures, and treatments needed to help the patient physically improve. This sense of helplessness in patients is reinforced by the medical treatment itself. In addition, patients lose their privacy during the dressing changes and physical examinations required. Art therapist Tracy Councill (2006) notes that giving pediatric patients control over their art productions—what to make, what materials to use, whether to keep their art or throw it away, whether to do art at all that day— encourages choice and control in the aftermath of trauma. Pediatric patients need opportunities to gain and maintain a sense of mastery over their situation and their environment.

Hospitalized patients also have unique feelings, perceptions, and experiences related to their medical injuries. Often their emotions and memories are either repressed due to fear of retaliation or embarrassment or overlooked by medical staff and/or parents. The role of art and play is to provide patients with a voice to be heard and be accepted and understood. Art and play give patients the opportunity to explore, gain mastery, and discover their own answers to psychosocial problems confronting them.

Developmental issues are particularly important in the treatment of psychological trauma in children and adolescents. Hospitalization for injuries can significantly affect the developmental tasks that children and adolescents must complete for healthy psychosocial growth throughout the lifespan. According to Thompson and Stanford (1981), children who are deprived of normal social and intellectual stimulation for long periods of time may display behavior consistent with developmental delays. Because traumatic injuries may require long hospitalizations with physical limitations, these injuries may hinder normal physical, cognitive, and social growth and development in children and adolescents.

Finally, parental involvement is critical in young children's lives, particularly after a traumatic event. According to Caffo and Belaise (2003) and Councill (2006), when patients and families work together creatively within the treatment setting, they can better mobilize inner resources such as hope and resilience. By working alongside others, the child and family employ familiar skills and strengths, experiencing themselves as normal, capable people instead of as passive patients. Children who are provided with structure, predictability, and a sense of safety within their family unit are less likely to develop posttraumatic stress after a trauma.

Most pediatric hospitals encourage family members to stay with patients to provide security, trust, and familiarity; however, in motor vehicle accidents, sometimes the parents are also injured. In all cases, the therapist's goal is to help patients remain connected to their families, even when separated, and to communicate with their health care providers. Patients who have survived an accident are often unable to articulate questions or concerns because of their injuries, and parents or caregivers may be too distressed to convey their feelings clearly. Because having accurate information is important to successful trauma recovery, therapists working with survivors of injuries encourage patients and their families to ask questions and, at times, may even become the liaison for patients and families in communication with health care providers.

TYPES OF TRAUMATIC INJURIES

Traumatic Brain Injury

Warzak, Allan, Ford, and Stefans (1995) report that 500,000 to 1.5 million Americans sustain traumatic brain injuries (TBIs) within any given year. Approximately 40% of all TBIs occur in pediatric patients, predominately caused by falls, motor vehicle accidents, and bicycle accidents. Brain injuries are categorized as mild, moderate, or severe depending on the amount of time the patient loses consciousness. Mild TBIs, also called concussions or minor head injuries, are classified as such when the person has loss of consciousness and/or confusion and disorientation for less than 30 minutes (Traumatic Brain Injury.com, LLC, 2004). Even if magnetic resonance imaging (MRI) scans are normal, the person may experience headaches, memory problems, mood swings, attention deficits, and frustration.

A moderate TBI occurs when a person loses consciousness from 20 minutes to 6 hours and has a Glasgow Coma Scale score of 9 to 12 (of a possible 15) points. This scale estimates the effects of the brain injury in terms of dependence on others, measuring motor response, verbal response, and eye opening (Traumatic Brain Injury.com, LLC, 2004). A severe TBI is defined as losing consciousness for more than 6 hours and having a Glasgow Coma Scale of 3 to 8 points. Both of these categories include deficits in attention, concentration, memory, speed of processing, language processing, and executive functions. Persons with moderate and severe brain injuries may exhibit increased perseveration, confusion, and impulsivity.

The Rancho Los Amigos Scale measures the awareness, cognition, behavior, and interaction of the injured person with the environment and is based on the premise that each patient will pass through the same stages of recovery; however, the rate of progress will vary from person to person depending upon the location of the injury, functions affected, severity of the injury, medical complications, and the person's physical health prior to the accident, to name a few influential factors (Johnson, 2006; Traumatic Brain Injury.com, LLC, 2004).

Traumatic brain injury affects the family as well as the patient through the patient's increased dependency in self-care activities, and the family's increased concern about the patient's physical safety and decreasing social interactions. Many brain-injured patients are not aware of deficits in cognition and judgment, yet the family recognizes the obvious changes in the behavior and emotions of their loved one, causing emotional distress in caregivers and siblings. Emotional disruption is ranked as the highest-rated obstacle by both caregivers and psychologists (Warzak et al., 1995).

Spinal Cord Injuries

According to Kokoska, Keller, Rallo, and Weber (2001), the leading mechanisms for cervical spine (C-spine) injuries in children of all ages are motor vehicle accidents. Spinal cord injuries are rare in children, constituting only 1 to 2% of all pediatric trauma victims due to the higher amount of mobility and elasticity of children's bodies (Parisini, Di Silvestre, & Greggi, 2002). Dr. Mark Proctor (2002) explained the young child's large head is disproportional to his or her body mass. Infants and toddlers have weak neck muscles, which increases the potential for their head to shift from their spine with great impact. Proctor added that, as the child reaches the age of 8–10 years, the spine matures to resemble an adult's. Injuries to the preteen or adolescent spinal cord are caused more often by motor vehicle accidents and sports-related injuries due to more risk-taking behaviors.

Spinal cord injuries are classified as either complete or incomplete, depending upon the amount of severing of the spinal cord. A complete spinal cord injury leaves the individual without feeling or movement below the point of the injury. Recent research has shown that some movement below the injury can be regained through gait-training techniques. An incomplete spinal cord injury can cause paralysis below the injured site, but this paralysis may be temporary as the swelling of the spinal cord decreases.

Injuries to the spinal cord also impact the autonomic nervous system, causing autonomic dysreflexia, which is common in patients with paralysis above the waist. Autonomic dysreflexia is defined as overstimulation of the sympathetic and parasympathetic functions of the nervous system, including episodes of uncontrollable sweating, increased blood pressure, and decreased regulation of body temperature. Each of these can be triggered by urine in the bladder, a wrinkle in the sheets under the patient, or other overstimulation not perceived by the patient.

Other aspects of spinal cord injury include the changes in patients' lifestyle and functioning. Patients with paralysis become more dependent on family members for daily care. Common self-care activities such as dressing, bathing, and picking up items off the floor may require the aid of another person, depending upon the location of the injury. The higher the C-spine injury, the more paralysis is experienced and the greater the patient's dependence. The financial and emotional burden also affects the patient and family members, especially if the patient was previously physically active or recognized for athletic abilities. These patients and family members will grieve over the loss of their dreams and hopes if the patients' physical abilities are permanently impaired.

Burns

Passaretti and Billmire (2003) reported that more than 30,000 inpatient admissions each year are related to pediatric burns. Eighty percent of these admissions are accidents caused by the children or adolescents. Traumatic burns can be the most detrimental injuries to sustain due to the physical and emotional pain experienced on a daily basis. The hospitalization can involve multiple surgeries, skin grafting, and tub debridement of the wounds. Extensive rehabilitation to maintain functioning of the limbs may require stretching of the skin, muscles, and ligaments. The burns cause physical and emotional scarring that remind the patient and family of the traumatic event.

Patients who experience a burn generally struggle with body image changes due to scarring or loss of a limb. Patients with burns to the face and hands generally suffer more psychologically than persons with other burned surfaces due to the visibility of their burns. Many of these children suffer from depression. Appleton (2001), who studied the effects of art therapy interventions with adolescents who sustained a burn requiring hospitalization, notes that the therapist's role in trauma intervention is to "offer media and provide a therapeutic opportunity for the expression of those deeply personal journeys to recovery" (p. 13).

INTERVENTIONS WITH ACCIDENT SURVIVORS

Councill (1999) notes that a visit from a therapist who brings familiar materials and play items and an invitation to create, instead of needles or pills to swallow, can be instantly comforting in a hospital setting.

Whether this first encounter between the therapist and patient leads to an expressive piece of artwork or just a few simple marks, art and play can establish a meaningful link to life outside the hospital and provide a concrete way to respond to the hospital experience. In this section, activities that help pediatric survivors of accidents express their feelings, explore psychosocial aspects of their injuries, and cope with symptoms of trauma are provided for practitioners who work in hospital settings.

Free Drawing

Many times therapists assume they know what children or adolescents are battling internally and expect that certain issues will present themselves in clients' artwork or play activities, but pediatric patients are unique in how they experience physical and emotional trauma. Free drawing—asking patients to draw anything they want to draw—allows patients to express what is important to them, posttrauma, and provides a nonstructured activity for authentic self-expression. Free play (nonstructured play with a specific selection of toys, games, and/or props) is similar in nature, allowing children to convey their personal experiences with traumatic injury.

Susan Bach (1990) notes the importance of free drawing or painting with seriously ill children. Bach's philosophy is based on the theories of psychoanalysis, particularly those of Carl Jung, and is founded on the belief that a child's spontaneous art is actually an expression of the self. After studying thousands of children's artworks, Bach concludes that the color, placement, and number of items in an image nonverbally communicate to the observer information about the self and/or the individual's medical condition. Free expression, in either art or play, allows for exploration and transformation of "conflicts and crises into healthy solutions, outlooks, and perspectives" (Malchiodi, 1998, p. 45). Allan (1988) stressed that the creative process can aid in processing information from the unconscious to the conscious and release the power of emotions related to a critical time.

For free drawing, the patient only requires a box of a variety of colored markers or oil pastels and an 8½″ × 11″ piece of white drawing paper. The therapist simply asks the patient to draw whatever he or she chooses to create (Figures 6.1 and 6.2).

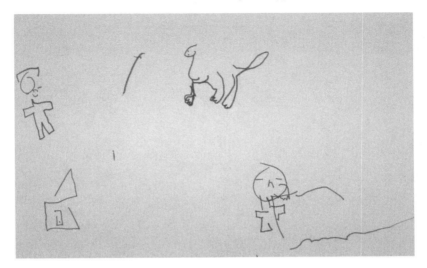

FIGURE 6.1. A 10-year-old male who was involved in a fatal house fire with his siblings kept his eyes closed for 3 days following the fire, complaining that they burned or hurt. The therapist asked the patient to draw whatever he wanted. With his eyes closed, the patient drew his house, a person with slits for eyes, another person, and his dog who died in the fire. He identified his house and his dog, but not the people, whom the therapist surmised to be himself and his sister, who unfortunately died of smoke inhalation the next day.

Narrative Drawing

"Narrative drawing" refers to asking patients to "draw what happened." Schreier and colleagues (2005) studied the effects of a specifically designed art therapy intervention on reducing PTSD symptoms shortly after patients' admission to the hospital for treatment and continued for 18 months postdischarge. The art therapy intervention involved patients drawing the traumatic event and telling their story to the therapist. According to Steele and Raider (2001), such exposure techniques provide patients with the ability to integrate traumatic memories into consciousness, reducing the power of the sensory stimuli to trigger traumatic responses. Narrative drawings give a child the space and time to process and reexperience the trauma within the boundaries needed to prevent retraumatization.

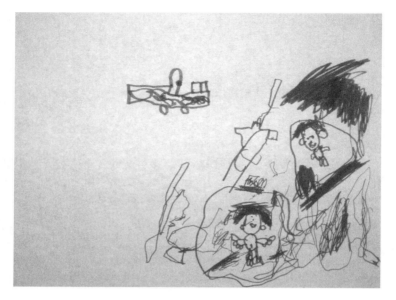

FIGURE 6.2. An 8-year-old male who survived a motor vehicle accident in which his mother died was asked by the therapist to draw whatever he wanted. He began to draw a car when the therapist noticed fresh blood on the paper. After looking at his hand, she found an open IV site and proceeded to put a bandage on it. During this time, the patient drew intensely over the blood spot with a brown marker, covering it completely. He then drew himself and his mother individually encapsulated, showing their separation. He added belly buttons to each figure and wrote "mom" above one of the figures. The blood that the child covered with brown marker may have reminded him of images from the site of the accident.

Zimmerman and Beaudoin (2002) described narrative therapy as using language to externalize the problem and empower the patient to change the story using his or her preferred values and goals. They describe the therapist's role as creating a context for change, not finding a solution. The storyteller finds the solution to the problem by retelling the story. In working with traumatized children and adolescents, the therapist listens to the story and may reflect new endings to stories depicted by the child in artwork, play, and/or storytelling. In the case of a child whose play activity generates increased distress in the child rather than stress reduction, a therapist may help the child explore other endings for "what happened" through art or play. For example, a therapist may guide a child traumatized by a car accident to engage in play with toys of paramedics and doctors or a toy operating room. The goal is to help the children not only convey the story of what happened, but also to experience other endings to the story—for example, being rescued instead of endlessly repeating the accident, an experience that may be emotionally retraumatizing (Figure 6.3a–f).

Levine and Kline (2007) add that repetition may "reinforce, rather than resolve, feelings and symptoms" (p. 179). They suggest asking the child to pause and check in with his or her bodily sensations and identify his or her feelings.

In most cases, therapists may not need to direct the patient to draw what happened; many patients do so spontaneously at some point during treatment; however, if the patient avoids discussing the traumatic event, then a directive to "draw what happened" may open the door to talking about the accident and related emotions. This directive provides children an invitation to freely share all the images and emotions related to the traumatic event. Collage materials, such as magazine images, provide another method for those patients who are either intimidated by drawing or who are physically unable to draw because of quadriplegia or other injuries. In these cases, the therapist can help the patient choose images for a collage or ask the patient to describe what happened through images chosen from a box of photographs or other items. Harrison and Grasdal (2003) describe a collage as taking old items and objects and making a new cohesive whole to help describe the artist and/or the current situation.

Timelines and Bridge Drawings

Timelines are another variation of the trauma story or narrative drawing and are effective with TBI patients who suffer from reduced memory, especially difficulty retaining new learning. Most TBI patients do not remember what happened to them or the traumatic event itself; therefore, a timeline, with the aid of a therapist, family, and friends, helps them sequence the events of the accident. Inclusion of goals and dreams for the future can help the patient gain a positive outlook about discharge and reentering life after the trauma.

Bridge drawings, mostly used for assessment, are similar to narrative drawing and timelines. Patients are directed to draw a bridge on

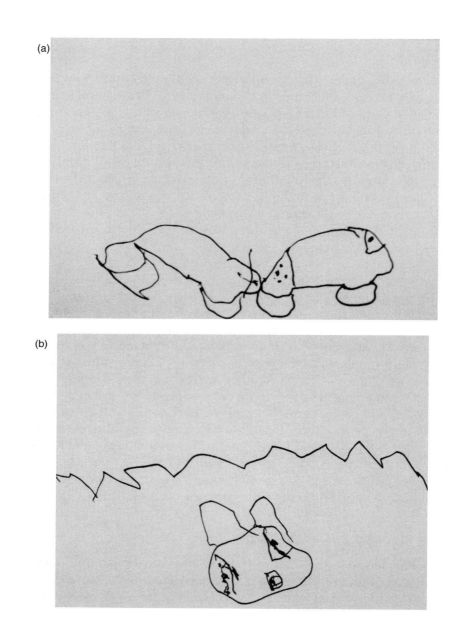

FIGURE 6.3a–f. An 8-year-old female was in a motor vehicle accident with her family, sustaining a serious hand injury. The therapist asked her to show what had happened. The patient drew the accident, beginning with the other car running her car off the road (a). The dots in the image represented her family members riding in the car. The next images showed the car in the

(c)

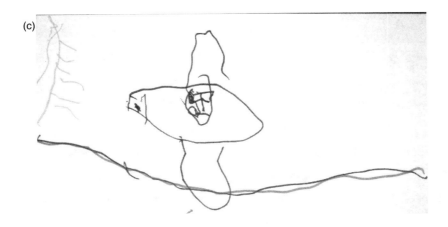

(d)

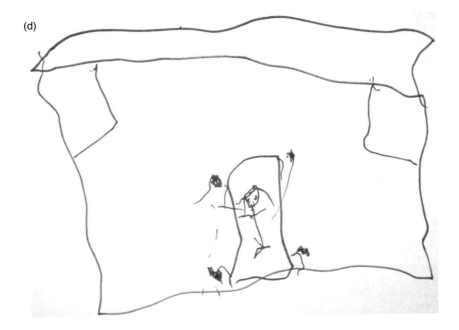

ditch (b), her flight to the hospital (c), and the stretcher and staff carrying her into the emergency room (d). She added an image of her and her brother in the room, surrounded by their family members (e). In each of these images, she mainly used a black marker. The therapist asked her to draw what would happen next. She chose brighter colors to illustrate her discharge home (f).

123

(e)

(f)

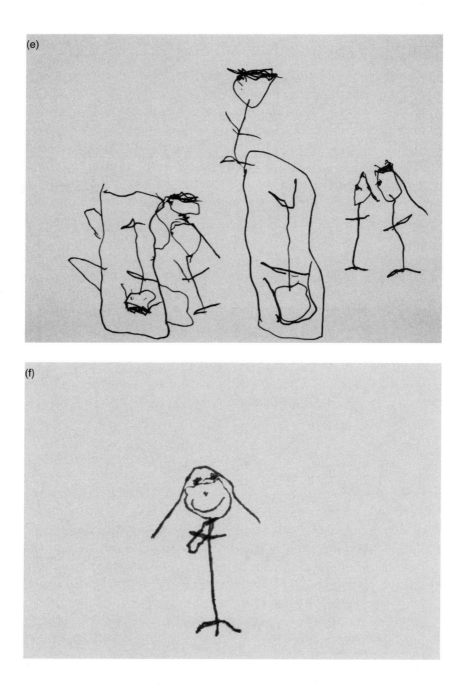

an 8½″ × 11″ piece of white paper using colored markers or pencils. Upon completion, patients are asked to describe the bridge and answer questions about where they came from, what is happening now, and where they are going. In my experience, most patients in rehabilitation settings tend to create only the bridge and no connecting land masses, possibly representing the ability or need to focus only on the current situation.

Masks

The word "mask" is taken from the Arabic term "maskhara," meaning to transform (Driessnack, 2004). Masks are present as a part of rituals on all continents, using basic elements and materials such as stone, wood, and leather. Driessnack stressed the importance of mask making in rituals and how masks are used to make rituals special and personal. In making a mask, an ordinary item is enhanced and taken into a realm different from the everyday. She described a case study of a young boy with cancer who chose to create a burial mask similar to the one on King Tut's tomb. By empowering the patient to create the mask, the therapist helped him move into the next realm.

Kruczek (2001) describes masks as a way for children and adolescents to develop their self-concepts and regulate their emotions. When children or adolescents experience medical trauma, they can develop feelings of helplessness. As a result, they may use adaptive coping skills to protect themselves from being too vulnerable in the hospital environment. Masks offer patients a means of strengthening their adaptive coping skills to meet the challenges of recovery. For example, masks can help children distance themselves from current stresses but still communicate feelings about their injuries. Mask making gives children permission to step back and look at how this character they have created would interact with them and others, safely convey emotions through dramatic play or storytelling, and explore what may be unfamiliar, frightening, or stressful.

Masks can be created in various media. More complex masks may use plaster and molds or the individual's face; other, simpler masks can be constructed from cardboard or paper. I prefer to use a preformed Styrofoam mask purchased from an arts and crafts catalogue. The patient is instructed to decorate the outside of the mask as desired using acrylic paints, feathers, sequins, pipe cleaners, yarn, buttons, glitter glue, and more. Once the outside of the mask is completed, the therapist then instructs the patient to decorate the inside of the mask using symbols of emotions, concerns, fears, hopes, dreams, or worries on the patient's mind. This decoration leads to discussion of issues the patient may have more difficulty acknowledging to him- or herself or expressing to others (Figure 6.4).

By creating images on the inside and outside of a mask, the patient is able to separate what is expressed to others and what is internal. Helping children and adolescents learn that some internal emotions may be expressed in external behavior can aid in increasing their self-awareness and self-regulation of behavior.

Often, children want to make more than one mask. If so, the therapist can use the masks in a role play of appropriate coping or other therapeutic interaction. The patient and therapist can attach wooden dowels to the masks to make them more interactive and easier to handle for patients with physical limitations. This intervention can also be utilized with the entire family in a group role play.

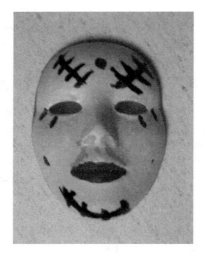

FIGURE 6.4. A 12-year-old male was involved in a motor vehicle accident with his father, mother, and sister. The patient sustained a broken leg and a few minor lacerations. His mother and sister suffered minor scratches and cuts. His father sustained a spinal cord injury resulting in paraplegia. The patient chose to create a mask with lacerations stitched closed. He described the red dot on the forehead as the hammer that "beat up" his father because it was loose in the truck when the vehicle rolled over seven times.

Sensory Activities

Because trauma memory is stored in the amygdala through images, sensations, and affect, various sensory techniques such as eye movement desensitization and reprocessing (EMDR) have been used to reduce arousal states caused by trauma. Steele and Raider (2001) created a technique that uses drawings to help reduce the emotional states of trauma and can be applied in work with some child survivors of accidents. The therapist works with patients' drawings as a way to discuss "the major sensations that follow trauma: fear, terror, worry, hurt, anger, revenge, accountability, absence of a sense of safety, powerlessness and victim versus survivor perceptions of self and the world" (p. 27). For example, when referring to a drawing of a car accident, the therapist may ask, "What is your biggest worry since the accident happened?" The patient may also be asked to make an image of a current worry or fear to visually compare it to the worries or fears associated with the original traumatic event. This technique helps counteract the sensory avoidance often seen in patients with posttraumatic symptoms.

Cohen, Barnes, and Rankin (1995) observe the need to substitute positive sensory experiences to reduce anxiety, such as touching soft clay, tasting a pear, or listening to soft music. Creating three-dimensional artwork in clay or assembling pieces of wood with glue also allows children to engage their senses through hands-on experiences with materials (Figure 6.5). In addition to using standard art materials, medical supplies and materials such as bandages, tongue depressors, cotton balls, gauze, medicine cups, and identification bands may also become part of the sensory experiences in a hospital setting.

Mandalas

Fincher (1991) writes that Carl Jung used the Sanskrit word "mandala" to describe the circular drawings he created and studied. Jung (1959) viewed the mandala as representing the whole personality of the creator at the present and considered the circle the most primitive shape in human existence. Ancient cultures around the world utilized the circle in their drawings and practices, such as sun and moon worship in ancient Egypt and Native American history. Tibetan mandalas are utilized for meditation, and in England and other European coun-

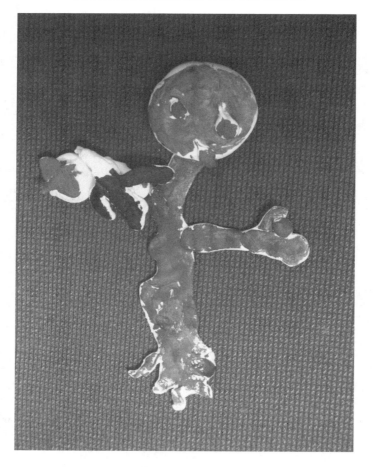

FIGURE 6.5. A 9½-year-old male came to visit his half sister in the intensive care unit after his father, his stepsister, and his half sister were in a serious motor vehicle accident. The 3-year-old half sister sustained a complete transection of her cervical spinal cord at the base of the skull. She was placed on a ventilator with the hope she would improve. In the art session, her brother chose to use Model Magic and began to sculpt a tree. He focused on the roots, moved up the trunk to the leaves, and then added apples. He carefully carved a cardinal and a nest. He placed a baby cardinal under each of the mother cardinal's wings in the nest. He also made an eagle, explaining how eagles can be bad and eat baby birds and other prey. He placed the eagle as though it were approaching the nest to steal a baby. When the therapist asked, "What happens next?" the artist answered, "We don't know yet." Clearly, the cardinal and eagle were metaphors for him, his mother, his half sister, and his half sister's impending death.

tries, the mandala aids in reaching desirable mental states, such as in circular labyrinths created on the floors in cathedrals (Fincher, 1991).

Judith Cornell (1994) notes that mandalas bring healing psychologically during a crisis of transition by allowing the fragments of the ego to find oneness. According to Cornell and others, the circle invites individuals to draw inward to the center, symbolically encouraging the artist to explore the inner being. The process of drawing or making a mandala is thought to provide a sense of centering or balancing within the psyche. In fact, mandala drawing has been studied as a method of self-regulation and relaxation. DeLue (1999) looked at the effects of creating mandalas on heart rate in school-age children. Her research demonstrates that, when focusing on making a mandala, children's heart rates decreased by an average of seven beats per minute. DeLue also observed that creating the mandala not only reduced the autonomic arousal in children, but also provided a means of centering their emotions and thoughts.

Curry and Kasser (2005) researched the use of mandalas, a plaid form, and a blank piece of paper to see if any helped reduce anxiety. They found working with the mandala and the plaid form more effective in reducing anxiety than the blank piece of paper. Mandalas and plaid forms provided the repetition called perserveration that aids in meditation. Curry and Kasser speculate that the mandala and plaid form provided structure for individuals with high anxiety or inner chaos and encouraged organization of thoughts and/or feelings through that structure.

CONCLUSIONS

Children and adolescents who sustain traumatic injuries may experience continued physical and emotional trauma throughout their hospitalization and medical treatment. Helping accident survivors requires offering opportunities to use art and play materials in what is often a challenging environment with diagnoses that may involve brain injury, disability, and even paralysis. Despite these aspects, trauma intervention in this setting involves many of the same goals as it does with children who have experienced other types of traumatic events. Although each patient is different, the goals of medical art and play are the same: to help child survivors to convey their feelings, thoughts, and worldviews and find hope and healing through creative self-expression.

REFERENCES

Allan, J. (1988). *Inscapes of the child's world.* Dallas, TX: Spring Publications.

Appleton, V. (2001). Avenues of hope: Art therapy and the resolution of trauma. *Art Therapy, 18*(1), 6–13.

Bach, S. (1990). *Life paints its own lifespan: On the significance of spontaneous pictures by severely ill children.* Einsiedeln, Switzerland: Daimon Verlag.

Caffo, E., & Belaise, C. (2003). Psychological aspects of traumatic injury in children and adolescents. *Child and Adolescent Psychiatric Clinics of North America, 12*(3), 493–535.

Cohen, B., Barnes, M., & Rankin, A. (1995). *Managing traumatic stress through art: Drawing from the center.* Baltimore: Sidran Press.

Cornell, J. (1994). *Mandala: Luminous symbols for healing.* Wheaton, IL: Quest Books.

Councill, T. (1999). Art therapy with pediatric cancer patients. In C. A. Malchiodi (Ed.), *Medical art therapy with children* (pp. 75–93). Philadelphia: Jessica Kingsley.

Councill, T. (2006). *Tracy's kids art therapy program training manual.* Washington, DC: Lombardi Pediatric Cancer Center Art Therapy Program.

Curry, N., & Kasser, T. (2005). Can coloring mandalas reduce anxiety? *Art Therapy, 22*(2), 81–85.

DeLue, C. (1999). Physiological effects of creating mandalas. In C. A. Malchiodi (Ed.), *Medical art therapy with children* (pp. 33–49). Philadelphia: Jessica Kingsley.

Driessnack, M. (2004). Remember me: Mask making with chronically and terminally ill children. *Holistic Nursing Practice, 18*(4), 211–214.

Fincher, S. (1991). *Creating mandalas: For insight, healing, and self-expression.* Boston: Shambhala Publications.

Harrison, H., & Grasdal, P. (2003). *Collage for the soul: Expressing hopes and dreams through art.* Gloucester, MA: Rockport Publishers, Inc.

Johnson, G. S. (2006). *About brain injury: Rancho Los Amigos Scale/the levels of coma.* Retrieved December 28, 2006, from *www.waiting.com/rancholosamigos.html.*

Jung, C. (1959). *The archetypes and the collective unconscious.* New York: Pantheon.

Kokoska, E., Keller, M., Rallo, M., & Weber, T. (2001). Characteristics of pediatric cervical spine injuries. *Journal of Pediatric Surgery, 36*(1), 100–105.

Kruczek, T. (2001). Inside-outside masks. In H. Kaduson & C. Schaefer (Eds.), *101 more favorite play therapy techniques* (pp. 70–74). Lanham, MD: Jason Aronson.

Kushner, H. (1981). *When bad things happen to good people.* New York: Avon.

Levine, P., & Kline, M. (2007). *Trauma through a child's eyes: Awakening the ordinary miracle of healing.* Berkeley, CA: North Atlantic Books.

Malchiodi, C. A. (1998). *Understanding children's drawings.* New York: Guilford Press.

Meiser-Stedman, R., Yule, W., Smith, P., Glucksman, E., & Dalgleish, T. (2005). Acute stress disorder and posttraumatic stress disorder in children and adolescents involved in assaults or motor vehicle accidents. *American Journal of Psychiatry, 162*(7), 1381–1383.

Parisini, P., Di Silvestre, M., & Greggi, T. (2002). Treatment of spinal fractures in children and adolescents: Long-term results in 44 patients. *Spine, 27*(18), 1989–1994.

Passaretti, D., & Billmire, D. (2003). Clinical experience: management of pediatric burns. *The Journal of Craniofacial Surgery, 14*(5), 713–718.

Perry, B., & Azad, I. (1999). Posttraumatic stress disorders in children and adolescents. *Current Opinion in Pediatrics, 11*(4), 310–322.

Proctor, M. (2002). Spinal cord injury. *Critical Care Medicine, 30*(11), 489–499.

Schreier, H., Ladakakos, C., Morabito, D., Chapman, L., & Knudson, M. (2005). Posttraumatic stress symptoms in children after mild to moderate pediatric trauma: A longitudinal examination of symptom prevalence, correlates, and parent–child symptom reporting. *Journal of Trauma-Injury Infection and Critical Care, 58*(2), 353–363.

Spinetta, J., & Spinetta D. (1981). *Living with childhood cancer.* St. Louis: C. V. Mosby.

Steele, W., & Raider, M. (2001). *Structured sensory intervention for traumatized children, adolescents and parents: Strategies to alleviate trauma.* Lewiston, NY: Edwin Mellen Press.

Thompson, R., & Stanford, G. (1981). *Child life in hospitals: Theory and practice.* Springfield, IL: Charles C. Thomas.

Traumatic Brain Injury.com, LLC. (2004). Retrieved December 27, 2006, from *www.traumaticbraininjury.com.*

Warzak, W., Allan, T., Ford, L., & Stefans, V. (1995). Common obstacles to the daily functioning of pediatric traumatically brain-injured patients: Perceptions of care givers and psychologists. *Children's Health Care, 24*(2), 133–141.

Zimmerman, J., & Beaudoin, M. (2002). Cats under the stars: A narrative story. *Child and Adolescent Mental Health, 7*(1), 31–40.

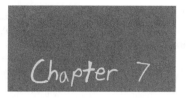

Chapter 7

Creative Approaches to Minimize the Traumatic Impact of Bullying Behavior

Diane S. Safran
Elysa R. Safran

Prior to the dramatic school shootings in the 1990s throughout rural and suburban towns in the United States, little attention was given to the deleterious impact of bullying behavior.[1] In response to school shootings such as the one at Columbine High School, research has proliferated on bullying behavior and school prevention/intervention programs for bullying. Focused studies evaluated overtly aggressive and violent behavior, teasing and practical jokes, and, ultimately, integrated the impact of subtler forms of relational aggression often found among girls. As a reaction to an increased awareness of the potentially horrific consequences of bullying behavior, some state laws now mandate the inclusion of a harsh "zero-tolerance" policy toward bullies

---

[1] Kentucky (E. Carter High School; Heath High School), California (Sacred Heart High School), South Carolina (Redlands High School), Tennessee (Richland High School), Washington (Frontier Jr. High School), Alaska (Bethel Regional High School), Mississippi (Pearl High School), Arkansas (Stamps High School; Westside Middle School), Pennsylvania (Parker Middle School), Oregon (Thurston High School), Colorado (Columbine High School), and Georgia (Heritage High School).

and the inclusion of anti-bullying programs in schools (Espelage & Swearer, 2003). While researchers concede that bullying behavior has psychological implications for both the bully and the victim (Swearer, Grills, Haye, & Cary, 2004), little research focuses on creative approaches one could utilize to minimize the causes and effects of bullying. Viable, psychotherapeutic interventions are especially needed within the context of working with bullies and their victims, who are often among the children and adolescents in individual and group psychotherapy. This chapter explores the prevailing definitions of bullies and victims, the prevalence and psychological implications of bullying behavior, and the creative approaches one might use to minimize the impact on children traumatized by enduring bullying encounters.

IMPACT ON THE SCHOOL ENVIRONMENT AND PREVALENCE OF BULLYING BEHAVIOR

According to Bosworth, Espelage, and Simon (1999), a single student who bullies can have far-reaching consequences in the school by creating a climate of fear and intimidation not only for his or her victims, but for other students as well. Many students between ages 8 and 15 ranked bullying as more problematic in their lives than discrimination, racism, or violence (Kaiser Family Foundation, Children Now, 2001). As early as 1995, a National Education Association report revealed that 160,000 students that year skipped class because they feared physical harm from peers at school (Borg, 1999; Juvonen, 2001; Juvonen & Graham, 2001). Studies conducted by the National Threat Assessment Center and the Department of Education, among others, found that in more than two-thirds of 37 shootings, the attackers' experience of feeling ongoing persecution in the form of bullying, threats, attacks, or injuries by others motivated their desire for revenge (Hazler & Carney, 2000; U.S. Secret Service, 2000; Vossekuil, Fein, Reddy, Borum, & Modzeleski, 2002). Twenty to thirty percent of U.S. schoolchildren (e.g., approximately 10 million) surveyed in a National Institute of Child Health and Human Development study reported involvement in some aspect of bullying during the school year that contributed to a climate of fear in their school (Juvonen, 2001; Nansel et al., 2001). Lack of intervention can lead to depression, anxiety, reduced self-esteem, or suicide in bullying victims (Juvonen & Graham, 2001; Swearer et al., 2004) and later diagnosed conduct disorders

(American Psychiatric Association, 2000), workplace violence, and verbal/spousal abuse in/by adult bullies (Garbarino & deLara, 2002).

Studies suggest that bullying is particularly acute in terms of frequency and severity in early adolescence (U.S. Department of Education, National Center for Educational Statistics, 2006), with seventh grade identified as the worst year, though bullies are most often first identified in elementary school (Pellegrini, Bartini, & Brooks, 1999). In several studies (Borg, 1999; Bosworth et al., 1999; Green, 1999) more than one-third of middle school students reported feeling unsafe at school because of bullying. Often, they did not report their fear, but internalized their distress because of their apprehension of being discovered by the bully or his or her friends, lacked the necessary skills for reporting, or were concerned that teachers and administrators would do nothing to stop the bullying (Hazler, 1996; Hazler, Miller, Carney, & Green, 2001; Hoover & Hazler, 1994; Juvonen & Graham, 2001; Slee, 1994).

Bullying behavior creates a tense and sometimes violent undertone in a school (Hoover, Oliver, & Thomson, 1993) that contaminates the educational environment and affects every child's learning (Olweus, 1994), sense of security, and well-being (Garbarino & deLara, 2002). Many students report silently suffering great physical and psychological pain, humiliation, and stress (Borg, 1999) and are traumatized as a consequence of undetected bullying behavior. The impact is long-standing, often leaving victims of bullying emotionally scarred. Most students report that they consider bullies to be a normal part of the school community (Smith, Twemlow, & Hoover, 1999), suggesting that bullying is enmeshed in the very fabric of a school's culture; however, bullying is not carried out in the school environment alone and, thus, one must evaluate the intricacies and impact of bullying behavior within the context of a social–ecological framework (Swearer & Espelage, 2004). Bullying should be examined not only within school and peer groups, but also within influential environments outside the school including the family and community and exposure to ideas transported through media and technology.

DEFINITIONS OF BULLYING

Dan Olweus (1978) originally defined bullying as the systematic use of physical and/or mental violence by one or several boys against another boy. He later added that a bully unrelentingly and persistently harasses another boy either physically or psychologically (Olweus, 1991). Deliberate negative actions that cause distress in a victim by a child who is physically or psychologically stronger and who repeats these behaviors across time were later added to the definition of bullying behavior (Olweus, 1994a, 1994b). Bullying behavior became recognized not as a single act, but rather as a systematic and intentional form of peer abuse as a means of achieving or maintaining social dominance (Arora, 1996; Olweus, 1996; Pellegrini, 2002; Pellegrini & Long, 2002; Smith, Madsen, & Moody, 1999). Later definitions added hurtful actions such as name calling, social exclusion, having money taken or belongings damaged, and hitting or kicking (Borg, 1999; Crick, 1997).

Behavioral and psychosocial measures describe bullying behavior as stemming from misconduct, belief systems supportive of aggression, feelings of depression, impulsivity, and a reduced sense of belonging to one's school (Bosworth et al., 1999; Green, 1999; Loeber & Hale, 1997). It was also thought that bullies embodied power and control through overtly aggressive means because their victims had insufficient social–emotional skills or were incapable of integrating into their peer group (Pellegrini & Long, 2002; Swearer et al., 2004). Researchers also determined that many of those children who bully were bullied themselves (Kumpulainen, Rasanen, & Henttonen, 1999; Swearer et al., 2004).

Most important, researchers added to the definition that bullying is intentional, unprovoked, and longstanding violence, psychological or physical, conducted by an individual or a group and that bullies are often older than or from the same age group as victims (Kumpulainen et al., 1999). Bullies have been defined as individuals who are frequently angry, hold beliefs supportive of violence, and do not feel a sense of belonging at school; they are considered disruptive and lacking in empathy (Duncan, 1999a, 1999b). Harryman (2004) describes the playground bully as one who makes the victim feel humiliated, stressed, undermined, isolated, overworked, ineffective, inefficient, or even guilty.

Newer research on bullying behavior has increasingly informed and developed studies on its intricacies, allowing theorists to better identify and delineate the forms in which bullying behavior, both direct and indirect, is manifested (Olweus, 1991). "Direct" bullying involves open attacks on a victim (Olweus, 1993) in the form of physical, verbal, or sexual abuse (Swearer et al., 2004). "Indirect" bullying is distinguished by social isolation, exclusion from a group, or non-selection for activities (Olweus, 1991; Sutton, Smith, & Swettenham, 1999a, 1999b) as well as through subtle methods such as social injustice and isolation (Bjoerkqvist, Lagerspetz, & Kaukiainen, 1992; Crick & Grotpeter, 1995; Espelage, Mebane, & Swearer, 2004; Simmons, 2002; Wiseman, 2002), including gossiping, spreading rumors, and ostracizing. Indirect bullying is done by both boys and girls. Unlike overt forms of aggression, which tend to diminish as children develop emotionally and physically, indirect forms of bullying are thought to continue and to become more sophisticated and subtle with maturity.

Borg (1999) summarized the salient features of bullying as involving attacks with the intention of inflicting negative consequences carried out by one or more perpetrators, occurring repeatedly and over a relatively long period of time, and directed toward a victim who is weaker than the perpetrator(s). All researchers converge around the point that bullying behavior can either be physical or psychological; is systematic (Brown & Gilligan, 1992; Crick & Grotpeter, 1995; Espelage & Swearer, 2003; Simmons, 2002; Swearer et al., 2004); direct (overt), indirect (covert), or relational; and endures over time. It is clear that the physical and psychological bullying more typical of boys differs dramatically from the relational aggression more characteristic of girls. These striking variations are important to consider in any discussion of bullying, its causes, its implications, and its interventions.

PSYCHOLOGICAL IMPLICATIONS OF BULLYING

According to Twemlow's (2000) research, it is possible to observe in victimized youth similar symptomatology to that of individuals who have experienced chronic domestic violence. He states: "This includes despairing acceptance of their victimization and development of an attitude of self-reproach, which may lead victims to feel they deserve to be taunted, teased, and harassed" (p. 746).

Due to their vulnerabilities, students diagnosed as having ADHD (attention-deficit/hyperactivity disorder), NVLD (nonverbal learning disability), LD (learning disability), or PDD (pervasive developmental disorder) are more susceptible to bullies (Safran, 2002). Many are extremely reactive, often thought of as being emotionally sensitive

(Shaughnessy & Lehtonen, 1998). Due to years of bullying, these students misperceive gestures, looks, and whispers as being directed toward them. In response to this misperception, they overreact. Many lack the appropriate interpersonal skills necessary for making and keeping friends. They become socially isolated and withdrawn or attract negative attention through inappropriate behavior (Safran, 2002). Their lack of social adaptation prevents them from understanding social missteps such as being too close or provocative to a peer or laughing inappropriately. Their vulnerabilities make them easy targets for bullies (Safran, 2002).

THEORETICAL PERSPECTIVES ON BULLYING BEHAVIOR

There are four theoretical perspectives on bullying behavior, which will be explained more fully in the following paragraphs. In sum, the first two models, the Social Skills Deficit Model and the Social Blindness Model, explain overt forms of bullying behavior, while the Social Intelligence Model and the Theory of Mind Model conceptualize indirect forms of bullying behavior. Although the Social Skills Deficit and Social Blindness Models focus on a bully's personal and social deficits, the Social Intelligence and Theory of Mind Models are conceptualized around strengths. The development of these theoretical perspectives stems from Sutton et al.'s research (1999a, 1999b), which suggests a need for greater insight into the psychological factors associated with persistent bullying or victimization. Other researchers raise the consideration of group processes, social skills, social information processing, and social perspective taking or mind reading ("Theory of Mind") abilities in children involved in bullying (Kaukiainen et al., 1999; Salmivalli, Kaukiainen, Kaistaniemi, & Lagerspetz, 1999); Sutton & Smith, 1999; Sutton et al., 1999a, 1999b).

Whereas aggression was once commonly thought to arise from biases or deficiences in the bully's ability to process social information effectively, researchers recognize the importance of evaluating the group context and social methods of bullying (Kaukiainen et al., 1999; Salmivalli et al., 1999; Sutton et al., 1999a, 1999b). Many have concluded that bullies may in fact have exceptional social intelligence (Kaukiainen et al., 1999). Although bullying is still considered an antisocial and aggressive act, researchers prompt critics not to consider all bullies as social "inadequates" but rather appreciate that some are skilled manipulators (Kaukiainen et al., 1999; Sutton et al., 1999a, 1999b) with strong social skills.

The *social skills deficit model* (Kaukiainen et al., 1999; Sutton et al., 1999a, 1999b) suggests that students who bully are not lacking in social skills but rather deliberately select strategies to maintain dominance and power in social relations (Smith et al., 1993). Bosworth et al. (1999) attributed the selection of aggressive acts as a lack of confidence in using nonviolent strategies and intention. This model (Sutton et al., 1999a, 1999b) encapsulates the popular theory that views bullies as physically powerful males who have little understanding of people and low intellectual ability, thus resorting to violence and aggression to maintain their status.

In the *social blindness model* (Kaukiainen et al., 1999), bullying behavior is attributed to the bully's inability to process social information accurately. Bullies also seem unable to make realistic judgments about the intentions of others, fail to understand the feelings of others, and have little awareness of what others may think of them (social blindness). According to Hazler (1996), these individuals see the event and its results from his/her own immature perspective (Crick & Dodge, 1994); they have difficulty processing and understanding how others may perceive the social situation. Consequently, they are unable to develop an appropriate working model of how to interact with others. The result is that often these individuals are antisocial or have social–cognitive deficits. In keeping with this model, bullying is assessed as an antisocial and aggressive act carried out in a social way in a social setting. The bully lacks empathy (Espelage et al., 2004)— the ability to take the others' perspective—or inaccurately interprets social cues as aggressive (Crick & Dodge, 1994), thought of as the "hostile attributional bias" (Espelage et al., 2004).

In the *social intelligence model* (Kaukiainen et al., 1999; Sutton et al., 1999a, 1999b), theorists distinguish between the interpersonal domain of intelligence and other cognitive abilities. They suggest that an individual's capacity to discern and respond appropriately to the moods, temperaments, motivations, and desires of other people indicates that his or her contextual–practical intelligence is an active adaptation to the environment. Consequently, socially intelligent individuals have the ability to draw upon their skills and subtly or covertly control social situations to suit their needs (Espelage et al., 2004). They are socially adept, but they use their social intelligence, in some cases, to hurt people. Attuned to social cues, these bullies can easily identify and act on weaknesses (i.e., instill fear) in their targets while remaining undetected by school authorities. These students can be very calculating in their bullying. They have metacognitive skills (goal setting, planning, monitoring, evaluating social actions, and empathy), as well as the ability or tendency to be vicariously aroused by the affective states of another person. They can recognize another's feelings and sympathize with them. These bullies have the ability to discriminate and label the affective states of others and to assume another's perspective and role and have both emotional capacity and responsiveness, and they are able to use these skills to their advantage. They use empathy, notably, to either inhibit or mitigate aggression (Sutton et al., 1999a, 1999b) in potentially subversive ways.

Indirect forms of bullying also require some understanding and social skills on the part of the bully. In order to make the victim feel left out, these bullies justify their social exclusion so that others will accept them (Sutton et al., 1999a, 1999b). The *theory of mind model* (Espelage et al., 2004; Kaukiainen et al., 1999; Sutton et al., 1999a, 1999b) asserts that some bullies will have the understanding, thought processes, and social skills to manipulate and organize others, inflicting suffering in subtle and damaging ways while avoiding detection. They have the ability to comprehend others' mental states in order to explain and predict behavior. Indirect forms of bullying also depend upon manipulating a fully developed infrastructure in a circuitous way. Often, the perpetrator goes unidentified or avoids the accusation of aggressive behavior because of the relational nature of the aggression (Kaukiainen et al., 1999; Sutton et al., 1999a, 1999b).

The possessor of such social skills (Sutton et al., 1999a, 1999b) has a superior advantage over followers and victims. Kaukiainen and colleagues (1999) believe that certain specific social–cognitive structures, such as normative beliefs and moral cognition, are inadequately developed in aggressive children who can use their social intelligence for both pro- and antisocial purposes. They may also use social skills and social intelligence to harm others for hostile purposes. The demands of the situation and aspects of one's personality (e.g., moral standards and level of empathy) determine the goals for which a person will use his or her social intelligence (Kaukiainen et al., 1999; Kumpulainen et al., 1999; Sutton & Smith, 1999a, 1999b).

Bjoerkqvist and colleagues (1992) asserted a developmental theory of aggression in which young children's aggression was considered primarily physical. With the emergence of more developed social skills, the use of indirect and manipulative aggression involving social intelligence made it possible to efficiently hurt others in nonphysical ways (Espelage et al., 2004; Pellegrini & Long, 2002, 2004). This theory reinforces the belief that direct methods of bullying decrease and relational elements of bullying in subtler forms increase with age and cognitive acuity. Having the capacity to understand the mental states and emotions of others, older children become more adept at effectively teasing; they can choose to utilize emergent social skills for peaceful interactions or for aggressive purposes. A sophisticated social cognition can be useful in avoiding detection, choosing the most effective time and method for each situation to maximize the victim's vulnerabilities and minimize the chance of being caught or hurt.

Findings further suggest that there is a correlation between highly developed social intelligence and an individual's facility with using indirect aggression, whereas theorists state that the use of direct forms of aggression (i.e., verbal/physical threats) is not associated with social intelligence (Espelage et al., 2004; Kaukiainen et al., 1999; Pellegrini & Long, 2004). In order for bullies to efficiently use aggression (e.g., understanding of human relations/skills applied in social settings), they must also be able to secure a favorable social position. They must be able to interpret the reactions of others and accommodate their behavior for the social manipulation not to backfire. These are demanding skills thought to emerge in later adolescence. Finally, not only does the bully's appearance of empathy mitigate his or her aggressive behavior, but the perpetrator of aggression must also have a certain amount of impudence and insolence in order to pull off the manipulation.

GENDER DIFFERENCES IN BULLYING BEHAVIOR

Gender differences are noted in both the prevalence of bullying and the types of behaviors used by children and adolescents who bully (Boulton, 1999; Crick, Bigbee, & Howes, 1996; Crick & Grotpeter, 1995; Crick & Grotpeter, 1996; Crick et al., 2001; Espelage & Swearer, 2003; Simmons, 2002), although recent research considers commonalities between genders (Espelage et al., 2004). Boys bully more often than girls and are more often the victims of bullying (Borg,

1999). They predominantly use direct forms of bullying, whereas girls tend to bully through indirect or social means (Boulton, 1999; Crick, 1995; Espelage et al., 2004; Simmons, 2002; Wiseman, 2002). Not all victims of bullying are outcasts, weaker, or overly emotional. Research on relational aggression indicates that bullying also occurs among girls within or outside popular cliques (Brown & Gilligan, 1992; Crick et al., 1999; Simmons, 2002).

Boys

More frequently, traditional views of bullying behavior are attributed to boys. Historically, when describing bullying behavior, researchers focused on the misconduct and anger of the bully. Bullies were often described as disruptive, lacking in empathy, and unpopular; however, a bully's powerful stance also seemed to gain him popularity, especially with aggressively oriented peers (Pellegrini et al., 1999).

Other notable characteristics of the male bully include: variable confidence levels, average-to-above-average self-esteem, and depressive features. Bullies are described as having high dominance needs, lacking problem resolution skills (Arbona, Jackson, McCoy, & Blakely, 1999), and being willing to resort to violence to resolve conflict (Espelage et al., 2004) because of their physical strength (Olweus, 1993). They appear not to consider the feelings of others, to enjoy their victims' pain, and are thought to be selfish and self-centered. Interestingly, Olweus (1994a, 1994b) found a relationship among impulsivity, anger, and bullying in boys; he suggested that, when angry, boys may impulsively lash out at victims who are emotionally and physically weaker as a means of relieving tension or frustration.

Girls

Ongoing research on relational aggression helps provide a fuller understanding of the intricacies of bullying behavior (Espelage et al., 2004). Early studies (Bjoerkqvist & Niemela, 1992; Crick & Grotpeter, 1995) found that, while girls are not averse to aggression, due to societal and cultural norms, they express their anger in alternative, relational ways. Unlike physical aggression, which is overt, relational aggression is covert and more difficult to detect.

As researchers' awareness of relational aggression grew, they more aptly delineated the forms it might take. "Alternative aggression"

(Simmons, 2002) has three forms: relational, indirect, and social. "Relational aggression" refers to acts that "harm others through damage (or threaten damage) to relationships or feelings of acceptance, friendship, or group inclusion" (Simmons, 2002, p. 126). Examples include purposefully ignoring someone as a means of controlling or punishing, revengeful social exclusion, displays of negative body language or facial expressions, sabotaging others' relationships, or threats to end a relationship unless a request is fulfilled. Perpetrators use their relationships with victims as a weapon (Simmons, 2002). By contrast, "indirect aggression" (Bjoerkqvist et al., 1992) allows the perpetrator to avoid confronting her target. Covertly, the perpetrator facilitates actions to use others as vehicles for inflicting pain on the targeted individual. In this way, rumors are spread, but one cannot easily identify the source, and the perpetrator is protected (Simmons, 2002). "Social aggression" is intended to damage the self-esteem or social status of the victim within a group by spreading rumors or excluding the victim from social events (Bjoerkqvist et al., 1992; Simmons, 2002; Wiseman, 2002).

Bullying behavior of girls is purposeful, planned, and subversive. Many girls display a demure, good-girl image, which maintains the invisibility of alternative aggression. Beneath the surface of sweetness lies a web of intricately woven alliances, secrets, and covert attacks. The intent is to elude teachers, administrators, and parents. Often, adults cannot reconcile the sweet persona with the reported villainness that victims claim the bullying girl to be.

Gilligan (1993) explained that women's development "points toward a different history of human attachment, stressing continuity and change instead of replacement and change" (p. 48). Relationships are primary in girls' lives. Thus, women and girls willingly engage in a social dance because relationships play an unusually important role in their social development (Gilligan, 1993). Early studies conducted by Crick (1995) found that relationally aggressive acts are more distressing for girls than they are for boys. Crick and Grotpeter (1995) using the Social Experiences Questionnaire (Espelage et al., 2004) sought to examine the implications of bullying within the relational sphere in an effort to unravel the complexity of bullying behavior. By doing so, Crick and Bigbee (Espelage et al., 2004) determined that relationally victimized children were most often girls, and that for many girls the psychological impact was devastating. Notably, in recent studies, researchers (Crick et al., 2001; Brown & Gilligan, 1992; Espelage et al., 2004; Pellegrini & Long, 2004) suggest that relational aggression can be used in different ways, some of which are socially appropriate means of navigating increasingly complex social situations, and experienced in differing degrees. Many girls are left unscathed. Others (Crick et al., 1996) explore the psychological implications of relational aggression on vulnerable adolescent girls. As relationships are central to girls' lives, the impact can leave some girls feeling lonely, depressed, and socially inadequate. Unlike boys, who describe a fear of entrapment or smothering, girls perceive isolation as dangerous in their lives; standing out and expressing one's true feelings of anger is equated with abandonment (Brown & Gilligan, 1992; Gilligan, 1993).

Consequently, the most painful bullying usually appears deep inside a close friendship and is fueled by secrets and shared weaknesses (Simmons, 2002). The relationship itself is often the weapon with which girls' battles are fought. As girls are socialized away from aggression and expected to be nice, they are unprepared to negotiate conflict in a healthy manner. Minor disagreements can call an entire relationship into question (Simmons, 2002). Girls will often remain in abusive friendships or continue involvement in cliques rather than risk social isolation (Brown & Gilligan, 1992; Gilligan, 1993; Simmons, 2002).

Comparison between Genders

Similarly to boys, girls employ "assistants" and "reinforcers" to justify bullying behavior and maintain their social power (Espelage & Swearer, 2004). Rather than the overt and direct way in which boys bully, girls tend to elongate the process by making the victim suffer for weeks or even months. Using a "mediator" the female bully displays her power of exclusion by making herself inaccessible for dialogue and alienating the victim from all association with her previous group of friends. The victim receives the silent treatment as long as the bully deems it necessary for her to be ignored. In some cases, the girl may be completely ousted from the group. A girl will spread rumors, "accidentally" bump into her victim in the halls, take her books, write notes and whisper about her or crank call her, send mean e-mail messages, or divulge previously kept secrets. Girls can be duplicitous if it means securing their position in a social clique. Most often, the bully uses other girls in her group to do the "dirty work" so as to position herself as innocent.

On the other hand, boys, alone or with the support of peers, insti-gate physical fights or the taunting of victims; these fights between friends often end with the last punch or cool off after a few days. For example, male bullies often back off if they tire of taunting or the victim stands up to them, revealing physical or emotional strength. In contrast, relational bullying is much more sophisticated. While both genders tend to pick on weaker peers, female bullies do not discriminate if their social power is in question. If a girl challenges the authority of the "queen bee" (Wiseman, 2002), she is targeted for her lack of subservience. Girls must find ways to redeem themselves if they want to regain the acceptance of the queen bee, even if they must silence their own needs and ultimately their voices. Subsequently, some girls have found that the only way to protect themselves from this bullying treatment is to remain silent.

As part of her qualitative research on bullying behavior in schools, Safran (2003) interviewed 11th-grade students who had been exposed to bullying behavior. The students Safran interviewed made the following remarks:

Girls say . . .

"There is often a leader, who promotes the competition and petti-ness between girls. . . . they egg people on because the leader is the queen of all the girls."

"Girls are petty and competitive. They're less comfortable with themselves, so they put other people down to make themselves feel better."

"Bullying is always mental. . . . girls are very mentally twisted."

"Victims are different in some way, whether it is their personality, physical characteristics, or clothing. A girl might be subjected to bullying if she is rebellious, smart, or intellectual, or if she is more timid and shy."

"I started having this eating disorder thing, which really was the result of being bullied and letting all these people push me around. I had stomachaches, too."

Boys say . . .

"Bullying for boys is considered a rite of passage. . . . coaches turn the other way. They look at it as part of the sport."

"The ringleader intends to embarrass, taunt, or hurt the victim physically or emotionally. Bullies like a good fight; however, if the victim does not respond most times the bully will find someone else to pick on."

"Boys who respond aggressively or overemotionally set themselves up to be bullied."

"Some students are bullied or teased because they express different sexual orientation or religious preferences."

Safran (2003) detected several emergent themes among boys and girls. Similar to the cases presented within this chapter, Safran found that male students in her study population generally picked on younger or smaller boys as a means of covering their own helplessness or insecurities or bullied out of boredom or the need to establish power. They are persistent, at times relentless, and enjoy confrontation. In contrast, girl bullies are cold and mean, self-involved, and overdramatize situations. They promote competition and pettiness by focusing on perceived differences among other girls to maintain their power and display retaliatory behavior. In conclusion, Safran found that female participants emphasized emotional characteristics and the relational nature of bullies and bullying behavior, while male participants emphasized physical intimidation or provocative behavior meant to annoy, tease, or instill fear.

WHO ARE THEIR VICTIMS?

The research describes victims of bullying as varying across a number of dimensions. Traditionally, researchers have divided victims into two groups: (1) passive and (2) aggressive/provocative. Passive victims tend to be physically slight, unassertive, and too reticent to retaliate (Schwartz, Proctor, & Chien, 2001). In the absence of bullies, they are often able to assimilate adequately, although they are not necessarily considered popular. Aggressive or provocative victims have a hostile style of social interaction, reminiscent of Dylan Klebold and Eric Harris, and tend to be highly emotional and hot-tempered. Emotionality results in aggressive behavior that is reactive rather than proactive, whereas bullies use aggression in a calculating and instrumental way. Victims in this group tend to use aggression only after losing control in response to a provocation. Aggressive victims are rejected by nearly all their peers and have few if any friends (Espelage & Swearer, 2004; Pellegrini et al., 1999; Sandstrom & Coie, 1999).

A victim's temperament makes him or her more susceptible to bullying or teasing (Duncan, 1999a, 1999b). Some individuals victimized by bullying are intimidated by others, complain about or tattle on peers, or have low self-esteem. They tend to be quiet and shy and often exhibit signs of nervousness and insecurity (Simmons, 2002; Smith et al., 1999). Victims tend not to retaliate and often display suffering, which inadvertently rewards a bully's behavior. Bernstein and Watson (1997) describe victims' interaction style as predisposing them to constant harassment. Children who are victimized often fail to engage in behavior that may help with self-protection. Those who are bullied daily demonstrate poor social and emotional adjustment; have greater difficulty making friends; and have low self-esteem, higher levels of insecurity, and greater feelings of sadness and loneliness (Bond, Carlin, Thomas, Rubin, & Patton, 2001; Swearer et al., 2004).

CREATIVE APPROACHES TO MINIMIZE THE IMPACT OF BEING BULLIED

The rest of this chapter concentrates on victims, those who are most vulnerable to bullying behavior. Creative strategies to ameliorate their symptoms will be discussed. These are students who, on a daily basis, experience bullying either physically or emotionally. They do not feel normal. They often feel like they do not fit in and isolate themselves on the playground or in the lunchroom, fearful of reoccurring bullying. Many of these students become patients within the mental health system exhibiting symptoms/behaviors related to stress and trauma, somatic complaints, affective disorders and anxiety that can lead to posttraumatic stress disorder (PTSD), and academic and/or social failure.

The Role of Art Therapy

Art therapy offers victims of bullies an opportunity to express themselves in a safe way. Emphasis is placed on their strengths and skills. School-based anti-bullying programs, while successful, often do not offer the opportunity to express deep-seated feelings. Although they are learning social strategies in the school environment, 90% of victims report psychological consequences, including a drop in grades, increased anxiety, and loss of friends or social life (Glew, Rivara, & Feudtner, 2000). Their feelings of insecurity and helplessness also dictate a psychotherapeutic intervention. The art therapist provides a venue for nonverbal self-expression. These students often are unable to verbally express their feelings of fear, worthlessness, confusion, and even rage. They often internalize these feelings as a way of coping with their daily trauma (Juvonen & Graham, 2001). Victims develop a lack of trust in school personnel who have been unable to protect them. For most students, repressed feelings emerge in his or her drawings allowing him or her an opportunity for self-actualization.

> A co-ed middle school art therapy group was presented with the task to draw a bully-proof school. Initially, the students became very excited, describing the school environment as "safer, quieter, being able to concentrate in classes, no need for counselors or psychologists, smaller class sizes which would be more conducive to learning and generally a happier place to be." What quickly followed was their inability to even imagine such an environment could exist. The students began to describe the necessity of surrounding the school with barbed wire, having armed guards in and outside the school, having special detectors to identify bullies, and so on. This discussion went on for many weeks. The group concluded that, without protection, the task was impossible.

A review of the literature does not reveal any school-based anti-bullying program that incorporates art therapy. All current school programs are behaviorally oriented (Hovard, Home, & Jeleff, 2001; Olweus, Limber, & Mihalic, 1999; Stein & Sjostrom, 1996; Smith & Brian, 2000; Wiseman, 2002). They are either single-sex or coed and led by school personnel who follow a "zero tolerance for bullying" curriculum (Vossekuil et al., 2002). The students seen in my practice, for a variety of reasons, are unable to participate in these programs. They are often too inhibited and afraid of retaliation. The daily trauma of attending school inhibits their ability to trust the school personnel facilitating the program. In some ways, attending a program in school contributes to symptoms of PTSD.

Therapists must understand symptoms of PTSD when treating victims of chronic bullying. In Steele's (2003) chapter "Using Drawing in Short-Term Trauma Resolution," he describes the use of art therapy as a structured trauma intervention that relies on reexposure to traumatic memories through drawing, developing a trauma narrative, and cognitive reframing (p. 142). Steele refers to DSM-IV-TR (American Psychiatric Association, 2000), which acknowledged that children could, in fact, experience PTSD and established the following criteria:

1. The person experienced, witnessed, or was confronted with an event or events that involved actual or threatened death or serious injury, or a threat to the physical integrity of self or others. An event need not lead to death for PTSD to be induced. Furthermore, injury need not occur; the threat to one's physical safety can be sufficient to induce trauma.
2. The person's response involved intense fear, helplessness, or horror. Intense fear (powerlessness) is the key reactions of trauma.

Steele's descriptions of the major components of intervention with children who have been traumatized include the following: reexposure to the trauma memories and experience, developing a trauma narrative or telling of the story, and cognitive reframing. Externalizing the story into a visual representation of the elements of that experience and cognitively reframing that experience into one that is manageable are the goals of successful trauma intervention. Drawing is a critical component of both reexposure and telling the story (Steele, 2003).

Case Study: Mike

Mike, like many socially inhibited boys, felt different from his classmates. He knew he was smart but not in a traditional way. He did not like team sports, but he was a superb skier. Mike loved art, mostly drawing. These traits, in a very conservative traditional school environment, set him apart from his male peers. He became a target of harassment and name calling, including being called a "homo." This went on for years. When I (D.S.S.) met Mike he was about to move up to middle school. He was extremely anxious, fearful that the constant bullying would increase. He became school-phobic, daily refusing to attend school. His parents and school personnel seemed unaware of the bullying situation. His sister, in a typical older sibling fashion, regularly teased him, and Mike's overreactivity confused his parents. He developed somatic symptoms; his pediatrician could not find physical ailments to explain these symptoms and suspected an emotional problem. Mike refused to divulge his secret—that "he was weak and had no friends."

He blamed himself for the daily attacks and became withdrawn and mute. When Mike came to me his vocabulary was reduced to a few grunts. He was unable to make eye contact, and his shoulders rolled in as if he were carrying the weight of the world. Following a traditional intake of projective drawings it was clear that Mike had secrets and that he was depressed. It was evident that he liked the idea of art therapy as a way to express himself. He saw art therapy as a viable means with which to express his innermost feelings, those he could not or dared not verbalize. The structured drawing assignments allowed Mike to fully express his submerged feelings of rage. We decided that it would be helpful for him to make an "angry book." What followed (after several months of developing a therapeutic relationship) was 13 weeks of individual art therapy sessions; each week he added another drawing to his book.

1. *Week 1:* In response to my suggestion "Draw how you feel about school," Mike drew a hand grenade (pin out) being tossed toward his school. He is not present in the drawing (Figure 7.1).

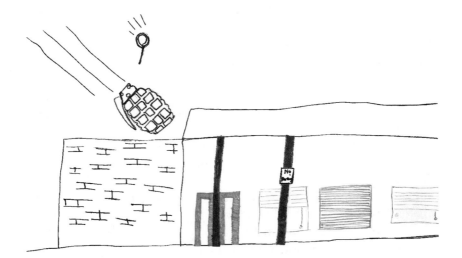

FIGURE 7.1. Mike throwing a hand grenade at his school.

2. *Week 2:* In response to my direction "Draw why you hate school," he made a collage of himself skiing and about to land on one of his tormentors. He labeled this drawing "DEAD MEAT!!"

3. *Week 3:* After reviewing his first two drawings he told me that he had other tormentors. I suggested that he draw a picture with one of them and himself interacting. This time he drew himself (arm only, in a ski glove) stabbing Dan with a ski pole. Dan is not in the picture, which contains only his name, blood, and an abundance of swear words.

4. *Week 4:* A repetition of the second and third week with another tormentor. Mike was becoming more animated and was able to talk about school events and students who had harassed him over the years.

5. *Week 5:* Mike had complained that his teachers were unaware of his situation, and they seemed to side with the bullies, seeing him as the problem. I asked him to draw what he would like to do to the teacher he was having the most difficulty with. Mike drew a fist, which he labeled "me," about to punch his gym teacher.

6. *Weeks 6 to 9:* Mike continued to draw himself (finally emerging as a tiny stick figure) stabbing, shooting, knifing, and even hitting his teachers. He began to smile, as he was able to displace his repressed feelings onto paper. His mother reported his change in attitude and willingness to attend school.

7. *Week 10:* I asked Mike if family members also harassed him. He then drew a picture of himself punching his older brother, who apparently constantly threatened him when their parents were not around. This secret brought concerns that if his parents found out his brother would retaliate. We discussed this dilemma in our session and concluded it would be prudent to wait until he was prepared to discuss this problem with his parents.

8. *Week 11:* I asked Mike to draw a self-portrait, as it was clear that through his drawings he was feeling more self-confident. Mike drew himself as a commando soldier in full army dress holding a gun and with a knife in a holster. He filled the entire paper (12" × 9"). He labeled his drawing, "Mighty Mike!" He told me that the kids in school were no longer hassling him. His attitude had changed remarkably. By depicting his daily trauma and telling his story he was emerging a stronger, more self-assured young man.

9. *Week 12:* Mike drew a picture of his house, with himself inside behind a Dutch door; the top part of the door was opened. He had

locked his sister out. She was saying, "I'm going to kill you!" He was laughing. A thermometer showed 90 degrees outside. He labeled the drawing, "Mighty Mike's revenge!" Mike had found a safe vehicle, through art (displacement), to retaliate. We discussed strategies of how to avoid being reactive to both his brother and sister. He was open to ignoring them. In fact, Mike was more animated and open to suggestions to bring about behavioral changes. He no longer felt like a victim.

10. *Week 13:* Mike came in with a desire to draw a picture for his book. He revealed how unhappy he was that his mother had recently returned to work. She was never home at the end of the school day. Mike drew himself as a large cleated shoe stamping out the dress shop where she worked.

Following this session we had a family meeting. Mike was able to talk about specific incidents at school where he was terrorized. He also talked about how he felt when his sister and brother teased him. Last, he revealed his feelings of abandonment when his mother returned to work. The family was able to empathize with Mike and recognize the growth he had made in the past 3 months. Mike left his book with me, asking me to share it with other students who suffered the effects of bullying behavior.

Art therapy provided a vehicle for Mike, a silent sufferer, to express his deepest secrets. Years of bullying had worn him down. He had become reclusive, angry, and depressed. Through the art process Mike was able to explore and ultimately express his narrative story. Although his artwork expressed violent thoughts, at no time was I concerned that he would act on them. He reexperienced the pain that he had internalized and was able to externalize his fury in his drawings. Through this process he emerged a more confident young man. He no longer fell victim to his siblings or school bullies. His family constellation changed with his willingness to share his experiences and feelings. As Shirley Riley (1997) observed, "the act of drawing is a form of externalization, visible projection of self, thoughts and feelings" (pp. 2–3). The more Mike drew, the more his symptoms diminished; his somatic symptoms disappeared altogether. Mike returned to school confident that he had mastered the strategy to walk away from bullies. He no longer presented symptoms of PTSD. He no longer felt helpless, but, like his drawing of "Mighty Mike," empowered.

Art Therapy Groups

Many students like Mike are seen in groups, meeting with similar-age students who are suffering from social inhibition. Most have been victimized by classmates and suffer low self-esteem. Allowing these students to participate in a social skills art therapy group with an emphasis on a cognitive-behavioral approach can be extremely successful. The idea behind art therapy groups is to provide an opportunity for children to meet their peers in a safe, controlled environment where they can achieve a successful social, emotional, and educational experience (Safran, 2002). This milieu provides an opportunity to explore issues of victimization while teaching strategies for emotional resilience.

Members are carefully screened to eliminate "group busters," persons who are not only victims but also bullies. Antisocial behavior is not tolerated in these groups. These students are seen individually with the hope that they can learn the skills to participate in a group.

Students are put in similar-age groups: elementary school, middle school, high school, and college. Some groups are coed and others single-sex, as determined by the diagnosis and needs of the individual members. Group size is limited to no more than 10 students. Initially, group members learn about art therapy and how it will be used to help them learn more about themselves and each other. In the case of group projects, learning skills to work as a group member are taught. All group members have suffered bullying. Many also are diagnosed with other mental health disorders. All have subscribed to the goal of learning how to handle bullies.

OBJECTIVE OF GROUP

The goals for each group participant are to develop an awareness of social cues and to increase self-esteem while developing self-awareness and self-advocacy skills. These students often feel like victims, rendering them helpless in maneuvering the social maze of friendship. They are, in fact, clueless as to why they have been picked on. If left untreated, these students suffer the impact of traumatization into their adult lives. As they have internalized feelings of rage and a desire for revenge, many become depressed and constricted. Participation in an art therapy group provides a unique place to safely express these extreme feelings.

ORGANIZATION OF GROUP

Respect is paramount. These students are suffering deeply, and they need to be believed. They have often experienced nonvalidation in their school environment. They have been made to feel it is their problem. Even family members unknowingly reinforce these feelings. This can become a vicious cycle: nonbelievers reinforce feelings of self-doubt and worthlessness, which frustrate the nonbeliever (often a parent or teacher). Everyone feels frustrated. Bullying is a hideous process that is often done in a veiled way, which reinforces the cycle.

Group rules of confidentiality and physical safety are established in the first group meeting, providing an environment that ensures no repetition of their school day experience. These rules are reviewed weekly to remind group members that this is a trusting and safe place to express their feelings.

The groups initially meet for 10 weeks; each session is 1 hour long. They are structured groups, which incorporate art therapy weekly, whether in the form of individual drawings or group projects (murals, "secret boxes," three-dimensional structures). Role playing and children's literature are also included as modalities to enhance and commiserate with the feelings victims of bullying behavior experience. Most groups are coed and led by an art therapist and a clinical psychologist.

Ten weeks is not enough time for most students to absorb the strategies that are offered to them during group sessions. Behavioral changes do not always follow cognitive skills (Braswell & Bloomquist, 1991). Practice and repetition of newly learned skills over a long time are necessary. Family members are encouraged to participate in family sessions to enhance the group experience. Many students will continue throughout the school year. This may become, for most, the one safe place to be with peers.

With younger children, who frequently relate to literature, appropriate books are introduced as a way to initiate discussion (see "Selected Children's Literature on Bullying" at the end of the chapter). Children frequently identify with the characters in these books, which leads to discussion and often the suggestion to draw their own story of being bullied, their feelings about the experience, and how they would handle the bully. Each participant makes his or her own book, then shares it with the others. This creative opportunity displaces feelings appropriately and allows participants to master feelings of helplessness and learn new strategies to conquer these feelings.

All group members are encouraged to bring in bullying situations that may have occurred during the week, which may lead to role playing, discussion, or drawing. Each group member has his or her own drawing pad (13" × 17" white paper).

Many of the group participants are highly defensive. For example, Ron, a middle school student, refused to make the connection between his provocative behavior and the bully's response. His whining and feelings of victimization were deeply rooted. Since kindergarten his peers had picked on him. His defensiveness was a result of chronic teasing. It was not until he drew a picture of his "revenge" (Figure 7.2) with himself saying, "shut up" repeatedly until he successfully provoked another student to respond by shouting, "Stop, stop, stop," that the other group members were able to help Ron identify his annoying behavior. Showing his drawing to his group members elicited questions like "Why do you do that?"; "Why don't you stop?"; and "Do you

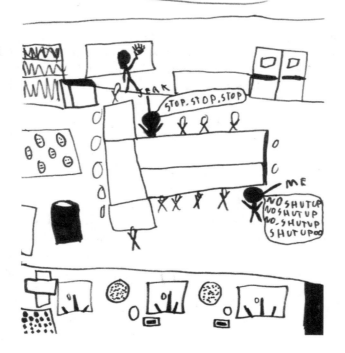

FIGURE 7.2. Ron's drawing of his "revenge."

realize how annoying you are?" Discussion followed on how his being provocative was one of the contributing factors resulting in others picking on him. Peer questioning and pointing out his behavior was much more successful than adults questioning his behavior and motivation. Ron was able to take suggestions like walking away instead of engaging to stop this negative cycle.

CASE STUDY: ERIC

For Eric, a slight, shy, anxious, highly intelligent 12-year-old middle school student, telling how he was physically and verbally attacked in school was a relief. He was able to draw the incident and describe it in great detail to his group members (Figure 7.3). He then drew a picture of what he would have liked to do to the bully who attacked him. The drawing, as described by Eric, was filled with violent imagery. He quickly expressed that he would never do these things and that by talking about them he felt the need for revenge less. Both therapists became aware of Eric's internalized rage, which proved helpful in his individual therapy. Initially, Eric told the group that he wanted his mother to call the school, but with the help of role playing within the group setting, it was determined that he would and could report the

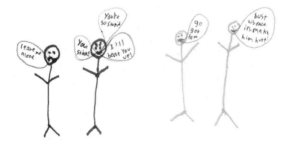

FIGURE 7.3. Eric—being bullied.

incident himself to enhance his power and control over the situation. The idea of being the reporter made him very anxious, and he developed somatic symptoms such as insomnia and chronic stomach- and headaches.

Like many boys who have been bullied, he intellectually understood why he was picked on, but it still hurt. The bully's friends verbally abused Eric for being a tattletale following his reporting the incident to his school counselor. None of Eric's friends came to his rescue. The art therapy group validated his feelings and shared similar occurrences, reinforcing his right to feel betrayed by his counselor and his friends. This group experience helped keep Eric from being retraumatized by the consequences of confiding in his school counselor.

Eric was able to give a graphic representation of a traumatic incident that he was reluctant to discuss. This allowed him to construct his traumatic narrative, which enabled his group members to empathize more with him. The drawing provided an impetus to tell his story (Malchiodi, 2001), while allowing for reframing and developing a strategy to manage his feelings of helplessness. The group, by validating the experience, reinforced his ability to take charge of the situation, rendering him empowered; he no longer felt helpless.

The Use of Drawing

The use of drawing for children like Eric provides a vehicle in a safe environment to express their trauma. Eric had been unable to tell his story, and drawing it aroused his feelings of being threatened, allowing him to reexperience the bullying incident. Following the drawing, Eric immediately became visibly relaxed and less anxious until it was suggested he take charge of the situation. An action-oriented solution, while the correct next step, was premature. Eric needed to rehearse, through role playing, the next step repeatedly in order to master his aroused feelings of anxiety. Once Eric "told on the bully, the bully's friends harassed him." Children experience bullies as terrorists, uncontrollable and unpredictable; however, they are more predictable than the victim understands. I realized that the bully's friends might harass Eric and prepared him for this possibility. Although prepared, he was still disappointed in the counselor to whom he revealed the incident, which reinforced his belief that he could not trust school personnel. Unfortunately, this is a very familiar experience for students who are victims of bullies.

Group Projects

Once group trust has been established, one should offer the opportunity to work on a project together. Group projects, such as murals, can evoke underlying feelings of tension and insecurity. Students are often hesitant to participate. Those who are the aggressive/provocative type of victim may attempt to take charge of the project in an inappropriate manner. Passive responders will go along without voicing their opinions. This process may quickly lead to a more definitive understanding for the therapist of why these students are objects of bullying and to group discussion with regard to each group member's role in the process.

An opportunity to take on a different persona can be offered through role playing as a useful and interactive means of exploring other members' identities. Sometimes writing and performing a play with members taking on different roles is less threatening. Using Polaroid pictures of each member glued onto popsicle sticks to make a puppet cast of themselves is fun and less threatening. Mural paper can be hung from the ceiling with a stage cut out. Members take turns directing the play, which involves retelling each participant's story of being bullied. In this way, they can evaluate by observation how their inappropriate behavior may have contributed to being bullied and/or offer appropriate strategies to deal with the bully. Learning can take place in an environment that is fun and conducive to self-awareness.

Case Study: Jamie

For Jamie, having obsessive–compulsive disorder (OCD) has presented its own issues. She revealed her OCD to her group through a drawing about why she thinks she is being bullied (Figure 7.4). As a high school student, she is acutely aware of and often misperceives others' responses to her. She felt safe in her group and was able to discuss not only her OCD, but also her hypersensitivity (extreme reactions to misperceived teasing). She was not the only group member with OCD; in fact, two other members revealed that they had the same issue as well as reporting incidents/feelings of being ostracized.

The group therapy setting offered both Jamie and the other group members a place to discover their similarities and to feel free to discuss their "secret" (OCD). More important, all group members were able to discuss openly the threat of daily bullying. Jamie's heightened anxiety

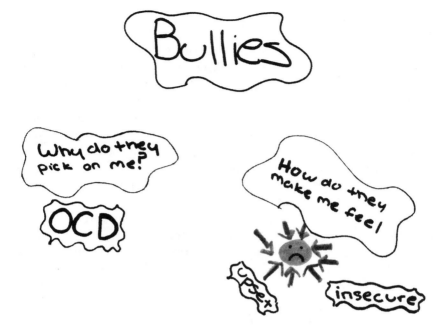

FIGURE 7.4. Jamie—revealing to group her OCD diagnosis.

about chronically being humiliated in school exacerbated her OCD symptoms. When a student like Jamie suffers persecution over a long period of time (since elementary school), he or she is more likely to develop symptoms of PTSD. Jamie became extremely somatic; she refused to attend gym, where the locker room had become a nightmare; and she cried easily, distrusted her school personnel, felt powerless, and became depressed. She even contemplated using drugs/alcohol as a way to fit in.

The support of the group and their suggestions lessened her fear of attending school. The other group members all drew similar pictures of being bullied and attributed it to their own differences: shyness, hyperactivity, smallness, being nonathletic, being depressed, dressing differently in a conservative private school, and being Jewish in a predominantly Christian public school. The need to celebrate their differences was encouraged, but, like wounded animals, they wanted to retreat from the provoking situation.

It took many months of group art therapy for change and empowerment to occur. Like Mike, group participants were offered the opportunity to express their unspoken feelings on paper and then to offer these illustrations of their despair and rage to their group members for discussion and validation of their feelings. A literature review was brought into the group, offering the high school students a heightened awareness of the enormous problem bullying behavior is throughout the United States and abroad. Children and adolescents often identify with what they read, finding comfort in knowing they are not alone in their suffering.

CONCLUSIONS

All students can be vulnerable to bullying behavior. Students with disabilities or disorders are predictably vulnerable (Safran, 2002). Would a student like Mike or Eric act on his internalized feelings of rage if he had not had the opportunity to express himself through art therapy? Statistics tell us that many victims of bullying become bullies. One can conjecture that the more opportunity is provided for self-expression the less need there is for revenge. Art therapy can provide a safe nonverbal platform for visual expression, sublimation, and displacement. Expressing victimization gives a student the opportunity to learn strategies to alleviate his or her feelings of helplessness.

Drawing allows students to reenact the trauma while lessening the experience of retraumatization. It also gives students a way to express angry feelings without the need to act on them. By sharing their narrative within their group of peers and therapists, students become more empowered to deal with bullies. Their pictures tell their stories, express their pain, and become a container for their intense feelings. Their drawings also offer them insight into their own feelings. Additionally, their drawings provide a depiction that captures these intense feelings, giving parents and school personnel a clearer image of their suffering and, hopefully, leading to successful school intervention.

Creative approaches alone, or in conjunction with school-based prevention/intervention programs, offer a viable means to minimize the impact of bullying behavior. Giving students a venue in which to safely explore internalized feelings of traumatization helps them become able to vocalize their pain, gain support and strategies, and learn to approach new bully situations from an empowered stance.

REFERENCES

American Psychiatric Association. (2000). *Diagnostic and statistical manual of mental disorders* (4th ed., text rev.). Washington, DC: Author.

Arbona, C., Jackson, R. H., McCoy, A., & Blakely, C. (1999). Ethnic identity as a predictor of attitudes of adolescents toward fighting. *Journal of Early Adolescence, 19*(3), 323–340.

Arora, C. M. J. (1996). Defining bullying. *School Psychology International, 17*, 317–329.

Bernstein, J. Y., & Watson, M. W. (1997). Children who are the targets of bullying. *Journal of Interpersonal Violence, 12*(4), 483–498.

Bjoerkqvist, K., Lagerspetz, K. M., & Kaukiainen, A. (1992). Do girls manipulate and boys fight?: Developmental trends in regard to direct and indirect aggression. *Aggressive Behavior, 18*, 117–127.

Bjoerkqvist, K., & Niemela, P. (Eds.). (1992). *Of mice and women: Aspects of female aggression*. San Diego, CA: Academic Press.

Bond, L., Carlin, J. B., Thomas, L., Rubin, K., & Patton, G. (2001). Does bullying cause emotional problems? A prospective study of young teenagers. *British Medical Journal, 323*, 480–484.

Borg, M. G. (1999). The extent and nature of bullying among primary and secondary schoolchildren. *Educational Research, 41*(2), 137–153.

Bosworth, K., Espelage, D. L., & Simon, T. R. (1999). Factors associated with bullying behavior in middle school students. *Journal of Early Adolescence, 19*(3), 341–362.

Boulton, M. J. (1999). Concurrent and longitudinal relations between children's playground behavior and social preference, victimization, and bullying. *Child Development, 70*(4), 944–954.

Braswell, L., & Bloomquist, M. (1991). *Cognitive-behavioral therapy with ADHD children*. New York: Guilford Press.

Brown, L. M., & Gilligan, C. (1992). *Meeting at the crossroads: Women's psychology and girls' development*. New York: Ballantine Books.

Crick, N. R. (1995). Relational aggression: The role of intent attributions, feelings of distress, and provocation type. *Development and Psychopathology, 7*(2), 313–322.

Crick, N. R. (1997). Engagement in gender normative versus non-normative forms of aggression: Links to social–psychological adjustment. *Developmental Psychology, 33*(4), 610–617.

Crick, N. R., Bigbee, M. A., & Howes, M. (1996). Gender differences in children's normative beliefs about aggression: How do I hurt thee? Let me count the ways. *Child Development, 67*(3), 1003–1014.

Crick, N. R., & Dodge, K. A. (1994). A review and reformulation of social information-processing mechanisms in children's social adjustment. *Psychological Bulletin, 115*, 74–110.

Crick, N. R., & Grotpeter, J. K. (1995). Relational aggression, gender, and social–psychological adjustment. *Child Development, 66,* 710–722.

Crick, N. R., & Grotpeter, J. K. (1996). Children's treatment by peers: Victims of relational and overt aggression. *Development and Psychopathology, 8,* 367–380.

Crick, N. R., Nelson, D. R., Morales, J. R., Cullerton-Sen, C., Casas, J. F., & Hickman, S. E. (2001). Relational victimization in childhood and adolescence. In J. Juvonen & S. Graham (Eds.), *Peer harassment in school: The plight of the vulnerable and victimized* (pp. 196–214). New York: Guilford Press.

Crick, N. R., Werner, N. E., Casas, J. F., O'Brien, K. M., Nelson, D. A., Grotpeter, J. F., et al. (1999). Childhood aggression and gender: A new look at an old problem. In D. Bernstein (Ed.), *Nebraska Symposium on Motivation: Vol. 45. Gender and motivation* (pp. 75–102). Lincoln: University of Nebraska Press.

Duncan, R. D. (1999a). Maltreatment by parents and peers: The relationship between child abuse, bully victimization, and psychological distress. *Child Maltreatment, 4*(1), 45–55.

Duncan, R. D. (1999b). Peer and sibling aggression: An investigation of intra- and extra-familial bullying. *Journal of Interpersonal Violence, 14*(8), 871–886.

Espelage, D. L., Mebane, S. E., & Swearer, S. M. (2004). Gender differences in bullying: Moving beyond mean-level differences. In D. L. Espelage & S. M. Swearer (Eds.), *Bullying in American schools: A social-ecological perspective on prevention and intervention* (pp. 15–35). Mahwah, NJ: Erlbaum.

Espelage, D. L., & Swearer, S. M. (2003). Research on school bullying and victimization: What have we learned and where do we go from here? *School Psychology Review, 32*(3), 365–383.

Espelage, D. L., & Swearer, S. M. (Eds.). (2004). *Bullying in American schools: A social-ecological perspective on prevention and intervention.* Mahwah, NJ: Erlbaum.

Garbarino, J., & deLara, E. (2002). *And words can hurt forever: How to protect adolescents from bullying, harassment, and emotional violence.* New York: Free Press.

Gilligan, C. (1993). *In a different voice: Psychological theory and women's development.* Cambridge, MA: Cambridge University Press.

Glew, G., Rivara, F., & Feudtner, C. (2000). Bullying: Children hurting children. *Pediatric Review, 21,* 183–189.

Green, A. H. (1999). The impact of physical, sexual, and emotional abuse. In J. D. Neship (Ed.), *The handbook of child and adolescent psychiatry* (Vol. 2, pp. 202–212). New York: Wiley.

Harryman, S. (2004). When bullies grow up. *ASCA School Counselor, 14,* 43–47.

Hazler, R. J. (1996). *Breaking the cycle of violence: Interventions for bullying and victimization*. Washington, DC: Accelerated Development.

Hazler, R. J., & Carney, J. V. (2000). When victims turn aggressors: Factors in the development of deadly school violence. *Professional School Counseling, 4*(2), 105–112.

Hazler, R. J., Miller, D. L., Carney, J. V., & Green, S. (2001). Adult recognition of school bullying situations. *Educational Research, 43*, 133–146.

Hoover, J. H., & Hazler, R. J. (1994). Bullies and victims. *Elementary School Guidance and Counseling, 25*, 212–220.

Hoover, J. H., Oliver, R., & Thomson, K. (1993). Perceived victimization by school bullies: New research and future direction. *Journal of Humanistic Education and Development, 32*, 76–84.

Hovard, N., Home, A., & Jeleff, D. (2001). Bully busting: A psychoeducational program for helping bullies and their victims. *Journal of Emotional Abuse, 2*, 181–191.

Juvonen, J. (2001). *School violence: Prevalence, fears, and prevention*. Santa Monica, CA: RAND.

Juvonen, J., & Graham, S. (Eds.). (2001). *Peer harassment in school: The plight of the vulnerable and victimized*. New York: Guilford Press.

Kaiser Family Foundation, Children Now. (2001). *Nickelodeon/Talking with kids about tough issues: A national survey of parents and kids*. Menlo Park, CA: Kaiser Family Foundation.

Kaukiainen, A., Bjorkqvist, K., Lagerspetz, K., Osterman, K., Salmivalli, D., Rothberg, S., et al. (1999). The relationships between social intelligence, empathy, and three types of aggression. *Aggressive Behavior, 25*, 81–89.

Kumpulainen, K., Rasanen, E., & Henttonen, I. (1999). Children involved in bullying: Psychological disturbance and the persistence of the involvement. *Child Abuse and Neglect, 23*(12), 1253–1262.

Loeber, R., & Hale, D. (1997). Key issues in the development of aggression and violence from childhood to early adulthood. *Annual Review of Psychology, 48*, 371–410.

Malchiodi, C. A. (2001). Using drawing as intervention with traumatized children. *Trauma and Loss: Research and Intervention, 1*(1), 21–28.

Nansel, T. R., Overpeck, M., Pila, R., Ruan, W., Simons-Morton, B., & Scheidt, P. (2001). Bullying behaviors among U.S. youth: Prevalence and association with psychosocial adjustment. *Journal of the American Medical Association, 285*, 2094–2100.

Olweus, D. (1978). *Aggression in the schools: Bullies and whipping boys*. New York: Wiley.

Olweus, D. (1991). Bully–victim problems among school children: Basic facts and effects of a school-based intervention program. In K. Rubin &

D. Pepler (Eds.), *The development and treatment of childhood aggression* (pp. 85–128). Hillsdale, NJ: Erlbaum.

Olweus, D. (1993). *Bullying at school: What we know and what we can do*. Oxford: Blackwell.

Olweus, D. (1994a). Annotation: Bullying at school: Basic facts and effects of a school-based intervention program. *Journal of Child Psychology and Psychiatry, 35*, 1171–1190.

Olweus, D. (1994b). Bullying at school: Long-term outcomes for the victims and an effective school-based intervention program. In L. R. Huesmann (Ed.), *Aggressive behavior: Current perspectives* (pp. 97–130). New York: Plenum.

Olweus, D. (1996). Bully/victim problems in school. *Prospects, 26*, 331–359.

Olweus, D., Limber, S., & Mihalic, S. (1999) *Blueprints for violence prevention: Bullying prevention program*. Boulder, CO: Institute of Behavioral Science, Regents of the University of Colorado.

Pellegrini, A. D. (2002). Bullying and victimization in middle school: A dominance relations perspective. *Educational Psychologist, 37*, 151–163.

Pellegrini, A. D., Bartini, M., & Brooks, F. (1999). School bullies, victims, and aggressive victims: Factors relating to group affiliation and victimization in early adolescence. *Journal of Educational Psychology, 91*(2), 216–224.

Pellegrini, A. D., & Long, J. (2002). A longitudinal study of bullying, dominance, and victimization during the transition from primary to secondary school. *British Journal of Developmental Psychology, 20*, 259–280.

Pellegrini, A. D., & Long, J. (2004). Part of the solution and part of the problem: The role of peers in bullying, dominance, and victimization during the transition from primary school through secondary school. In D. L. Espelage & S. M. Swearer (Eds.), *Bullying in American schools: A social-ecological perspective on prevention and intervention* (pp. 107–117). Mahwah, NJ: Erlbaum.

Riley, S. (1997). Children's art and narratives: An opportunity to enhance therapy and a supervisory challenge. *The Supervision Bulletin, 9*(3), 2–3.

Safran, D. (2002). *Art therapy and AD/HD: Diagnostic and therapeutic approaches*. London: Jessica Kingsley.

Safran, E. (2003). *Bullying behavior: Perspectives of eleventh-grade high school students*. New York: New York University Psychoeducational Center.

Salmivalli, C., Kaukiainen, A., Kaistaniemi, L., & Lagerspetz, K. M. (1999). Self-evaluated self-esteem, peer-evaluated self-esteem, and defensive egotism as predictors of adolescents' participation in bullying situations. *Personality and Social Psychology Bulletin, 25*(10), 1268–1278.

Sandstrom, M. J., & Coie, J. D. (1999). A developmental perspective on peer rejection: Mechanisms of stability and change. *Child Development,* 70(4), 955–966.

Schwartz, D., Proctor L. J., & Chien, D. H. (2001). The aggressive victim of bullying. In J. Juvonen and S. Graham (Eds.), *Peer harassment in school. The plight of the vulnerable and victimized* (pp. 147–174). New York: Guilford Press.

Shaughnessy, M., & Lehtonen, K. (1998). *The emotionally sensitive adolescent.* Albuquerque, NM: U.S. Department of Education.

Simmons, R. (2002). *Odd girl out: The hidden culture of aggression in girls.* New York: Harcourt.

Slee, P. T. (1994). Situational and interpersonal correlates of anxiety associated with peer victimization. *Child Psychiatry and Human Development,* 25, 97–107.

Smith, P. K., & Brian, P. (2000). Bullying in schools: lessons from two decades of research. *Aggressive Behavior,* 26, 1–9.

Smith, P. K., Madsen, K. C., & Moody, J. C. (1999). What causes the age decline in reports of being bullied at school?: Towards a developmental analysis of risks of being bullied. *Educational Research,* 41, 267–285.

Smith, J., Twemlow, S. W., & Hoover, D. W. (1999). Bullies, victims and bystanders: A method of in-school intervention and possible parental contributions. *Child Psychiatry and Human Development,* 30(1), 29–37.

Steele, W. (2003). Using drawing in short-term trauma resolution. In C. A. Malchiodi (Ed.), *Handbook of art therapy* (pp. 139–151). New York: Guilford Press.

Steele, W., & Raider, M. (2001). *Structured sensory interventions for traumatized children, adolescents, and parents: Strategies to alleviate trauma.* New York: Edwin Mellen.

Stein, N., & Sjostrom, L. (1996). *Bullyproof: A teacher's guide on teasing and bullying for use with fourth- and fifth-grade students.* Washington, DC: National Educational Association.

Sutton, J., & Smith, P. K. (1999). Bullying as a group process: An adaptation of the participant role approach. *Aggressive Behavior,* 25, 97–111.

Sutton, J., Smith, P. K., & Swettenham, J. (1999a). Bullying and "Theory of Mind": A critique of the "social skills deficit" view of anti-social behavior. *Social Development,* 8(1), 117–127.

Sutton, J., Smith, P. K., & Swettenham, J. (1999b). Social cognition and bullying: Social inadequacy or skilled manipulation? *British Journal of Developmental Psychology,* 17, 435–450.

Swearer, S. M., & Espelage, D. L. (2004). Introduction: A social-ecological framework of bullying among youth. In D. L. Espelage & S. M. Swearer (Eds.), *Bullying in American schools: A social-ecological perspective on prevention and intervention* (pp. 1–12). Mahwah, NJ: Erlbaum.

Swearer, S. M., Grills, A. E., Haye, K. M., & Cary, P. T. (2004) Internalizing problems in students involved in bullying and victimization: Implications for intervention. In D. L. Espelage & S. M. Swearer (Eds.), *Bullying in American schools: A social-ecological perspective on prevention and intervention* (pp. 63–83). Mahwah, NJ: Erlbaum.

Twemlow, S. (2000). The roots of violence: Converging psychoanalytic explanatory models for power struggles and violence in schools. *Psychoanalytic Q, 69,* 741–785.

U.S. Department of Education, National Center for Education Statistics. (2006). *Digest of Education Statistics,* 2005 (NCES 2006-030). Washington, DC: U.S. Government Printing Office.

U.S. Secret Service. (2000). *Safe school initiative: An interim report on the prevention of targeted violence in schools.* U.S. Secret Service National Threat Assessment Center, U.S. Department of Education. Washington, DC: Department of the Treasury.

Vossekuil, B., Fein, R. A., Reddy, M., Borum, R., & Modzeleski, W. (2002). *The final report and findings of the safe school initiative: Implications for the prevention of school attacks in the United States.* Washington, DC: U.S. Secret Service and the United States Department of Education.

Wiseman, R. (2002). *Queen bees and wannabees.* New York: Three Rivers Press.

SELECTED CHILDREN'S LITERATURE ON BULLYING

Best, C. (2001). *Shrinking Violet.* Illustrated by Giselle Potter. New York: Farrar Straus & Giroux.

Bosch, C. (1988). *Bully on the bus.* Seattle, WA: Parenting Press.

Bruchac, J., & Bruchac, J. (2001). *How chipmunk got his stripes: A tale of bragging and teasing.* Illustrated by Jose Aruego & Ariane Dewey. New York: Dial Publishing.

Carlson, N. (1997). *How to lose all your friends.* New York: Puffin.

Caseley, J. (2001). *Bully.* New York: Greenwillow.

Cohen-Posey, K. (1995). *How to handle bullies, teasers and other meanies: A book that takes the nuisance out of name calling and other nonsense.* Illustrated by Betsy A. Lampe. Lake Zurich, IL: Rainbow Books.

Crary, E. (2000). *Heidi's irresistible hat.* Seattle, WA: Parenting Press.

Crary, E., & Megale, M. (1996). *My name is not dummy.* Seattle, WA: Parenting Press.

Depino, C. (2003). *Blue cheese breath and stinky feet.* New York: Simon & Schuster.

Falukner, M. (2000). *Black belt.* New York: Knopf.

Gedig, B. (1999). *Simon's hook: A story about teases and put-downs.* Illustrated by Laurie Barrows. Felton, CA: GR Publishing.

Hammerseng, K. (1996). *Telling isn't tattling*. Illustrated by Dave Garbot. New York: Parenting Press.

Harker, L&T. (2000). *Stop picking on me*. New York: Barron's Educational Series.

Keats, E. J. (1998). *Goggles*. New York: Viking Children's Books.

Lester, H. (1999). *Hooway for Wodney Wat*. Boston, MA: Houghton Mifflin.

Lovell, P. (2001). *Stand tall, Molly Lou Melon*. Illustrated by David Catrow. New York: Putnam.

McCain, B. (2001). *Nobody knew what to do: A story about bullying*. Illustrated by Todd Leonard. New York: Albert Whitman & Co.

Moss, M. (1999). *Amelia takes command*. Middletown, WI: Pleasant Company Publications.

Moss, P., & Lyon, L. (2004). *Say something*. Gardiner, ME: Tilbury House.

Naylor, P. (1994). *The king of the playground*. Illustrated by Nola Langner Malone. New York: Aladdin.

O'Neill, A., & Huliska-Beith, L. (2002). *The recess queen*. New York: Scholastic Press.

Romain, T. (1998). *Cliques, phonies, and other baloney*. Minneapolis, MN: Free Spirit.

Romain, T. & Verdick, E. (1999). *Bullies are a pain in the brain*. Minneapolis, MN: Free Spirit.

Shapiro, L. (2004). *Betty stops the bully*. Vienna, VA: CTC Publishing.

Wells, R. (1980). *Hazel's amazing mother*. New York: Greenwillow Press.

Chapter 8

Trauma, Loss, and Bibliotherapy

The Healing Power of Stories

Cathy A. Malchiodi
Deanne Ginns-Gruenberg

In *The Healing Power of Stories*, Taylor (1996) observes that "we tell stories because we hope to find or create significant connections between things. Stories link past, present, and future in a way that tells us where we have been, where we are, and where we are going" (p. 1). Stories, legends, myths, and tales are an important part of human history that give meaning to life and provide guidance and wisdom. More recently, psychology has embraced storytelling in the form of narrative and other postmodern therapies, underscoring its reparative nature and ability to "restory" one's life.

Creative interventions such as drawing, movement, writing, or play therapy often capitalize on the power of storytelling to give meaning to nonverbal self-expression; however, the purposeful use of books in therapy, known as bibliotherapy, and specific storymaking techniques are effective interventions in and of themselves in work with children who have experienced traumatic events. Children who are grieving a loss, struggling with divorce or foster care, or recovering from abuse or neglect can all benefit from the sensitive use of books in therapy.

This chapter gives a brief overview of how to use children's books in intervention, providing specific suggestions for children's literature relevant to various traumatic events, loss, and bereavement. Guidelines for using books in therapy are offered, emphasizing how children's books can enhance trauma intervention when used appropriately and sensitively. In particular, we recommend books that can be used with experiential activities to enhance bibliotherapy in work with children experiencing trauma or loss.

BIBLIOTHERAPY

The word "bibliotherapy" is derived from the Greek words "biblio," meaning book, and "therapeia," meaning healing. The sharing of stories is older than literacy; early storytellers used language to illuminate individual and collective experiences, to convey universal emotions, and as a form of healing (Berns, 2004). The use of books in therapy emerged from the human proclivity to identify with characters in stories and with the stories themselves. For this reason, the books used in bibliotherapy convey specific themes, evoke connection with characters, and communicate how others have confronted and solved problems. According to Pardeck and Pardeck (1993), good literature naturally provides individuals with models to help them cope with dilemmas and handle real-life situations. Although bibliotherapy extends to work with adults, it generally refers to the use of books with children. Fairytales, fiction, nonfiction, poetry, and autobiographies are used in bibliotherapy to bring about change in affect or behavior. Therapists often choose specific books for use with children who have experienced trauma or loss, based on the goals of intervention.

Gladding and Gladding (1991) describe two different types of bibliotherapy: reactive and interactive. Reactive bibliotherapy involves the child reading specific stories or books; if they have been appropriately selected, the child will identify with the character or story and will have increased understanding and insight after reading the book. Interactive bibliotherapy involves discussion between the therapist and child client to facilitate, reinforce, and integrate concepts gained from reading a particular story.

Many therapists feel that bibliotherapy is a method only to be undertaken by professionals who are trained psychotherapists and understand the application of literature as an intervention. Others see bibliotherapy in a broader context and believe that books are natural agents of healing and that nonprofessionals can effectively utilize books to help others. Additionally, many individuals use books for self-help or to learn more about themselves (Rudman, Gagne, & Bernstein, 1993).

In this chapter, we define bibliotherapy as the application of specific literature within a therapeutic context. In this sense, bibliotherapy is an important method in helping children understand traumatic experiences, learn new adaptive coping skills, and consider different perspectives (Vernon & Clemente, 2005). It is the selection of reading material with special relevance to the child's situation (Jackson, 2001). In the case of trauma, one may choose books with themes relating to the crisis the child has experienced.

Like other creative activities, reading a book can recall early memories of connection, attachment, and emotional closeness associated with early childhood. Nursery rhymes, for example, involve tone of voice and repetition of sounds and words. Because rhymes are repeated many times, they form associations with positive relationships with parents and caregivers. Reading can also involve calming rituals and self-soothing experiences. For children, the time before bedtime often involves reading or being read to, a tradition that helps children prepare for separation from parents and sleep. Additionally, childhood stories are usually read over and over, leading to familiarity, comfort, and security in knowing how the story ends. Stories may be read at specific times of year, as family traditions, or on cultural or religious holidays.

A PERSONAL EXAMPLE

One of us (Malchiodi, 2001) relates the following demonstration of how stories can heal, even after the experience of the September 11, 2001, terrorist acts:

A few days after the terrorist acts, I had an experience that reaffirmed the importance of appropriate and timely intervention to transform and stabilize. I was conducting an art and play session with a small group of children at a local residential treatment center. The children had all watched television broadcasts of plane crashes, fireballs, and the Twin Towers of the World Trade Center falling. They were anxious and fearful, overhearing adults' and caregivers' worries and concerns. Because I, too, felt the effect of the television images I had witnessed, I told the group that I was having a hard time understanding why people would do such terrible things to others they did not even know. I also wondered out loud how everyone else was feeling and asked the children to make a drawing of how they were feeling today.

Predictably, all the children drew images about feeling sad or afraid and talked about seeing the devastation they had witnessed on television that week. Pictures of explosions, wounded people, airplanes, buildings on fire, and "bad men" emerged. Many children asked about what had happened to the people who died and if something like this could happen to their school or to someone's house. We spent time talking about how these feelings were normal and that other children and adults were having a lot of the same feelings.

I then asked if anyone in the group could think of a story—a book or a fairytale—that was like "the bad day when the planes crashed into the buildings." Because events of violence and terror are often confusing to children, I wanted to try to find a child-appropriate way of helping the group explore and express their experiences. One 8-year-old boy volunteered that it reminded him of *The Grinch Who Stole Christmas*. The acts of terrorism in the preceding days indeed felt a lot like someone had come and stolen all the presents under the tree and ruined everyone's fun. The terrorists had taken all that was good in life that we had come to expect—joy, peace, and freedom—and left us with fear, uncertainty, and sadness.

We decided to read the story out loud and make drawings about the Grinch and his bad deeds. But what was most remarkable about this simple experience was the ending of the group that day. In the spirit of the story, the children wanted to hold hands and sing songs like the citizens of Whoville who, despite the loss of Christmas presents and roast beast, found a sense of appreciations in each other at a time of crisis. (p. 9)

Reading the story of the Grinch was a small step in mastering trauma for these children, but the experience demonstrates that stories naturally enhance the healing process. In the case of these children, they had not only witnessed disaster on television, but also had experienced personally traumatic events during their young lives. Working with this particular familiar story helped empower them to express their fears, worries, and questions, find comfort and meaning for their emotions, and feel hope through sharing a story with universal themes.

This brief example illustrates many of the unique goals of bibliotherapy with children who have experienced trauma or loss. Stories help children find some distance from their emotions by talking about characters and find a focus outside themselves. The retelling of the story of the Grinch increased the sense of companionship between group members and the therapist, validated thoughts and feelings, and enhanced empathy. In subsequent sessions, the children in this group were able to identify similarities between their lives and the lives of the story's characters, both of whom had experienced sadness, betrayal, and loss. Successful bibliotherapy moves children from their personal crises toward recovery through placing feelings and memories in a larger framework beyond the self.

GUIDELINES FOR BIBLIOTHERAPY WITH CHILDREN

The purposeful use of books in trauma intervention enhances and guides discussion of painful feelings and memories. It helps children realize that they are not alone in their experiences and often answers their questions in a developmentally appropriate way. The experience of sharing a story with child clients can be equally rewarding to therapists because it brings a creative and relational dimension to treatment.

To use bibliotherapy effectively with traumatized children, therapists should consider the following:

1. *Preview all books.* Therapists must read all books they plan to use with child clients. Prereading helps one spot any text or illustrations that may be inappropriate or inadvisable. Previewing a book's content is also important to discover if the theme or characters are culturally relevant to the child and to evaluate whether the material is too simple or too complex. When selecting books for bibliotherapy, illustrations should be carefully previewed for content and effect on children. First, are the pictures engaging? Can they be readily understood by child audiences/readers? If the book is to be used in a group setting, can participants easily see the illustrations? With regard to affect, do the characters appear menacing? Do illustrations invite anx-

iety or fears, or do they calm and soothe? Would individual children have fears about the characters depicted in the story? For example, while *When Dinosaurs Die* (Krasny & Brown, 1998) is a wonderful book for addressing death-related issues, it would not be the initial book of choice for a child terrified by dinosaurs or monsters in nightmares.

2. *Consider the relevance of the book or story to the child's current situation.* Books and stories should relate to the child's current situation, although they do not have to address that situation directly. For children who may be resistant to talking about their experiences, stories with metaphors or symbolic characters, rather than realistic descriptions, can ease fears while providing the opportunity to safely explore how characters deal with crises or conflicts. Children who are severely traumatized may prefer to communicate indirectly and may not be ready to communicate directly about how their situations relate to the book's characters or theme.

3. *Introduce why the book is relevant.* A therapist may introduce why he or she is reading a particular book to a child, but he or she does not need to talk about the child's specific situation in introducing the story. In fact, with traumatized children, it is often best to talk about the story's characters. For example, in the story of *No-No and the Secret Touch* (Patterson & Feldman, 1993), a story about sexual abuse, the therapist can explain that the story is about how adults sometimes touch children in places that they should not. Often, sensitively framing the contents of a book or story and relating how the story can help children serves as a catalyst to future disclosures of personally painful experiences, conflicts, or memories as therapy unfolds.

4. *Consider developmental needs.* Be sure that the book is developmentally appropriate and is suitable for the child's vocabulary and reading skills. In other words, the therapist must be knowledgeable about the child's cognitive abilities and comprehension, if possible, and what types of books and literature are appropriate for various age groups. In times of crisis and loss, attention spans are limited for children of all ages, so the amount of time they are able to focus on the words of the books must be considered. In work with traumatized children, less complicated plots are often more helpful in the long run.

5. *Engage the imagination and senses.* Well-written, well-illustrated books involve young readers or listeners, are emotionally and cognitively absorbing, and stimulate creative thinking. Animal characters with human attributes stimulate the imagination, allow for emotional

distance, and encourage projection. For example, *The Adventures of Lady* (Pearson & Merrill, 2007) is a story about a squirrel orphaned by Hurricane Charley and explores the animal's feelings of sadness, loneliness, and hope. Children may spontaneously initiate creative play about these characters or be encouraged to express how the animals in the story felt, either verbally or through art, movement, or pantomime. Acting out or drawing these experiences empowers children to more closely identify with characters and imagine new solutions, reinforcing the idea that they, too, can surmount obstacles.

6. *Choose books that provide comfort and reassurance.* Traumatized children often experience intrusive thoughts, hyperarousal, and avoidance of painful feelings and memories. Books that gently, yet realistically reassure children and offer strategies for self-soothing and coping are ideal for these children. Books can give traumatized children hope and confidence through stories' themes and characters. For some children, reading true stories or essays written by others their own age can be effective. Children readily identify with what others who have had similar experiences say and find these stories empowering because they are by "real people." Finally, in working with traumatized children, consider alternating heavy and light reading. For example, start with a book with a relevant message and follow it with a story that is humorous, fun, and easy to read.

BIBLIOTHERAPY AS TRAUMA INTERVENTION

The following books are recommended for use in bibliotherapy with traumatized children, based on our experiences. To help therapists choose the appropriate literature for work with their child clients, books are categorized by specific use, with brief descriptions of their contents and characters.

Learning about Trauma Intervention

Brave Bart (Sheppard, 2001) is the story of a cat that has been traumatized. He learns from his trauma therapist, Helping Hannah, that his thoughts and feelings after a trauma are common and normal (Figure 8.1). A number of trauma-related issues are explored throughout the story, including posttraumatic stress disorder triggers, the importance of asking for help and group support, and the process of recovery.

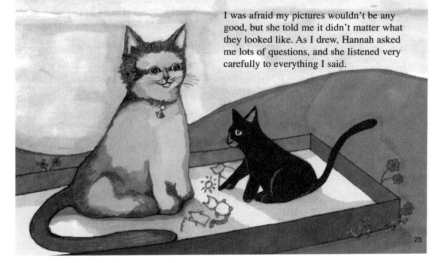

At first, I was afraid to talk to Helping Hannah. She asked me to tell my story by drawing pictures in the sand with my paw of what had happened.

I was afraid my pictures wouldn't be any good, but she told me it didn't matter what they looked like. As I drew, Hannah asked me lots of questions, and she listened very carefully to everything I said.

23

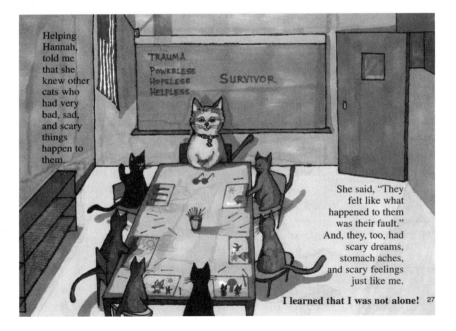

Helping Hannah, told me that she knew other cats who had very bad, sad, and scary things happen to them.

TRAUMA
POWERLESS
HOPELESS
HELPLESS
SURVIVOR

She said, "They felt like what happened to them was their fault." And, they, too, had scary dreams, stomach aches, and scary feelings just like me.

I learned that I was not alone! 27

FIGURE 8.1. Two pages from *Brave Bart* (Sheppard, 2001). Copyright 2001 by the National Institute for Trauma and Loss in Children. Reprinted by permission.

While some children relate well to human characters, animal characters are appealing and engaging to traumatized children, especially those who may be mistrustful of other children and adults. Children identify with the animal characters in this story, learn about therapy, and are encouraged to believe that they, too, can surmount the issues that confront them.

Trauma Symptom Management

Children can benefit from good books that help them learn to identify and express their feelings, and there are many outstanding books on this subject. *When Sophie Gets Angry—Really, Really Angry* (Bang, 1999) is the story of Sophie, who gets angry and breaks things. *Sometimes I'm Bombaloo* (Vail, 2002) tells the story of Katie who, when she gets angry, stops being Katie and turns into "Bombaloo." The book covers fighting with siblings, using time-out to calm down, and apologizing after becoming "Bombaloo." *Alexander and the Terrible, Horrible No Good, Very Bad Day* by Judith Viorst (1987) focuses on Alexander, who wishes he could move away from his problems after a series of things go wrong in his life. *Double Dip Feelings* (Cain, 2001) gives children permission to have more than one feeling at the same time. For children who have contradictory feelings about traumatic events or losses, this book is particularly helpful.

Children who are traumatized feel less isolated when learning others share their situation or problem. Author Inger Maier has written a valuable series of books that address common fears children face and include a positive outcome for the situation or circumstance the characters face. One of her books, *When Fuzzy Was Afraid of Losing His Mother* (2005), focuses on separation anxiety and encourages children to identify with Fuzzy and his dilemma. In this story, a mother sheep and her little lamb, Fuzzy, do not give up on problems but create solutions together. Fuzzy faces his fears by creating "pictures in his head" (p. 10) and repeating helpful phrases his mother told him, emphasizing a positive outcome and providing ideas for mastery. Children particularly enjoy creating puppet scenarios related to the story of Fuzzy and his mother.

To help children cope with nightmares, two excellent resources are *Jessica and the Wolf* (Lobby, 1990) and *Annie Stories* (Brett & Chess, 1988). *Jessica and the Wolf* is a story that demonstrates different methods of coping with bad dreams, including reworking a nightmare to give it a healthier, more positive ending. *Annie Stories* is a collection of stories on numerous topics in which the author actually provides footnotes for the caregiver. This helpful information explains the rationale for specific strategies that characters demonstrate through their actions.

Natural and Manmade Disasters

In the days after September 11, 2001, children, especially those most exposed to the terrorist attacks and those whose previous traumatic experiences increased their sense of vulnerability, craved experiences that provided comfort and familiarity. While books that address themes related to disaster can be important in work with children, simply providing well-known and well-loved stories that evoke positive memories is effective.

Edie Julik's *Sailing through the Storm* (1999) was useful in classrooms after 9/11. A sailboat on the water of life is "happily sailing along in calm, blue water. Suddenly there is a big boom. Someone has been hurt, and everything changes. Violence has happened to you, or to someone you know, or even someone you have never met" (p. 12). This interactive book serves as a springboard to initiate discussion and expressive activities. The metaphor of sailboats on the water of life is an empowering tool that offers a sense of hope. Speaking directly to children, the story captures a wide range of emotions, including feeling like your "little sailboat is going to sink" and moves in a positive direction, encouraging children to express those scary feelings. *Sailing through the Storm* affirms the power to make a difference and sail toward the ocean of peace.

September 12th We Knew Everything Would Be All Right, written and illustrated by first-grade students in Missouri (Byron Masterson School, 2002), was an excellent story for restoring feelings of normalcy to children. The book opens with, "On September 11, 2001, many bad things happened. September 12th was a new day. We knew everything would be all right because . . . " (p. 5). At this point in the story, children can create their own illustrations and stories about the importance of consistency, routines, and self-soothing activities. Children may be encouraged to use props or drawings to express how they "know everything will be all right." This particular book can be used in a multitude of situations, such as divorce, accident, or disaster.

Moving or Displacement

Children are subjected to moving for a variety of reasons, and moving to a new community, school, and home can be a stressful event, depending on the reasons for the move or displacement. In many situations, a parent's job change or military transfer is the reason; in other circumstances, the move may be associated with a disaster (fire, hurricane, or other natural or manmade disaster), divorce, or other changes. Recently, therapists witnessed mass displacement of families with children during the evacuation of New Orleans and the Gulf Coast region of the United States when Hurricane Katrina destroyed thousands of homes.

Shadow Moves (Sheppard, 2002) is one of the few children's books to address the trauma of moving, describing all the worries that preschool and school-age children typically have during and after a move to a new location. The main character, Shadow, gets help from a neighborhood friend who helps Shadow understand the fears that everyone has about a move, such as who will take care of her, who will play with her, and what it will be like at her new school. In particular, this book addresses making new friends and how to remain friends with previous acquaintances and neighbors.

The Storm (McGrath, 2006) is one of several books published on the topic of Hurricane Katrina. In this book, children share their stories, drawings, and paintings, providing honest reflections of what it was like to live through a powerful storm. Evacuation, displacement, and loss of property are just a few of the topics covered. The book ends with a theme of hope and recovery, reinforcing concepts of resilience and posttraumatic growth.

Relaxation and Stress Reduction

Because the management of trauma symptoms involves affect regulation, stress reduction and relaxation are important components in any trauma intervention. Fortunately, there are good children's books that therapists can use to help child clients learn to reduce anxiety and practice relaxation skills to self-regulate and decrease uncomfortable symptoms of distress and hyperarousal.

Cool Cats, Calm Kids (Williams, 1996) is a popular book on stress management and relaxation skills that children enjoy. There are nine examples of "cat-recommended" stress reduction techniques, such as

"Hold your head high," and "Hang in there." Children enjoy participating in the movement exercises illustrated throughout the book, and therapists can encourage young readers to come up with their own recommended stress reduction activities after reading the book.

Additionally, soothing audiotapes or CDs played at bedtime can help decrease anxiety and stress levels. Books like *Starbright, Moonbeam,* and *Earthlight* (Garth, 1991, 1993, 1997) provide calming imagery and affirmations for elementary school-age children. *Ready, Set, Relax* by Jeffrey Allen and Roger Klein (1996), a favorite of many play therapists and trauma specialists, is an outstanding tool with calming scripts for the active imagination. These are followed by specific activities and questions for discussion. The scripts, put to music, are available both in a CD and cassette format called *Ready, Set, Relax* (Allen & Klein, 1996) and are valuable for all ages.

BIBLIOTHERAPY, DEATH, AND BEREAVEMENT

Although developmental factors ultimately affect how children deal with the death of a significant person, it is important to acknowledge that all children handle loss differently. Some children cry, some may be anxious or angry, some are distracted, many will suppress feelings, and others may even laugh. Before reading any stories to children who are grieving, therapists can reassure them that there is no single way children cope with death or loss. Talk with children about any cultural or religious beliefs they may have and be sensitive in the use of stories that are culturally relevant or appropriate. It is generally advisable not to use books that contain euphemisms such as "passed away" or "fell asleep." Young children may confuse death with sleep or become afraid that they will die when they fall asleep at night. While the term "passed" is commonly used in the southeastern United States, it is not understood by children unless they have learned it as part of their cultural or community beliefs about death.

It is also important to query children and their caregivers about how the deceased died because the details may provide information important in choosing stories. Therapists should know the age of the children at the time of the loss, their relationship to those who died, how they died, and how children learned about the death. Knowing as much as possible in advance can help in selecting the best books for successful intervention based on developmental aspects, situational factors, and individual needs.

Death of a Family Member or Friend

Death, whether it is the loss of a relative or friend, is one of the most difficult and traumatic experiences for any child. Noting the importance of stories about death and loss, Bettelheim (1976) writes, "Modern stories written for young children mainly avoid existential problems, although they are critical for all of us. The child needs most particularly to be given suggestions in symbolic form about ways he may deal with these issues and grow safely into maturity. 'Safe' stories mention neither death nor aging, the limits of our existence, nor the wish for eternal life. The fairy tale, by contrast, confronts the child squarely with the basic human predicaments" (pp. 7–8). Fairytales do touch upon basic universal principles, including death, loneliness, isolation, and loss. A number of authors of contemporary children's books have also created stories to address these issues.

When Dinosaurs Die (Krasny & Brown, 1998) is a book that children of all ages will return to many times, but is an ideal book to share with children in the elementary grades when one of their classmates has experienced a death. Dinosaur characters express the common questions and concerns that children have regarding death. The story itself provides young people with some practical suggestions in answer to the question of what to do when someone dies or when someone's parent or family member dies. Different beliefs about death and loss are included in the story and are presented in a sensitive, non-threatening manner. Although it is geared to younger children, it can be used with older children and adolescents by saying, "I know this book looks like it is for younger children, but teens frequently mention how helpful it has been."

Mick Harte Was Here (Park, 1995) validates common feelings young people experience after a death and may help their peers empathize with them. The story is told from the point of view of a teen whose 12-year-old brother was killed in a bicycle accident.

I Know I Made It Happen (Blackburn, 1991) is a story about believing one is responsible when bad things occur. In this story, adults explain that bad things do not happen just because a child thinks or wishes them to, and children learn that it helps to share their feelings and to know that the death of a loved one is not their fault. A *Terrible Thing Happened* (Holmes, 2000) also helps children understand their feelings about death through the story of a raccoon named Sherman Smith. Sherman becomes afraid, angry, and disruptive at school until his teacher, Ms. Maple, helps him understand his feelings through play and drawing.

There are also books that therapists can use to help children prepare for the death of a parent or family member. *The Christmas Cactus* (Wrenn, 2001) describes how a granddaughter and grandmother come to terms with the grandmother's impending death around the holidays. As an expression of love, the child brings her grandmother a Christmas cactus as a gift. When the grandmother sees the plant, she explains to her granddaughter that the cactus waits all year for Christmas, the one time of year when it blooms, and shares that we all live and grow for a lifetime and, at the end of our lives, we "bloom." The message is one of transformation, not ending, and imparts an experience of positive remembrance during a holiday when memories of the deceased are often painful.

Finally, *Tear Soup: A Recipe for Healing after Loss* (Schweibert & DeKlyen, 1999) uses the metaphor of making soup to explain bereavement. This story is designed for older children and adolescents, but is also useful with adults and families because of its message. Grandy, the main character, has just suffered a loss and faces her suffering by making "tear soup," filling up a pot with her tears, memories, and wishes. In essence, she knows that making tear soup is uncomfortable, messy, takes longer than one expects, affirming the feelings and experiences that everyone encounters when they face loss. The strength of this book in intervention with children who have experienced the death of a family member or friend is in its honesty about emotions, particularly grief, anger, and confusion.

Death of a Pet

Corr (2004) notes that the most important message for therapists concerning a child's loss of a pet is to acknowledge the intimate relationship of the child and the pet. For many children, particularly those who have experienced abuse or neglect, the loss of a pet is a devastating experience and one that represents a significant emotional loss, especially if the pet has died suddenly and unexpectedly as in an accident. Books like *Tough Boris* (Fox, 1994) show children that even

Tough Boris, a fearless and scary pirate, has deep feelings when he cries over the death of his pet parrot. The purpose of his story is to give young readers permission to cry when a death occurs.

There are also many good activity books that address the death of a pet. *Saying Goodbye to Your Pet: Children Can Learn to Cope with Pet Loss* (Heegaard, 2001) provides pages on which to draw and helps 5- through 12-year-old children learn to express their feelings and cope with loss through experiential work. *They're Part of the Family: Barkley and Eve Talk to Children about Pet Loss* (Carney, 2001) is part of a series of activity and coloring books in which Barkley and Eve, two Portuguese water dogs, talk about death and related topics. It relates three brief stories: about a dog who developed an illness and was euthanized, a turtle who was found dead one morning, and a cat who was killed in an accident. This book helps children understand what it physically means when a pet dies and the importance of memories when feeling sad about a pet's death. Large pages encourage children to draw and, with the guidance of a therapist, this book can help children explore their experiences and feelings about a pet's death.

Coping with Death through Books and Creative Activities

While all books mentioned in this section can be adapted to creative use of art, drama, or play activities, some additional books are worth mentioning in this regard. *Sadako and the Thousand Paper Cranes* (Coerr, 1977) is about a memorial activity based on the death of a Japanese girl, Sadako, who died of leukemia in 1955, as a result of the atomic bombing of Hiroshima. The story explains the legend of the crane that was supposed to live for a thousand years and that good health is given to a person who folds 1,000 origami paper cranes. Sadako and her family begin to fold cranes, but Sadako dies before the project is completed and her classmates take over the task in her memory. Through this story, children learn a specific activity (origami cranes) to commemorate a loved one as well as how another culture remembers its deceased through a specific ritual for self-healing.

Someone Special Died (Prestine, 1993) and *Anna's Scrapbook: Journal of a Sister's Love* (Aiken, 2001) validate the memories of a person who has died through encouraging children to create a tangible record of the deceased. For example, *Anna's Scrapbook* reproduces a child's fictional diary, but also includes blank pages for readers to use as a scrapbook for writing and photographs. *Sweet Memories* (Stillwell, 1998) describes a series of projects such as scrapbooks, memory boxes, and other activities to help children and their families cope with death and preserve their memories of their loved one. In all cases, these books reinforce that creation of a ritual or object is important to the process of healing from a significant loss and empower both the child and therapist to engage in active coping as part of the recovery process.

WORKING WITH STORIES

Discussing stories offers children the opportunity to express their feelings about characters and reflect themselves in those characters. Like art expressions, toys, or puppets that can be used for their projective qualities, the situations and characters in carefully selected books can be capitalized on in much the same way, particularly with children who may not wish to talk about their feelings directly. Some questions that may help children explore a story and its characters include:

- Are you like any of the story's characters?
- Do any of the characters remind you of someone?
- Who would you like to be in the story?
- Is there anything you would like to change about the story?
- How would you change the characters, what happened, or how the story ended?
- What is your favorite part of the story?
- Did anything in the story ever happen to you?
- What do you think will happen to the characters in this story tomorrow, in a few weeks, or a year from now?

In general, in working with traumatized children therapists should encourage the free flow of associations and ideas, respecting all expressions equally and noting child clients' unique perspectives on stories' plots, resolution of conflicts, and thematic messages. Therapists can use children's responses to stories and story characters to discuss sensitive issues from a third-person point of view, providing psychological distance and helping bring emotional relief.

Finally, stories offer alternate solutions to problems that children may have not been able to imagine because of beliefs, worldviews, or events in their own lives. Children often become repetitive in their thinking and reactions, including how they tell stories about their experiences. Often, conflicts are left unresolved and children remain "stuck" with negative feelings, thoughts, and perceptions. Using specific books allows therapists to present children with new possibilities for endings to stories that have reinforced sadness, anxiety, fear, or hopelessness.

CONCLUSIONS

Webb (2002) observes that "although stories will not keep children from hurting, they may keep them from hurting for the wrong reasons, and from feeling strange and alone" (p. 328). While this chapter does not represent an exhaustive list of all literature that is useful to trauma intervention with children, it provides a valuable foundation for choosing books for therapeutic purposes. Overall, bibliotherapy can help children normalize trauma and loss and, in doing so, "restory" their lives through experiencing how others have faced adversity or loss. More important, therapists can capitalize on the use of books to help child clients learn that recovery is possible after traumatic events, imparting hope and anticipation for a brighter future.

REFERENCES

Aiken, S. (2001). *Anna's scrapbook: Journal of a sister's love*. Omaha, NE: Centering Corporation.

Allen, J., & Klein, R. (1996). *Ready, set, relax*. WI: Inner Coaching.

Bang, M. (1999). *When Sophie gets angry—Really, really angry*. New York: Blue Sky Press.

Berns, C. (2004). Bibliotherapy: Using books to help bereaved children. *Omega: Journal of Death and Dying, 48*(4), 321–336.

Bettelheim, B. (1976). *The uses of enchantment: The meaning and importance of fairy tales*. New York: Knopf.

Blackburn, L. (1991). *I know I made it happen*. Omaha, NE: Centering Corporation.

Brett, D., & Chess, S. (1988). *Annie stories*. New York: Workman Publishing.

Byron Masterson School. (2002). *September 12th we knew everything would be all right*. New York: Tangerine Press.

Cain, B. S. (2001). *Double dip feelings*. Washington, DC: Magination Press.

Carney, K. (2001). *They're part of the family: Barkley and Eve talk to children about pet loss*. Wethersfield, CT: Dragonfly Publishing.

Coerr, E. (1977). *Sadako and the thousand paper cranes*. New York: Putnam.

Corr, C. (2004). Pet-loss in death-related literature for children. *Omega: Journal of Death and Dying, 48*(4), 399–414.

Fox, M. (1994). *Tough Boris*. New York: Harcourt Brace.

Garth, M. (1991). *Starbright: Meditations for children*. San Francisco, CA: HarperCollins.

Garth, M. (1993). *Moonbeam: New meditations for children*. San Francisco, CA: HarperCollins.

Garth, M. (1997). *Earthlight: New meditations for children*. Sydney, Australia: HarperCollins.

Gladding, S. T., & Gladding, C. (1991). The ABC's of bibliotherapy for school counselors. *School Counselor, 39*(1), 7–13.

Heegaard, M. (2001). *Saying goodbye to your pet: Children can learn to cope with pet loss*. Minneapolis: Fairview Press.

Holmes, M. (2000). *A terrible thing happened*. Washington, DC: Magination Press.

Jackson, S. (2001). Using bibliotherapy with clients. *Individual Psychology, 57*, 289–298.

Julik, E. (1999). *Sailing through the storm: To the ocean of peace*. Lakeville, MN: Galde Press.

Krasny, L., & Brown, M. (1998). *When dinosaurs die*. New York: Little, Brown.

Lobby, T. (1990). *Jessica and the wolf: A story for children who have bad dreams*. Washington, DC: Magination Press.

Maier, I. (2005). *When Fuzzy was afraid of losing his mother*. Washington, DC: Magination Press.

Malchiodi, C. A. (2001). Editorial. *Trauma and Loss: Research and Intervention, 1*(2), 8–9.

McGrath, B. (2006). *The storm*. Watertown, MA: Charlesbridge.

Pardeck, J. A., & Pardeck, J. T. (1993). *Bibliotherapy: A clinical approach for helping children*. New York: Routledge.

Park, B. (1995). *Mick Harte was here*. New York: Random House.

Patterson, S., & Feldman, J. (1993). *No-no and the secret touch*. Fulton, MD: National Self-esteem Resources.

Pearson, I., & Merrill, M. (2007). *The adventures of a lady: The big storm*. Book Surge.

Prestine, J. (1993). *Someone special died*. Torrance, CA: Frank Schaeffer.

Rudman, K., Gagne, K., & Bernstein, J. (1993). *Books to help children cope with separation and loss: An annotated bibliography* (4th ed.). New Providence, NJ: R. R. Bowker.

Schweibert, P., & DeKlyen, C. (1999). *Tear soup*. Portland, OR: Griefwatch.

Sheppard, C. (2001). *Brave Bart*. Grosse Pointe Woods, MI: National Institute for Trauma and Loss in Children.

Sheppard, C. (2002). *Shadow moves: A story for families and children experiencing a difficult or traumatic move*. Grosse Pointe Woods, MI: National Institute for Trauma and Loss in Children.

Stillwell, E. (1998). *Sweet memories*. Omaha, NE: Centering Corporation.

Taylor, D. (1996). *The healing power of stories*. New York: Bantam Doubleday Dell.

Vail, R. (2002). *Sometimes I'm Bombaloo*. New York: Scholastic.

Vernon, A., & Clemente, R. (2005). *Assessment and intervention with children and adolescents: Developmental and multicultural approaches* (2nd ed.). Alexandria, VA: American Counseling Association.

Viorst, J. (1987). *Alexander and the terrible, horrible no good, very bad day*. New York: Aladdin Paperbacks.

Webb, N. B. (Ed.). (2002). *Helping bereaved children: A handbook for practitioners* (2nd ed.). New York: Guilford Press.

Williams, M. (1996). *Cool cats, calm kids: Relaxation and stress management for young people*. San Luis Obispo, CA: Impact.

Wrenn, E. (2001). *The Christmas cactus*. Omaha, NE: Centering Corporation.

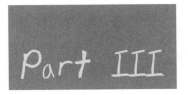

CREATIVE INTERVENTIONS
WITH FAMILIES AND GROUPS

Chapter 9

Creative Crisis Intervention Techniques with Children and Families

Lennis G. Echterling
Anne Stewart

Not far from our community is a cornfield that has been transformed into a maze, filled with dead ends, blind spots, and disorienting twists and turns. The cornfield maze is a wonderful metaphor for how children and families find their way through life's challenges, whether the challenges are anticipated developmental tasks, unexpected family changes, or natural or manmade disasters. In the cornfield, some children cling to their parents as they enter the maze, but most run ahead, exuberant and enthusiastic about this new adventure, skipping along, laughing, and shouting. When they reach a turning point or stray too far ahead, children typically return to the security of their parents. They grab an adult's hand, accompany him or her for a few steps, share impressions about their surroundings, wonder about possible options, and then rush headlong down the path once again. The children rely on their own problem-solving capacities and their caregiver's reassurance and guidance to playfully create a pathway through the maze.

    To gain an appreciation for the power of creativity and the resources you have to use in times of confusion and chaos, take a look

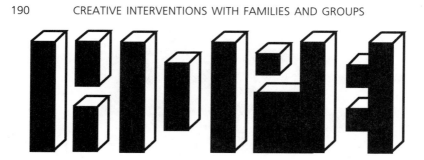

FIGURE 9.1. Create a vision of hope.

at Figure 9.1. At first glance, it may appear to be a maze like the corn-field, except this one doesn't seem to have any particular beginning or end—just a meaningless assortment of block-like shapes. Neverthe-less, your challenge is to find something meaningful here. You may feel the same sense of doubt and apprehension that you have when you look at one of those Magic Eye pictures and cannot see any hidden fig-ures, but as you explore the terrain of this puzzle, keep in mind that you can rely on your internalized base to find hope. As you may recall from your own experiences of creativity in times of chaos, you do not need to force the process. Instead, just relax and focus your eyes on one specific point in the figure. It doesn't matter where as long as you stay focused. By keeping your attention tuned into one spot for 20 or 30 seconds, something meaningful seems to pop out of the chaos—you create a unified vision of hope. If you didn't have much luck with that strategy, you can also gain some perspective by moving 4 or 5 feet away from the figure. What word appears?

CHALLENGES OF CREATIVE
CRISIS INTERVENTION

In other chapters in this volume, you have learned creative techniques that you can readily apply to your traditional therapeutic relationships with traumatized children. Typically, your counseling and therapy work takes place at appointed times, during regular working hours, for 50-minute sessions, in professional offices that provide a sense of safety and privacy, and with therapeutic tools that are not easily portable. You are surrounded by trappings such as diplomas, certificates, and books that speak to your legitimacy as a therapist. Moreover, you normally have the opportunity to complete a comprehensive assessment, develop a treatment plan, and establish therapeutic goals before you decide how you will apply these interventions.

In this chapter, we focus on crisis intervention, in which the circumstances are often dramatically different from the typical therapy session. "Crisis intervention" is any rapid, brief collaboration to assist someone in surviving and resolving a crisis (Echterling, Presbury, & McKee, 2005). The creative techniques we describe can be used in the immediate wake of a crisis event and under adverse conditions. In the midst of the chaos and confusion of a personal or community crisis, encounters with survivors are likely to be unscheduled and take place any time, day or night. They often occur in a nontraditional setting, such as a disaster assistance center, emergency room, or temporary shelter. Without any diplomas on the walls, the therapist must rely solely on actions to demonstrate his or her ability to help, and the intervention may last a couple of minutes or go on for several hours.

Wherever and whenever crises confront children and families, you nevertheless can offer creative interventions with materials you are able to take with you. The purpose of this chapter is to help you engage children and families in creative experiences that promote reaching out, making meaning, taking heart, and moving on to resolve their crisis. The techniques we describe require minimal materials, can be done with little or no special preparation, and can be implemented in virtually any setting, however primitive the conditions. The activities can take any form of creative expression—playing, drawing, singing, sculpting, dancing, or making music. Whatever the form, the active, potent ingredient in every technique is you.

Outside a temple compound in Sri Lanka, one of us (A.S.) conducted play-based activities with child survivors of the 2004 tsunami. Neither the children and families nor the therapists had any of their/ our familiar surroundings or tools. As the therapists entered the gated temple area, we were introduced to the caregivers and children and listened to the children perform songs about daily life and their hopes for the future. We then participated in play-based activities to enhance the children's ability to identify adaptive coping behaviors, to focus, and to regulate their emotions. We taught and sang songs about healthy coping with engaging gestures, including the sign language gestures for "I love you." A few days later we returned to the temple, where children came running to greet us, laughing, smiling, shouting our names, and signing "I love you." The intervention was unconventional, powerful, and genuine.

We believe that crisis intervention competencies are vital elements of effective mental health practice, but this does not mean that each practitioner should provide services in the midst of a disaster area. It is neither necessary nor advisable for all therapists to be on the scene of a crisis. Most therapists offer excellent services to traumatized children and families in more traditional settings and do not choose to work under primitive or unconventional conditions. As with all the services you provide, in times of crisis it is important to critically evaluate your knowledge, skills, and abilities as you determine your professional response. We recommend that you consult with colleagues and refer to your discipline's professional practice standards and code of ethics to inform your decision making. It is imperative that you do not compromise the well-being of your current clients, students, employer, or employees as you make your decision about how to respond. Of course, it is necessary to consider the impact of how you choose to respond on your family and other personal relationships. Last, carefully consider your tolerance for discomfort, ambiguity, distractions, and confusion. If you are willing to accommodate to these circumstances, then you may be a good match for providing interventions in the "ground zero" type of environment.

THE CONCEPT OF CRISIS

There is an important distinction between the concepts of trauma and crisis. "Trauma," which comes from the Greek word for wound, refers to a serious psychological injury that results from a threatening, terrifying, or horrifying experience. Psychological traumas can have a profound impact on a person's cognitive abilities, emotional reactivity, behavior, and even neural functioning (Le Doux, 1996; Perry, 2001). (For more information about child trauma and brain development, see the work of Bruce Perry at *childtraumaacademy.com*.) However, studies have found that resilience is much more common than was once believed (Ryff & Singer, 2003). For example, Kessler, Davis, and Kendler (1997) documented that the majority of children who experienced severe traumas, such as sexual assault or death of a parent, did not develop psychiatric disorders such as posttraumatic stress disorder (PTSD). In fact, many people report posttraumatic growth (PTG) (Tedeschi, Park, & Calhoun, 1998). Concepts such as trauma can be useful by calling attention to a particular phenomenon, but they may limit our focus and reduce our attention to supporting healthy striving if we rely only on trauma to provide our entire conceptual framework.

The concept of crisis provides a useful complement to that of trauma. "Crisis" comes from the Greek word for decision, and its Chinese symbol combines the figures for danger and opportunity. A crisis is a pivotal moment of decisive change that involves both peril and promise. Not everyone in crisis is dealing with trauma. For example, a refugee child facing the crisis of entering an American school is going through a major turning point in life that presents both dangers and opportunities; however, that child is not likely to be traumatized by this particular event. On the other hand, orphaned and homeless Sri Lankan children who managed to survive the tsunami were not only suffering trauma, but also facing a crisis. At this brief but crucial point in their lives, how they and their communities dealt with this traumatic event had far-reaching consequences, either positive or negative.

The purpose of crisis intervention is not to achieve a cure. Instead, it is to promote resilience by supporting the potential for hope and resolve that survivors possess. Because you intervene at such a crucial point in a child's life and a family's history, a seemingly small intervention can make a profound difference for years to come.

SYSTEMIC CONSIDERATIONS

In crisis work with children, you will want to keep in mind several important points regarding families. First, you may be intervening with an individual child, but the family is always present psychologically. Children bring along their families in their hearts and minds; family beliefs, expectations, voices, images, and histories are fixtures of a child's inner world. As a crisis intervener, you need to respect and build on this family context, especially when you are working with the child alone.

A second significant point is to recognize and appreciate the exciting and dramatic changes that are taking place in family constellations across the United States and throughout the world. In your work with children, you will encounter families that do not conform to the stereotyped and traditional models of the past. Same-sex partners, stepfamilies, single parents, blended families, and other forms are becoming more common. In fact, the conventional family of a married man and woman living together with their biological children is now the minority.

Third, families form a dynamic system. If one member is in crisis, then the entire system is likely to be in turmoil. Like individuals, family systems in crisis face both dangers and opportunities. If they fail to resolve a crisis, families may come away with a sense of alienation from one another, in a state of confusion and chaos, and on the verge of disintegration. If they cope successfully, families can emerge from crises feeling closer, having a greater sense of commitment to one another, and working more effectively as a system. The stakes for both individuals and systems are high.

Another important consideration is that families also function within the context of other systems. Your most important intervention may be to connect a family in crisis to those systems with the particular resources that can address their needs, such as social services, formal counseling and therapy, and financial support. Related to this consideration is the fact that these broader systems may also be in crisis. Violence, catastrophic accidents, natural disasters, and acts of terrorism can throw entire schools, churches, neighborhoods, communities, and societies into a state of crisis. You will need to design your creative interventions and, likely, broaden your ideas about your role with the child and family to accommodate these different conditions.

Finally, just as you take into consideration the developmental level of the child when you intervene, you also need to recognize the stage of the family's development in the family life cycle. As families grow and change, they negotiate many developmental tasks and face turning points (Kanel, 2003) that produce a range of emotions— anxiety, joy, heartbreak, compassion, and hope. Families rarely seek crisis intervention for such developmental crises as marriage, birth, and empty nest, and are more likely to contact you regarding specific situational crises that confront them. You will find it helpful to keep these broader developmental crises in mind as you work with families. These issues form the backdrop to the precipitating event and provide the context for exploring possible resolutions that lead to both personal and family growth.

BASIC PRINCIPLES

Before focusing on specific techniques, we want to mention several basic principles of effective crisis intervention. First, always intervene with LUV. The acronym LUV stands for Listen, Understand,

and Validate, the foundation of any successful helping relationship (Echterling et al., 2005). As you practice LUV and the other principles, we encourage you to reflect on your own theoretical orientation. Evaluate the degree to which these principles of crisis intervention are congruent with your understanding of the emotional life of children and families as well as your conceptualization of your role. When you offer LUV, you are actively *listening* to the child's verbal and nonverbal messages, communicating your empathic *understanding* of the child's thoughts and feelings, and *validating* unconditionally the child's innate worth. When someone does not feel heard, understood, and accepted, then your creative interventions, however elegant, can appear to be only scheming manipulations or, at best, meaningless gimmicks. You are not the expert with all the answers, the sage who dispenses advice in troubled times. Instead, by offering your supportive presence, you offer a safe space, a psychological refuge in this threatening storm. Fundamentally, an intervention takes place whenever a person in crisis is able to make contact with someone who cares. Your LUVing encounter with a child in crisis is the most powerful intervention of all.

Another basic principle of crisis intervention is to recognize and value the resilience of children and families—to presume that they are survivors, not pathetic and passive victims. When you encounter young people in crisis, you may feel tempted to be the knight in shining armor who rescues them from any emotional turmoil, but your job is more like the carpenter's assistant, helping children and their families to use the tools they may be overlooking as they begin to rebuild their lives. Of course, people in troubled times feel overwhelmed and distressed, but they also possess undiscovered strengths, overlooked talents, and unnoticed resources. As children and families begin to experience empowerment, recognize their untapped capabilities, and reconnect to sources of sustenance and nurturance, they build the scaffolding for a successful resolution to the crisis.

CREATIVE INTERVENTIONS

Children and families are more likely to be resilient when they reach out to others for support, make meaning of the crisis experience, take heart by managing their emotions, and move on by actively coping with these challenges (Echterling et al., 2005). Therefore, we have organized our recommended creative interventions according to these four essential processes that promote resilience and facilitate successful resolution.

I. Reaching Out

Especially in times of crisis, people are not islands. Research on social support has shown that relationships offer survivors many vitally important resources, such as affection, advice, affirmation, and practical assistance (Reis, Collins, & Berscheid, 2000). Although the experience of victimization can initially provoke a sense of isolation and alienation, survivors quickly turn to others (Berscheid, 2003). The purpose of these interventions is to help children and families connect with one another to find support, comfort, and nurturance as they embark on the journey toward resolution. An underlying, and often overlooked, assumption of these techniques is that children are also resources in times of crisis. Providing children with the opportunity to make a positive difference during troubled times can promote their own sense of resilience.

From My Heart to Your Heart

This group activity is a playful and quick way to connect children to others and promote a sense of community after a disaster. Begin by inviting the children to pair up. Demonstrate how you want them to encounter one another by acting out the words as you chant. You can begin this introductory activity by saying, "From my heart to your heart, I wish you well," while pointing to your own heart and then pointing to the heart of your partner. Then go on to other body parts, such as, "From my elbow to your elbow, I wish you well," while connecting to another person at the elbow. Respecting personal privacy, you can facilitate a playful encounter among participants by leading them through other connections—toe to toe, knee to knee, shoulder to shoulder, hand to hand, and ear to ear. In Sri Lanka after the tsunami, children found this welcoming activity an appealing way to connect with a team of international interveners. Because the activity relies on gestures to communicate, you can use it even if you do not speak the same language. (This activity is based on the song, "I Wish You Well," on the CD by Bailey and Hartman (2002) entitled *It Starts in the Heart*.)

Helping Hands

You can easily adapt this intervention to use with individuals, families, or even large groups. Briefly talk about how all of us need and offer helping hands to one another. Give each person a pencil and paper and invite them to draw the outline of one of their hands. In each finger, they then can make a drawing or write the name of a person, thing, or organization that has helped them through the crisis so far. The survivors can also make another helping hand to describe five ways that they have been a resource to others. If no materials are available, survivors can just show their hands and describe the help they have received from and given to each other.

This activity invites children to explore how they have been making a positive difference during this difficult and painful time. It encourages them to become conscious that they are playing an active role in contributing to the resolution of the crisis.

Rituals and Routines

Families and broader systems have many traditions that bring people together, affirm their collective identity, and celebrate their roots. As a crisis intervener, you can explore with children and families the customs that offer structure, meaning, and connectivity in their lives. You can then help them to be creative in designing new rituals and routines that preserve, as much as possible, these traditions while accommodating to new circumstances. These experiences—whether they are special occasions, such as birthdays and holidays, or daily routines, such as greetings in the morning and bedtime rituals—offer children and adults a sense of connectedness and normalcy.

For example, after Hurricane Katrina, school counselors in Pascagoula, Mississippi, implemented a communitywide project to help children and families reach out to one another at Halloween. The disaster had destroyed many homes, left dangerous debris scattered throughout the city, and made it impossible for many families to purchase costumes and candy for their children. To promote a sense of community, the high school students and other volunteers organized "Trunk or Treat." They arranged for children to receive donated costumes and publicized that families could bring their little trick-or-treaters to the community's high school parking lot, where more than 70 decorated cars had trunks of candy to disperse. Children and families were able to celebrate a traditional holiday, experience a sense of normalcy, and reach out to one another in a safe space.

Making Meaning

When children and families are in crisis, they are also experiencing a crisis of meaning (Janoff-Bulman, 1992). Using creative activities to tell their crisis stories offers them an opportunity to begin to give form to raw experience, gain some sense of cognitive mastery over the crisis, and make important discoveries about possible resolutions. Children tell their stories in a variety of ways—talking, playing, drawing, sculpting, singing, and writing—but whatever form their stories take, the process helps children create meaning from the destructive event that has taken place.

The themes that emerge from these stories eventually shape the storytellers' sense of personal identity and family legacy. In other words, the narratives that children and families create do more than organize their life experiences. They affirm fundamental beliefs, guide important decisions, and offer consolation and solace in times of tragedy (Neimeyer, 2000). Using the following creative activities, you can help children transform their crisis narratives into survival stories. In the process, you not only facilitate a successful resolution to a particular crisis, but also give them the opportunity to go on to thrive in their lives.

Art of Surviving

Children often become absorbed in using art to give form to their life experiences. When those life experiences are painful, frightening, or tragic, many spontaneously draw pictures of the crises they face and the ordeals they suffer. You can also invite children to give expression to their own resilience during these troubled times. Drawing pictures about their perseverance, resourcefulness, and creativity gives children an opportunity to recognize their strengths and contributions to the resolution process. They can also use drawings to portray the help that others gave them, the lessons they have learned from this experience, and the ways that they are stronger now that they have survived.

Children's art may take many forms. It could be a scene showing how they escaped danger, a depiction of something new that they have learned, a portrait of themselves as survivors, an illustration of how they helped others, or an example of how they overcame an obstacle. For example, when asked to draw a picture of a lesson that he had learned from coping with a flood to offer advice for other children who might be faced with a similar experience, a boy drew a rainbow over a river and wrote the caption, "You will be surprised what you can live through." You may invite them to design a poster showing what children could do to be better prepared for a disaster or what children could tell themselves as they face a crisis.

When you have a conversation with children about their art, you want to empathize with their victimization and be curious about their survival. In other words, acknowledge the crisis and ask questions to create opportunities for them to talk about their endurance, courage, compassion, joy, and hope. You can say, for example, "I notice that this boy and his mama are smiling at each other in your picture. How are they able to smile even though their house was destroyed?" Or you might wonder, "What is this girl feeling as she helps with cleaning up after the fire?" Such questions invite children to become more aware of the depth and richness of their own resilience.

Family Crisis Crest

This activity can be done with one child, a group of children, or an entire family. With individuals or groups, you can invite them to work alone to create their own family crisis crests. If you are working with a family, you can invite them all to collaborate in designing a single crest to share. See Figure 9.2 for an example of a blank template that you can use. One segment of the crest could be an animal that symbolizes family traits that have helped them through challenges. Another section could display a flower, tree, or plant that represents the family's roots and potential for growth. A third part could show a symbol, such as a mountain or threatening scene, that portrays the crisis event. Finally, the fourth portion of the crest could be a sign or symbol that expresses the family's hope for the future. Below the crest is a space for the family's motto, which should summarize one of the family's basic values.

Survival Diary

Many older children keep diaries or journals, finding satisfaction in the process of transforming their life experiences into words. In trou-

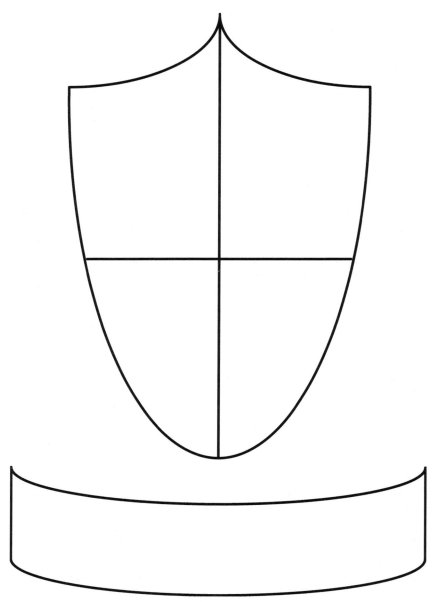

FIGURE 9.2. Template for family crisis crest.

bled times, you can invite children to give voice not only to their crisis narratives but also to their stories of survival. Instead of focusing on the details of the crisis event, you can encourage children to elaborate on how they have been facing these challenges, managing the many changes in their lives, and making sense of what is happening. The theme here is that children may have been victims of a crisis, but they are now survivors who have shown determination, courage, and compassion.

Through the child's disaster diary, you can hear the child's story, see the representations of the disaster, recognize its impact, and acknowledge the ways the child made it through this challenge. As with any encounter with someone in a crisis situation, you will want to leave the child on a positive note, feeling a greater sense of hope and resolve.

Playing to Strengths

Many children act out their crisis experiences and demonstrate their resilience through their play. Moreover, adult survivors find play to be a wonderful opportunity to experience their own vitality and to savor the joys of life in spite of the sorrows and hardships of tragic events. Through play, children and families recreate themselves by expressing their feelings, enhancing their self-esteem, gaining self-control, acting out possible resolutions, and reinvigorating themselves. Play is one of your most powerful crisis intervention tools.

Play offers several significant benefits. By supporting children's independent play and creating specialized play-based interventions, you can normalize reactions, invite children to try out new coping strategies, modify cognitive distortions, increase self-soothing, enrich relationships, enhance social support, and leave children and families with a sense of hope (National Child Traumatic Stress Network—Terrorism and Disaster, Branch, 2005). Although you typically will not have the luxury of a well-stocked play therapy room when you do crisis work, you can create a portable bag of toys and other materials for play-based intervention (Landreth, 2002). As you can see in Figure 9.3, you can assemble an impressive variety of materials to help people express themselves through different forms of art, engage in nurturing and family-life behaviors, play out fantasies, enact rescue operations, and vent feelings of aggression and destruction. Keep in mind that

EXPRESSIVE ARTS
    Crayons, colored pencils, markers
    Drawing and construction paper, scissors, pipe cleaners
    Balloons, bubbles, queen-size sheet

NURTURANCE AND HOME LIFE
    Baby bottle, cups, dishes
    Cardboard box dollhouse, furniture
    Doll family, including baby doll

FANTASY
    Magic wand
    Royalty- or magical-themed puppets or figures

RESCUE
    Telephone
    Emergency vehicles and workers, airplane
    Construction blocks
    Bandages, medical kit

DESTRUCTION AND AGGRESSION
    Popsicle sticks, egg cartons, or sheets of bubble wrap
    Nonrealistic plastic dart gun, rubber knife
    Toy soldiers and aggressive puppets

YOU !

FIGURE 9.3. Basic materials in a tote bag for creative crisis intervention.

although these toys can be a helpful aid in your creative crisis interventions, the most important tool is you. The fields of crisis intervention and play therapy are growing and changing rapidly, so you must make a commitment to obtain and maintain your skills through periodic education and training in order to effectively intervene with children and families.

Taking Heart

As a crisis intervener, your job is not to provoke emotional catharsis. Instead, you should help children regulate their emotions by reducing distress, soothing themselves when they are upset, enhancing feelings of resolve, and staying in the zone (Echterling et al., 2005). Successful athletes talk of being "in the zone" when they are performing at their best. At these times, they are energized yet focused, emotionally charged yet poised. Children and families are more likely to survive troubled times if they are in this ideal state of emotional arousal. The purpose of the following creative interventions is to help children and their families to take heart and manage their emotions productively.

Crisis is a time of intense emotions, but a common assumption is that individuals in crisis have only negative feelings, such as fear, shock, and grief. Recent research has demonstrated that they actually experience not only painful crisis reactions, but also feelings of resolve (Larsen, Hemenover, Norris, & Cacioppo, 2003). These feelings of resolve include courage, compassion, hope, peace, and joy. Acknowledging and giving expression to the gamut of emotions, both negative and positive, can promote a positive crisis resolution (Stein, Folkman, Trabasso, & Richards, 1997). In other research, Emmons, Colby, and Kaiser (1998) explored how some survivors were eventually able to transform their losses into gains. They found that, even during the crisis experience itself, these future thrivers were able to take pleasure in savoring the few desirable events that took place, appreciating discoveries that they had made and celebrating small victories. The following creative activities can help a child regulate emotions by reducing distress and enhancing feelings of resolve.

Sharing Your Worries

One way to help children regulate their emotions is to involve them in activities in which they use long, slow, deep breathing. For example, you can give balloons to children and other family members, ask them to imagine a worry or concern they would like to blow into the balloons, and have them allow the tension to flow into the expanding balloons as they slowly exhale. (You may need to inflate the balloon for young children.) This activity combines the relaxing process of deep breathing with the imagery of externalizing a concern. Once children and family members have inflated their balloons, they can play with them however they like, illustrating how they can share their worries and have fun along the way. They may want to toss them in the air, play catch with one another, or bounce the balloons.

If you are working with a group or family, you can add another creative activity that involves a sheet. Gather the participants around a sheet that you have spread on the floor. Invite them to place their balloons on the sheet, grasp the edge of the sheet, and lift it as a group in order to carry these worries together. The group may want to work together to guide all the balloons to the center or one of the corners of the sheet. They can collaborate to raise and lower the sheet while walking in a circle. They will enjoy shaking the sheet to toss their worry balloons into the air. At the end of the activity, some may decide to keep their balloons, exchange them with others, or even pop them.

Blowing Bubbles

Another breathing activity for emotional regulation can involve blowing bubbles, using commercial products, homemade materials, or even imaginary ones. You can begin by asking children what happens if they blow too hard when trying to blow bubbles. Then invite them to participate in the activity, either real or imagined, of softly, slowly, and gently blowing air to create bubbles. You may also want to encourage children to say one thing to themselves that helps them keep their hopes afloat as they prepare to blow bubbles.

Singing a Song of Resolve

Children love to sing, and one song you can offer them in times of crisis is a form of self-talk and reassurance that they can use later to regulate their emotions by themselves (Shelby & Bond, 2005). To the tune of "Twinkle, Twinkle, Little Star," you can lead children in the following song:

> I am safe and I am strong.
> Take a breath [take a deep breath and exhale] and sing this song.
> I am growing strong each day.
> Everything will be okay.
> I am safe and I am strong.
> Take a breath [take a deep breath and exhale] and sing this song.

When you sing the words "Take a breath," you can model slow, deep breathing for the children. You can also engage the children in acting out the other lines by making a muscle to show strength and giving a culturally appropriate sign for things being "okay."

Expressing Collective Resolve

Families and communities often spontaneously give expression to their collective resolve. These expressions may include tying yellow ribbons to trees, wearing bracelets, flying the flag, and building spontaneous shrines at the scene of a traumatic incident. Other examples include family activities, street performances, displaying survivors' drawings, painting murals, making posters, collecting survivors' stories, and participating in commemorations. Such public expressions can create a powerful synergy because their performance requires an audience. One of the classic symptoms of PTSD is a flashback, when some reminder triggers the traumatic experience. The power of these expressions of collective resolve is that they can become triggers for resolution to reconnect survivors to their experiences of success and triumph in coping with the crisis.

IV Moving On

Crises rob children and families of their dreams for the future at least temporarily. As a crisis intervener, you can use these activities to help them envision new possibilities by inviting them to create positive goals. Once articulated, goals serve as beacons that light the way for the journey to resolution. In this section, we describe creative activities that can help children and families begin the process of rebuilding their lives. Once they begin to see a future, survivors gain a sense of direction and hope, become more motivated, and increase their momentum toward resolution. Studies have found that people who strive to attain positive goals have higher levels of well-being than those who merely try to avoid negative goals (Emmons, 1999).

Keep in mind that even though children and their families may not have resolved a crisis, somehow they have successfully survived it. You can invite children and families to explore the achievements that they have already accomplished. By drawing attention to these instances of taking flight, dealing with challenges, and finding refuge, you can assist survivors in discovering unknown strengths, appreciating unrecognized resources, and achieving a sense of hope. These strengths and resources form the foundation for a successful resolution.

Out of the Ashes

Begin this activity by giving everyone a small piece of paper and a pencil. Invite them to name or draw the crisis event that they experienced. Then, in a safe container, burn the paper and mix the ashes into a piece of modeling clay. Invite the participants to think of one of the hopes they have for the future. Using what they have learned and discovered in dealing with their crisis so far, the participants can mold a symbol of hope from the ashes and the clay.

Growing Garden

The growing garden activity is a story you create about flowers that grow up to live in a lovely garden. One version of the story follows, but feel free to improvise.

> Tell the children to pretend to be tiny flower seeds under the soil [children curl up in a little ball with their legs tucked under them]. The sun warms the soil and the rain falls down on the seeds [tap your fingers on the children's heads and shoulders]. The seeds soak up the rainwater and begin to get bigger and bigger [children uncurl] and a stem begins to sprout [children raise one hand over their head and continue to uncurl]. The stem grows and grows and leaves appear on it [children slowly stand up and spread their arms for leaves]. Then a lovely blossom begins to bloom on the flower [children make big bright smiles]. A big storm comes, and the rain and wind come to the garden [children sway and bend]. The storm ends, the sun appears, and all the flowers admire the strong and beautiful flower friends in their neighborhood garden [children nod and smile at one another].

This activity highlights for children the resilience and adversity living things can withstand and the support friends and family provide.

Rebuild Your Village

This activity is particularly useful when there has been significant or widespread destruction in an area. First, acknowledge the disaster that has occurred and the loss of familiar homes, parks, schools, or neighborhoods. Share that you know many people are busy planning ways to rebuild and that you are interested in the children's ideas about how to rebuild. Children can create their village using objects from the immediate area (scan for safety) or by using blocks. A version of this activity can also be done with children and families who have lost their home, school, neighborhood, etc.

Hope Quilting Bee

This activity is like an old-fashioned quilting bee in which different members contribute their personal material, which the entire group then sews into a collective patchwork. You can use different colored construction paper, crayons, pencils, and tape to connect the pieces into a hope quilt. Begin the activity by inviting members to draw the things that give them hope in this troubled time. What are their hopes and dreams for the future? If they could look into a magic mirror that showed what they would look like, how they would feel, and what they would be doing 6 months from now, what would they see? What can emerge from this process is a complex and rich portrait of collective survival.

CONCLUSIONS

At the beginning of this chapter, we used the metaphor of a maze to discuss the dynamics of children and families in times of crisis. Exactly which turn survivors decide to take in troubled times is uncertain, but we can use play-based intervention to help them to find comfort, make meaning, take heart, and move on to follow the path that courage, hope, and compassion lead them down.

REFERENCES

Bailey, B. A., & Hartman, J. (2002). I wish you well. Loving Guidance website. See *It starts in the heart*, CD recording. Retrieved July 23, 2007, from *www.beckybailey.com*.

Berscheid, E. (2003). The human's greatest strength: Other humans. In L. G. Aspinwall & U. M. Staudinger (Eds.), *A psychology of human strengths: Fundamental questions and future directions for a positive psychology* (pp. 37–47). Washington, DC: American Psychological Association.

Echterling, L. G., Presbury, J., & McKee, J. E. (2005). *Crisis intervention: Promoting resilience and resolution in troubled times*. Upper Saddle River, NJ: Merrill/Prentice Hall.

Emmons, R. A. (1999). *The psychology of ultimate concerns: Motivation and spirituality in personality.* New York: Guilford Press.

Emmons, R. A., Colby, P. M., & Kaiser, H. A. (1998). When losses lead to gains: Personal goals and the recovery of meaning. In P. T. P. Wong & P. S. Fry (Eds.), *The human quest for meaning: A handbook of psychological research and clinical applications* (pp. 163–178). Mahwah, NJ: Erlbaum.

Janoff-Bulman, R. (1992). *Shattered assumptions: Towards a new psychology of trauma.* New York: Free Press.

Kanel, K. (2003). *A guide to crisis intervention* (2nd ed.). Pacific Grove, CA: Brooks/Cole.

Kessler, R. C., Davis, C. G., & Kendler, K. S. (1997). Childhood adversity and adult psychiatric disorder in the U.S. National Comorbidity Survey. *Psychological Medicine, 27,* 1101–1119.

Landreth, G. (2002). *Play therapy: The art of relationship* (2nd ed.). Muncie, IN: Accelerated Development.

Larsen, J. T., Hemenover, S. H., Norris, C. J., & Cacioppo, J. T. (2003). Turning adversity to advantage: On the virtues of the coactivation of positive and negative emotions. In L. G. Aspinwall & U. M. Staudinger (Eds.), *A psychology of human strengths: Fundamental questions and future directions for a positive psychology* (pp. 211–225). Washington, DC: American Psychological Association.

Le Doux, J. (1996). *The emotional brain: The mysterious underpinnings of emotional life.* New York: Simon & Schuster.

National Child Traumatic Stress Network—Terrorism and Disaster Branch. (2005). *Tips for helping school-age children.* Retrieved July 23, 2007, from *www.nctsnet.org/nctsn_assets/pdfs/pfa/TipsforHelpingSchool-AgeChildren.pdf.*

Neimeyer, R. A. (2000). Searching for the meaning of meaning: Grief therapy and the process of reconstruction. *Death Studies, 24,* 541–558.

Perry, B. D. (2001). *The neuroarcheology of childhood maltreatment: The neurodevelopmental costs of adverse childhood events.* In K. Franey, R. Geffner, & R. Falconer (Eds.), *The cost of maltreatment: Who pays? We all do* (pp. 15–37). San Diego, CA: Family Violence and Sexual Assault Institute.

Reis, H. T., Collins, W. A., & Berscheid, E. (2000). The relationship context of human behavior and development. *Psychological Bulletin, 126,* 844–872.

Ryff, C. D., & Singer, B. (2003). Flourishing under fire: Resilience as a prototype of challenged thriving. In C. L. M. Keyes & J. Haidt (Eds.), *Flourishing: Positive psychology and the life well-lived* (pp. 15–36). Washington, DC: American Psychological Association.

Shelby, J., & Bond, D. (2005, October). Using play-based interventions in Sri

Lanka. Association for Play Therapy Annual Conference, Nashville, TN.

Stein, N., Folkman, S., Trabasso, T., & Richards, T. A. (1997). Appraisal and goal processes as predictors of psychological well-being in bereaved caregivers. *Journal of Personality and Social Psychology, 72*, 872–884.

Tedeschi, R. G., Park, C. L., & Calhoun, L. G. (Eds.) (1998). *Posttraumatic growth: Positive changes in the aftermath of crisis.* Mahwah, NJ: Erlbaum.

RESOURCES

All Family Resources
www.familymanagement.com

All Family Resources is a comprehensive website that provides information and services to enrich families. The topics include aging, providing child care, communicating, parenting, and dealing with catastrophes.

Association for Play Therapy
www.a4pt.org

The mission of this interprofessional association is to promote the value of play, play therapy, and credentialed play therapists. The Association for Play Therapy works to advance the psychosocial development and mental health of all people by providing and supporting those programs, services, and related activities that promote the therapeutic value of play across the lifespan.

Creating Hope and Resolve in Troubled Times (CHARTT)
collegeprojects.cisat.jmu.edu/chartt

The CHARTT website describes a model of crisis intervention and offers mental health providers and survivors of disaster information about effective techniques for discovering strength, helping others, and building bonds that promote hope and resolve.

Federal Emergency Management Agency (FEMA)
www.fema.gov

The FEMA website contains education and training materials and modules for emergency personnel, teachers, clergy, and parents. See also FEMA for Kids at *www.fema.gov/kids*. This is a fun and interactive site for children to learn about disaster preparedness and response through stories, games, and activities.

National Child Traumatic Stress Network
www.nctsnet.org/nccts

The mission of the National Child Traumatic Stress Network is to raise the standard of care and improve access to services for traumatized children and their families and communities throughout the United States. The website offers a wide variety of resources for caregivers, teachers, and mental health providers.

National Institute of Child Health and Human Development
www.nichd.nih.gov/publications/pubs.cfm?from=

This site provides an activity book for African American families to use to help their children cope with crises.

National Institute of Mental Health (NIMH)—Helping Children and Adolescents Cope with Violence and Disasters
www.nimh.nih.gov/publicat/violence/cfm

This portion of the NIMH website describes the impact of violence and disasters on children and adolescents, with suggestions for minimizing long-term emotional harm.

Substance Abuse and Mental Health Services Administration (SAMHSA)
www.mentalhealth.samhsa.gov/dtac/default.asp

This site provides up-to-date information about disasters as well as a guide to "psychological first aid" in times of crisis.

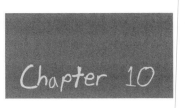

Chapter 10

Working Creatively with Children and Their Families after Trauma

The Storied Life

Ann Cattanach

THE STORIED LIFE

This chapter describes creative ways to support families with members who have experienced traumatic events. The approach is narrative, and the aim is to explore with the family a story about their lives encompassing the trauma as a part of their family history.

Most of my work is with families who have adopted children, enhancing the attachment process. This means integrating children's past experiences, some of which might include traumatic stress, into the family history and exploring new ways of being in a family, hopefully finding safety instead of harm. Some children who are adopted have been abused, while others have experienced the loss of caregivers.

When a tragedy envelops a family, they try to make sense of it. As time passes, the story shifts and moves in detail until some stories merge into the culture of the time and become folktales or folk memories to be shared with the community. An example of such a story is the Scottish tale of the "three times seven" sons of Morrison. Facts merge with magic to form some sort of consolation. An intolerable loss has threads of hope and is transformed into a story belonging to a family and a culture.

THE SEVEN SONS OF MORRISON IN COLD WINTERS WHEN THE ICE WAS THICK

It was a very long, cold, hard winter and all the lochs were frozen. It seemed that all the folk of Dalbeattie were skating on the ice or taking part in curling matches, sliding their curling stones along the ice.

There were three families of Morrisons, each with seven sons, all competing in the curling. They laughed and skated and whacked their curling stones all day long. The daylight faded, and all the Morrisons left the ice with their friends and began to walk back to their farms through the deep snow.

As they walked they heard the cries of curlers on the ice, and looking back towards the loch they saw crowds of fairy revelers playing on the ice. They were laughing and shouting as they slid their curling stones across the ice.

The Morrisons returned to the shore and watched. The fairies were having a wonderful time, playing and drinking, singing and sliding on the ice. They were all dressed in luminous green clothes. The fairy women began to dance as the men played their curling matches. All the three times seven sons of Morrison wanted to join in but were too frightened until one of them couldn't contain himself and sped off across the ice to join the fairy folk. All three sets of brothers joined the fairies on the ice, but their friends were too afraid or perhaps too prudent to join the fairy throng. They watched enviously from the shore.

Then suddenly, above the noise and the laughter, came the sound of a great crack, and from end to end of the loch the ice split open. In an instant the fairies had vanished and all 21 Morrison men plunged into the deep black waters of the loch. They were drowned in an instant in front of their friends watching from the shore.

And for many centuries travelers passing the loch near the midnight hour have seen the fairy dancers dressed in green and among them the three times seven sons of Morrison on steeds of milk-white foam. They gallop among their fairy folk with spears of sedge and swords of rush. Before the morning they are gone. No blade of grass crushed, no drop of dew disturbed as they gallop away.

The Morrisons' tragedy was made into a fiction in their community. The pain of losing 21 young men from the same family was too much to bear, so it became embedded in a fictional story that brought comfort to those left to experience the grief of so many young men drowned. The sons of Morrison are immortal, their tragic story told around the fire of a winter evening as a warning to others about the dangers of ice on the loch and an expression of loss when a whole generation of young men were lost to their community.

NARRATIVE THERAPY IN PLAY THERAPY

Narrative therapy can be used in play therapy as a way of helping children express and explore their experiences. Engel (1995) states that every story a child tells contributes to a self-portrait that he or she can look at, refer to, think about, and change and that this portrait can be used by others to develop an understanding of the storyteller. The stories we tell, whether they are about real or imagined events, convey our experience, our ideas, and a dimension of who we are.

White (2005) lists a series of concepts that describe his key ideas of narrative therapy. He states that the primary focus of a narrative approach is people's expressions of their experiences. The narrative expressions of both adults and children act as interpretations, and through these interpretations people give meaning to their experiences that seems sensible to themselves and to others. White concludes that meaning does not exist before the interpretation of experience.

White believes that expressions are constitutive of life; they structure experience and inform future understanding. Expressions have a cultural context and are informed by the knowledge and practices of life that are culturally determined. The structure of narrative provides the principal frame of intelligibility for people in their day-to-day lives. It is through this frame that people link the events of life in sequences that unfold through time according to specific themes.

The basis of narrative therapy when used in play therapy is to explore the stories children present in play and facilitate an exchange of ideas and thoughts about the stories. This approach means that the relationship between child and therapist is one of co-construction, sharing ideas and listening to each other to find the story that best supports the child in what he or she wants to say. The therapist's listening response is a continuous inquiry about the material presented in a play session. This developing narrative always presents the therapist with the next question. This is a "not knowing" position; the therapist's understanding is always developing.

When using narrative therapy in play therapy, the therapist and child construct together a relationship and a space where the child can develop a personal and social identity by finding stories to tell about him- or herself and the lived world of that self. The partnership agreement between child and therapist gives meaning to the play as it happens. The stories created in this playing space may not be "true" but often will be genuine and powerfully felt and expressed. Some of these stories can, with the child's permission, be shared with the child's caregivers to help bond their relationships. In his book *Into the Silent Land* (2003), Paul Broks, a neuropsychologist, suggests that we build a story of ourselves from the raw materials of language, memory, and experience. Hopefully, child, therapist, and caregivers can share the raw materials to encourage new patterns of positive growth.

SOCIAL CONSTRUCTIONIST STANCE

My work with children also uses themes developed in social construction theory. Burr and Butt (2000) state that postmodern thought proposes that we will never be able to penetrate "the real" with our imperfect perceptions and constructions, but we are naturally sense-making beings who interpret events and confer meanings upon things. They posit an objective world that is revealed to us through our senses. There is a split between the objective world and our subjective reality, and the world we experience is between subject and object. What we experience is both made and found. So we are limited both by events in the world and by our constructions of those events. We might describe this as the "lived " world. The perceived world is not a more or less perfect replica of objective reality; instead, we produce constructions that serve our purposes and help us in our projects.

This social constructionist view of the world is a hermeneutic approach. Hermeneutics is the activity of interpreting and explores how meaning is constructed through language discourse, story, and narrative. In this form of analysis, the world appears as we interpret it and the search for meaning is ongoing. Knowledge is a socially interpreted event constructed through relationships and conversation with others. Anderson and Goolishian (1992) state that a therapist working in a hermeneutic way lets the client's story unfold until a coherent theme or new meaning emerges from the dialogue. The therapist is curious to know more about what is being said—that is, how a client makes meaning that engages the future or "not-yet-said" narrative. Therapeutic conversation involves a mutual search for understanding in which the therapist and client talk "with" not "to" each other. This not-knowing hermeneutic stance means the therapist supports the child client in finding his or her own meaning in understanding his or her own problem.

TOYS AND STORYMAKING

When I work with a child, I define a space as the playing space. Very often, I use a blue mat, and the child and I sit together with toys on the mat. In the playing space, you can say what you want but not hit or hurt. Much of my work takes place in the children's home, so it is important to define the playing space and to make sure that the end of play is clear; once the mat is folded, we return to reality.

It is also important to carefully select toys to facilitate storytelling. I have a huge bag of "slime" and other messy materials and a bag of assorted figures including animals, aliens, and humans. The figures are made of a jelly-like substance and are easy to stretch. Many children make their first stories with the slime and figures, often depicting a scary, chaotic place. I also have a box of assorted small figures that facilitate storytelling—people, soldiers, dragons, witches, farm animals, wild animals, and the like. There are soft toys, dolls, and drawing and painting materials. The child chooses what toys he or she will use from one bag at a time, mostly. In this special space, using the toys and objects, the child and the therapist create a relationship and co-construct the play led by the child.

WORKING WITH FAMILIES
WITH ADOPTED TRAUMATIZED CHILDREN

Children who come to live in a family that wants to adopt them arrive with a story about themselves and their life. They might understand parents as violent abusing people who terrorize each other and hurt children. They might understand the role of the father as the man who comes to their room late at night to touch and tickle, which is nice but scary, or the role of the mother as someone who is so out of it on drugs that there is nothing to eat and the house is cold.

This baggage of hurt and trauma goes with the child to the new home, and the struggle is for the new family to understand and help the child trust enough to begin to find a place in the family. While the child might need a space to express his or her pain, it is important to work with the whole family if the appropriate attachment is to be made.

I make a contract with the family, usually to see the child for play therapy, then to meet the parents with the child to share issues and stories that might have emerged through the play. What is shared with the parents is negotiated with the child, and often the whole family plays around the stories that the child has used previously with me. I work with the narratives that are present in the relationship of the child and the caregivers and we explore helpful stories and unhelpful stories, what the family might want to change, and what they need to keep as their history develops together. When working with families who are seeking to find ways to attach to each other it is important for the therapist to facilitate this process by helping both parents and child to negotiate with and speak to each other about the meanings and understanding they have of family life.

Understanding the Experiences of the Adopted Child

The adoptive parents have a story about the life experiences of the child they wish to adopt. They are desperate to take away the pain and hurt of a traumatic past. One way to help parents/caregivers understand how their child might be feeling is to ask them to make up a story using the toys in the same way the child has played or perhaps to draw a picture on the same theme the child has drawn. Mimicking the story of Mary, one of my clients, by playing it as she had gave her caregivers insight into her mistrust and anger at the way adults behave when they are drinking. Here is Mary's story:

> Once upon a time there was a wicked witch and a wicked dragon.
> They lived together.
> They put the birdie in the cage.

They hurt the birdie and hit it.
They drank a lot.
They hurt the dog and the baby.
The wicked witch is dead.
Mary killed her.
She put the animals in the cage and shot the animals.
They are all dead.

Mary instructed her adoptive parents how to place the toys to act
out the story. She was in command. Her new parents felt her mistrust
as they narrated her story back to her using the toys and the environments she had made. Mary felt they had validated her experience and
was proud that they wanted to play it. After they shared this event,
Mary skipped out of the room, into the garden, and climbed onto the
swing; we could hear her singing as she flew higher and higher. Her
parents were saddened by their recreation of the story but understood
her perceptions of the world more. They also realized that, in playing,
Mary had relieved some of her burden, leaving her to enjoy singing
and swinging in the garden. She was beginning to trust her parents
with her history, which left her free to explore the world about her.

Another way of helping a family is to create new rituals together,
shifting the child's distrust of nurture and care. Simple attunement
play between caregivers and child, sharing stories, rhymes, jokes, and
riddles can bond the family together. We often play a game of choosing rhymes to go with new rituals, the family trying them out to see
which they like best. One rhyme perhaps describes how a child might
feel in a new home:

As I walked by myself
And talked to myself
Myself said unto me,
Look to thyself
Take care of thyself
For nobody cares for thee.

I answered myself
And said to myself
In the self-same repartee,
Look to thyself,
Or not to thyself
The self-same thing will be.

The family might also like nurture rhymes, such as:

Warm hand, warm,
The men have gone to plough.
If you want to warm your hands,
Warm your hands now.

Brush hair, brush,
The men have gone to plough.
If you want to brush your hair,
Brush your hair now.

Wash hands, wash,
The men have gone to plough.
If you want to wash your hands,
Wash your hands now.

It is easier to encourage a child to begin to care for him- or herself through a fun rhyme than through nagging. Skipping rhymes are skillful and with actions make great play. Making the actions can be inventive (How do you wriggle like jelly?) and can become a family mime.

Jelly on the plate
Jelly on the plate
Wiggle-waggle, wiggle-waggle
Jelly on the plate.

Sausage in the pan
Sausage in the pan
Turn it round, turn it round
Sausage in the pan.

Paper on the floor
Paper on the floor
Pick it up, pick it up
Paper on the floor.

Baby in the pram
Baby in the pram
Pull her out, pull her out
Baby in the pram.

Burglars in the house
Burglars in the house
Kick 'em out, kick 'em out
Burglars in the house.

There are many little rhymes and sayings that can become part of
family history. In Scotland, we have a snow rhyme:

The folk in the east
Are plucking their geese,
And sending their feathers
To our town.

We also have rhymes about soccer:

My old man's a scaffie [scavenger].
He wears a scaffie's hat.
He took me round the corner
To see a football match.

The ball was in the centre.
Then the whistle blew.
Skinny passed to Fatty
And down the wing he flew.

Fatty passed to Skinny.
Skinny passed it back.
Fatty took a dirty shot
And knocked the goalie flat.

Where was the goalie
When the ball was in the net?
Hanging to the floodlights
Wi' his trousers round his neck.

You might also use a toast to the family:

Here's to you and yours
And here's to me and mine
And if ever me and mine
Meets in wi' you and yours
Me and mine'll be as good

To you and yours
As you and yours
Has been to me and mine.

These rhymes and play are special rituals to show how a family can share affection and love and remind each other of the ties that bind. I remember my father repeating

Night, night, sleep tight.
Don't let the bugs bite.

to me before bedtime, and although he is long dead, I see his smiling face as I write.

OVERCOMING A SPECIFIC TRAUMA: PETER'S STORY

Some children may have experienced a specific trauma that has subsequently disturbed the family dynamic, and the therapist can explore with the child and caregivers how to shift some of the stress and find new ways of coping in the family. Peter was 6 years old when I met him. His parents were separated and, in a fit of anger and despair, his father had come to the house, taken Peter and his mother, and kept them hostage for 3 days. During that time he had assaulted Peter's mother and threatened both of them with a gun. He was subsequently arrested and was now in prison.

I saw Peter and his mother for the first time some weeks after the event because they were finding it difficult to cope with such a shocking incident. Peter's mother took out her anger on Peter, and he felt blamed and responsible for his father's behavior. He felt he should have rescued his mother and protected her from his father's violence. During my talks with Peter's mother when she felt angry with him, I told her the story of "The Missing Axe."

THE MISSING AXE

A man whose axe was missing suspected his neighbor's son.
The boy looked like a thief, walked like a thief, spoke like a thief.
But the man found his axe while digging in the valley,

And the next day he saw his neighbor's son.
The boy walked, looked, and spoke like any other child.

We began to talk about Peter as a small child threatened with a gun by his father and how she had felt trying to protect both Peter and herself. His mother started to think of him as he was—a small child, not an adult who should have protected her. Peter began to talk about the incident, and we were able to work out together what would have been possible in such circumstances and what would not have been possible due to Peter's father being bigger and stronger and holding a gun. Peter said that he had jumped on his father's back several times to try to stop him. He repeated this often, seeking confirmation that he had done his best. In play Peter evolved a story about Peter Pan and Captain Hook. I was Captain Hook, and he was Peter Pan. We both had swords and were fighting each other; although Captain Hook was bigger and stronger, Peter Pan was quicker and more agile and managed to outwit Captain Hook and win the fight.

We played this scene many times throughout our meetings, and as Captain Hook I admired Peter Pan's agility and ability to outwit me. This play was helpful to Peter because it fulfilled his wishes and gave him a sense of power and control that he had not experienced when his father was violent. He was able to think positively about what he had actually managed by jumping on his father's back and trying to stop his father from hurting his mother. He became reconciled to the idea that he had done what he could. It was only after playing this scene that Peter was able to describe what had really happened. Some children do not wish to talk about the real experience, but stay in the play they have made, where we co-construct solutions within the play.

I spoke with Peter's mother about his feelings of helplessness, and she began to think about what Peter had done and how frightening it must have been for him. She began to talk to Peter about his bravery in jumping on his father's back. They began to watch a video of Peter Pan together, and Peter told her our Peter Pan story. They began to play together, and she remembered the story of the three musketeers, whose motto was "One for all, and all for one." They played the two musketeers, and both mother and son felt more powerful as they played together, them against the world. Laughter returned to the house. The memories of violence still lurked in dark places and uncertain times, but the bond between mother and son remained strong, both accepting that they had done their best.

CONCLUSIONS

Reconstituted families or families that have experienced a trauma such as abuse or domestic violence need to find ways to incorporate past and present history to integrate together and bond with each other. It is helpful for adults to share through play and storytelling what it might feel like to be a new member of the family. Talking about the past with the child does not have the same emotional value as experiencing the child's play or storytelling. The child's story brings adults more directly into the child's world and can create bonds of attachment through mutual respect for their lived experiences.

Folktales and other stories are important in helping understand the universality of many experiences, even the harshest, and finding a story that mirrors certain aspects of one's life can be a consolation. I end with the story of "The Three Brothers," which describes one brother's traumatic loss of home and then his triumphant return. The return home is the dream of many refugees.

THE THREE BROTHERS

There were once three brothers who belonged to the Arapaho Indian tribe. They were all good hunters, but the youngest brother always had the best luck hunting. The older brothers became very jealous of him.

"Let us kill Little Eagle," said the eldest brother, "and then the other hunters will stop jeering at us." So Wild Bear, the eldest, and Red Horse, the middle brother, decided to take Little Eagle hunting and lose him in the forest so far away from home that he would not be able to find his way back.

When the tribe was out hunting the three brothers went off together as usual. The two wicked brothers pushed further and further into the forest, drawing Little Eagle away from the rest of the tribe. Suddenly, when Little Eagle was examining some animal tracks, the two wicked brothers attacked him from behind, and he fell senseless to the ground. As they were about to kill him, they heard the cries of the other hunters, and they hurried off in that direction to make it appear that nothing had happened. They told the rest of the tribe that Little Eagle had gone off to track a wonderful animal and would rejoin them later.

Little Eagle lay in the bushes all night because his brothers had given him such a terrible beating.

One of the Enchanted Beings who guide the affairs of men found him and brought him back to consciousness. But he was still badly injured and could not see, so the Enchanted Being guided him to the tents of some friendly Indians.

These Indians were blood brothers of the Arapaho, and he spent many months with them. His wounds healed, but he still did not remember what had happened. He did not know his name or who he was. So he stayed with his new friends and was accepted by the old chief, who felt sorry for him.

Little Eagle became known as Two Persons to represent the man he had been and forgotten and the man he was now.

In time, Two Persons became a great hunter and was admired by the young men of his adopted tribe. They were not jealous, as his brothers had been.

Sometimes Two Persons wondered who he was. He knew he was an Arapaho because of the way the beads were sewn on his shirt, his leggings, and the small pouch he wore on his belt.

The chief had a daughter called Blue Stone. She fell in love with Two Persons, but she knew that it was impossible for him to ask her hand in marriage because he was a nameless man with no tent of his own.

Two Persons brought food for the tribe and could eat with the men with no shame, but, although he loved Blue Stone, he felt powerless to approach her.

One night the Enchanted Being came to him in a dream and told him of his past. He told him his name and where he was born and what his brothers had done to him. He said it was time for Little Eagle to return to his tribe but first he must ask for the hand of Blue Stone and take her back with him as his wife. He said that his brothers no longer wanted to kill him. The Enchanted Being gave Little Eagle instructions for the journey.

The next day Little Eagle went to the old chief and told him the whole story. He asked for Blue Stone to be his wife if she were willing. The chief knew his daughter's mind and agreed. So Little Eagle took Blue Stone's hand, and they went to collect a few herbs as the Enchanted Being had instructed in the dream.

Little Eagle's home was far away, and the journey took a long time. When they got to the place where he had been born, they found that the people in his tribe were stricken by a mysterious illness. It was called the spotted sickness and was, in fact, smallpox brought by some of the first white men to come to their land.

Little Eagle and his wife knew what they must do. They boiled the herbs they had brought and made an infusion that they gave to the sick. Some lived and some died, but the medicine helped many to recover.

Little Eagle's two brothers, Wild Bear and Red Horse, were changed in their appearance by the smallpox, but the medicine helped save their lives.

The brothers begged Little Eagle to forgive them for their cruelty to him in the past. They knew he had saved their lives with the medicine he had brought.

Little Eagle forgave them, and when they were well and strong again they went out hunting together. The two brothers rejoiced that Little Eagle was alive and that they had not killed him.

The Enchanted Being looked after Little Eagle and preserved his life so he became a great hunter honored by the tribe and loved forever by his wife Blue Stone.

REFERENCES

Anderson, H., & Goolishian, H. (1992). The client is the expert: A not-knowing approach to therapy. In S. McNamee & K. J. Gergen (Eds.), *Therapy as social construction* (pp. 25–39). London: Sage.

Broks, P. (2003) *Into the silent land*. London: Atlantic Books.

Burr, V., & Butt, T. (2000). Psychological distress and postmodern thought. In D. Fee (Ed.), *Pathology and the postmodern* (pp. 186–206). London: Sage.

Engel, S. (1995). *The stories children tell*. New York: Freeman.

White, M. (2005). *An outline of narrative therapy*. Available at *www.massey.ac.nz*.

White, M., & Epston, D. (1990). *Narrative means to therapeutic ends*. New York: Norton.

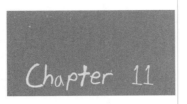

Vanquishing Monsters

Drama Therapy for Treating
Childhood Trauma in the Group Setting

Craig Haen

What drew me to the story and what I wanted to show people,
is that even in the midst of trauma, children play.
—MAURICE SENDAK (cited in Fosha, 2001)

My first internship during my clinical training as a drama therapist was
spent working with adult clients in a day-treatment setting. When I
initially sat in on group therapy sessions, I found myself amazed at the
frequency with which clients spoke about their painful childhood
memories. The memories of traumatic events seemed to have a particularly tenacious grasp on these adults, locking them into their pasts as
they continually tried to rework the experiences. Indeed, recent
research speaks to the tremendous power trauma wields over the
human psyche—resistant to intervention and slow to fade, rendering
it a truly pernicious disease of the mind (Bonne, Neumeister, &
Charney, 2003; van der Kolk, 2002, 2003a). Research also suggests
that some of the greatest hope for improving the quality of life for
young people who have been traumatized lies in the early implementation of trauma-specific treatment during childhood (Perry, 2006; Silva

et al., 2003). Therapists who work with this population are continuously charged with the difficult tasks of engaging and building trust with clients whose ability to connect with an adult and to process what has happened to them is often compromised.

Drama therapy is a creative arts therapy modality that integrates role play, stories, improvisation, and other techniques derived from theatrical performance with the theories and methodology of psychotherapy. The result is an embodied, experiential process that draws on the client's capacity for play, utilizing it as a core route for accessing and expressing internal conflict, achieving insight, rehearsing alternative choices, and cognitively reworking habitual patterns of response to stressful situations. In essence, drama therapy works with and through the client's imagination, making it an advantageous process for therapists who treat traumatized children. In van der Kolk's (2005) words, trauma is "a failure of the imagination" in which the past overtakes the present and the client becomes plagued by his or her own internal imagery, unable to foresee other possibilities for him- or herself. As Bloom (2005) wrote, "It is this ability to create possibility, to envision alternative universes, that must be unfrozen if an ill child is to re-enter the stream of life" (p. xvi).

In a previous article (Haen, 2005b), I described a game that spontaneously developed during my work with young children who lost parents in the terrorist attacks on the World Trade Center. In this game, one child pretended to be a monster and chased the other group members around the room. Upon catching them, he would attack them in the most grotesque fashion, gnawing at their limbs and eating their body parts. This game seemed a clear metaphorical representation of the traumatic deaths of their parents, whose bodies had been similarly torn to pieces. Eventually, the group members were able to work with me to develop a safe space under a table where the monster was not welcome. In this space, they were able to discuss the things that made them feel safe in real life. After they had sufficiently connected with one other and internalized the safe space, they went back out to face the monster. Together, they vanquished him, taking control of the game and experiencing a collective sense of accomplishment.

This clinical vignette provides an illustrative example of the drama therapy process with traumatized children. The first stage of this process involves externalization, in which the trauma itself is projected, separated from the client, so that it can be viewed from a safe distance. During this externalization process, some children feel the need to embody the perpetrator/traumatizing agent, as did some of the group members who chose to play the role of the monster. In the second stage, a psychological safe space is built within the group, either obliquely through the group process or more tangibly, as we did in this game, concretizing the metaphor through the creation of an actual secure base in the room. In the third stage, connection, the members begin to join together as a working group, finding strength, validation, and purpose. Finally, the monster is vanquished. Group members find ways to gain mastery over their traumatic material, to combat and contain it. In defining these stages, I am not articulating a progressive model, as each of these stages may evolve at any point in the process and groups may return to them time and again, as children's recovery is often cyclical. Indeed, in the aforementioned group, a great deal of work was done on creating safety before the members felt ready to invite a monster into their play.

In this chapter, I illustrate how drama therapy processes can be used for externalization and containment of trauma material, as well as for the purposes of creating safety and building connection in the group therapy medium. Group therapy has a long history in the treatment of children and holds a particular place in trauma treatment as the group setting helps combat some of the isolation that is created as a result of exposure to trauma (Nader, 2004). It is important for readers to understand that these techniques are not provided for application in a cookbook fashion. Rather, they are presented as additional tools on which a group leader can draw. The most resonant interventions are those that reflect the therapist's attuned response to clients' needs and that emerge naturally from the group process (Nash & Haen, 2005).

ON THE EFFICACY
OF DRAMA THERAPY INTERVENTION

Coalescing largely in the 1960s and 1970s, drama therapy is a relatively young discipline when compared to some of its counterparts in the mental health field. As Landy (2003) articulated, there are far more practitioners in drama therapy than there are researchers. The vast majority of research in the field is qualitative in nature, providing case studies, theoretical advances, and assessment tools. In the area of trauma, there have been a handful of quantitative studies of drama therapy in the treatment of adults. These studies (Johnson, Lubin, James, & Hale, 1997; McKenna & Haste, 1999) show preliminary evidence for greater efficacy of trauma treatment when drama therapy is utilized as part of the treatment framework than when there is no creative arts therapy used. A careful reading of recent research advances in the fields of traumatology, developmental psychology, neurobiology, and attachment studies provides strong support for drama therapy as a treatment method for traumatized children. The findings of studies from these parallel fields illuminate treatment goals that drama therapy is uniquely suited to achieving, making it a promising practice in the realm of trauma treatment.

GROUP TREATMENT OF TRAUMATIZED CHILDREN: A SERIES OF RETURNS

Galatzer-Levy (1991), in writing about therapy with adolescents, stated, "The central goal of adolescent psychotherapy is to renew the adolescent's capacity to grow and develop. Health is the ability to engage in further development, not a state from which symptoms are absent. When treatment goes well, however, youngsters take away even more than the resumption of development. They learn something of how to approach and rectify situations that cause them difficulty later on" (p. 86). Galatzer-Levy's perspective is readily applicable to trauma treatment with children. Trauma has the effect of freezing young people in their psychological, social, and biological growth (Haen, 2005b). Therapy, particularly in the initial stages, must help return children to their normal developmental pathways. As the effects of trauma are multifaceted, treatment usually involves a series of returns.

A Return to Safety

One of the great paradoxes of trauma treatment is that the therapist is working with clients to face emotions and thoughts related to the very events that have caused them harm and from which their bodies and minds are working to protect them (Hegeman & Wohl, 2000). Children's exposure to trauma can rupture their notions of safety at a time when they often lack the developmental capacity to verbalize cohesively what has happened to them or how they feel about it (Haen, 2007). Even when traumatized children are able to put their experiences into words, the feelings of hyperarousal and internal dys- regulation that result from the physiological imprints of trauma can render the treatment experience a failure. While children may gain insight and develop a narrative that organizes the experience, their internal reactions continue to leave them feeling unsafe (Perry, 2006; van der Kolk, 2003a).

Research points to the need for clients to be able to establish psy- chological distance from the affectively charged trauma material so that an internal sense of safety can be achieved. In van der Kolk's (2003b) words, "To help traumatized individuals process their trau- matic memories, it is critical that they gain enough distance from their sensory imprints and trauma-related emotions so that they can observe and analyze these sensations and emotions without becoming hyper- aroused or engaging in avoidance maneuvers" (p. 187).

Drama therapists, whether they treat traumatized children or not, regularly utilize distance as a central concept. By working through metaphor, story, and role, the client is able to address a problem from a place that is safely removed from reality. From a position of sufficient distance, the traumatized child can process information cognitively and view the situation more clearly (Kellermann, 2000; Landy, 2003; Lindahl, 2002). As the child internalizes the therapist's interventions, she learns to negotiate distance for herself, gradually responding to her internal distress in a self-protective yet active way. Casson (2004) articulates this process: "This play with distance creates the space between therapist and client: space for the growth and expansion of the self. Such play enables us to discover that we can feel, think, move, achieve control, let go of control, choose, negotiate, change, lose and find self and other" (p. 125).

Providing distance opens the door for trust to develop. When children begin to trust the therapist and the group, they can step into a process that requires taking emotional and psychological risks that are often in opposition to the internal, self-protective barriers they have established (Pitruzzella, 2004). In new groups of young children, I frequently bring in a stuffed animal, usually a dog, who functions as my veritable co-therapist. As a warm-up, the kids pass the dog around and tell him how they are feeling or what they would like to talk about that day. By introducing this small piece of projective work, the inten- sity of being in the group and talking to a therapist is lessened.

Distance is also achieved through the method used in creating characters. For example, I always have children who are engaging in dramatic play create characters with names other than their own or those of anyone in the group, so that these characters can function as separate from the actors. Defining the boundaries of the dramatic space also helps establish distance. The "stage" can be physically marked in the performance space through the use of furniture, tape, a circle of participants, and so on. The process of entering into a scene is also important in distancing the action from reality. I often use the device of having the group collectively shout, "One, Two, Three, Action!" to serve as a catalyst for the scene to begin.

Trauma practitioners regularly talk about developing a safe space in treatment, a mental image that clients can return to when they begin to experience distress in therapy or in life. Rothschild (2000) refers to this imagined safe space as an anchor. The notion of a safe space harkens back to childhood attachment, in which safety is learned through the experience of dyadic regulation with a trusted caregiver (Meares, 2005; Siegel, 2003). In the caregiver–child relationship, safety is communicated largely through visual and sensory aspects of interaction—breath, touch, soothing sounds, facial expressions, singing, and prosody—leading to a felt sense of security that the child can summon when distressed (Holmes, 2001). Similarly, the building of a safe space in drama therapy can be actualized in the creation of that space in the room, allowing the client not only to verbalize what it is like, but also to feel it in reality (Burmeister, 2000; Mulkey, 2004). In Pitruzzella's (2004) words, "Dramatic work is, to a greater extent, an establishment of boundaries" (p. 141).

During group sessions, particularly when it appears that the group members are becoming dysregulated, I often ask the children to find a space in the room. Once there, I ask them to imagine themselves in a place that feels safe and to create a pose of themselves in that place. One by one, I tap them and allow them to show and talk about what they are doing in that space, what it looks like there, and how it is similar to and different from the space of the group.

A lasting sense of safety is one that is sustained over time through treatment experiences in which the child is able to summon trauma memories while simultaneously engaging in newly generated experiences of groundedness, trust, and self-efficacy (Carbonell & Parteleno-Barehmi, 1999). The result of this pairing is that the trauma memory gradually becomes associated neurologically with greater degrees of calm and internal regulation (Perry, 2006; Siegel, 2003). Van der Kolk (2005) asserts that theater is adept at providing this pairing for children because, by engaging in stances of power, freedom, and safety, they gain "the physical experience of how things can be different."

In groups with older children from traumatized families, I often invite one member to create a "family portrait," casting other group members in a bodily sculpture that represents how the portrait maker perceives things to be in his family. I then ask the group member to step in for himself in the picture and to speak about how it feels to be in the picture. Next, I ask him to step out of the picture and to make adjustments to it to show how he wishes it would look. He then steps back into the picture to talk about how it feels to be in the revised version of the family. This activity can be adapted for younger children or group members who need greater distance by asking them to create a fictional family in which there are problems or a family of animals, wizards, or any other fantasy characters. In addition to providing the impetus to voice desires for change, the family portrait allows the child to experience these differences and highlights the internal sensations that develop as a result. In addition, it allows him to step out of character and view the scene from a safe cognitive place. This facilitated movement between experience and reflection is often cited as a reason that "bottom-up" treatments like eye movement desensitization and reprocessing (EMDR) are demonstrating efficacy for traumatized clients (Shapiro, 2001).

Finally, by working with children's imaginations, drama therapists can help them learn to regulate their fantasies. There are many drama therapy rituals for containment that can assist in teaching mastery over trauma material. Among the ones I use most frequently with children are the magic box (Johnson, 1986) and the magic shop (Emunah, 1994). In the former, a magic box is brought down from the ceiling, and the group members take turns putting something from their lives that they would like to get rid of in the box, where it can be safely kept. The box is then packed away through closing and locking the lid and other group efforts. In the latter example, the group members bring something frightening from their lives into a magic shop, where they trade it in for something they need.

The second exercise works with the idea of transformation, which usually resonates with traumatized children. The group can be accessed to transform overwhelming, violent images into safe ones (Haen, 2005a; Haen & Brannon, 2002). The children might be asked to wave a magic wand to turn a monster into a mouse. They might be taught to use an imaginary remote control to change the channel on a violent show to another show that is fit for family viewing. Like Mulkey (2004), I have sometimes engaged groups in which members have been abused in pushing their perpetrator out of the room or in building a jail to contain scary memories while they are in the group session. These rehearsed pieces of mastery can be extended outside of the group setting into learning how to alter intrusive thoughts, nightmares, and other internally generated imagery.

A Return to the Body

Trauma is also a highly biological phenomenon with enduring effects on the body (Bonne et al., 2003; De Bellis, 2001; De Bellis et al., 1999; van der Kolk, 2002, 2003a). When trauma happens to young people, it occurs at a time of rapid growth and development. The collision of these two powerful forces often results in the child's discomfort being present in the body and being aware of bodily sensations (Young, 1992). During my time spent working on a children's psychiatric unit, I encountered many traumatized children who went into hiding in their own bodies or waged war against them: sexually abused girls who attempted to disguise their developing feminine features; recipients of physical abuse who disengaged from physical activities and resisted any kind of touch or sensory stimulation; witnesses of traumatic deaths who stopped eating so that they would not grow up; and abused and neglected children who engaged in self-harm.

Creative arts therapists have long appreciated the importance of engaging the body in the therapy process. Indeed, all of the creative arts therapies involve some degree of kinesis and bodily rhythm (Malchiodi, 2003). Drama therapy works with degrees of embodiment, from the small, controlled movement involved in manipulating miniature toys or projective objects to the partial embodiment of taking on a role utilizing a puppet to the more intimate, less distanced experiences of full-body role play, sculpting, and mask work (Haen, 2007). In addition to increasing the child's comfort with embodiment, engagement in drama therapy in a group setting can help gradually sensitize children to the experience of being looked at, a particular trigger for children who have endured abuse or bodily injury.

Often, simple drama games can begin this process. Because these games are fun, many children readily engage despite their fears. One game in particular that I have used to get children and adolescents warmed up to the drama therapy process is Exploding Red Light, Green Light. This game is played similarly to the children's game red light, green light, in which players must attempt to be the first to reach the leader, who calls out "green light" to indicate when players can start moving and "red light" when they must stop. When the leader catches a child moving after she has called out "red light," she says that child's name and that child must return to the starting line. In this version of the game, while returning to the line, the child is asked to "explode." Many versions of explosions are celebrated, from uttering the words "Boom!" or "Kapow!" to letting out a noise of frustration to yelling at or challenging the leader. This simple game introduces group members to the concept of freezing and self-control, as well as to the idea of expressing emotion through sound and movement. When the leader encourages explosions directed toward herself, she gives permission and a context for the expression of anger and resistance in a contained structure. By engaging in this game, children are being brought safely into their bodies.

Sculptures have endless applications and are easy introductions to role play, as well as to being in the body. I have asked group members to physically take on brief, individual poses that reflect different feelings and situations. I have also asked groups to create sculptures together to reflect pertinent themes. One group of preadolescents would begin each drama therapy session by casting group members to create a picture from their day, from which full scenes would later be built. In another group that took place in a school, the members engaged in a game called Wax Museum in which they created a series of thematically similar sculptures for another group member to walk through as though visiting a wax museum. Like Exploding Red Light, Green Light, some of the focus of the game is on the participants moving when the person walking around is not looking. In this group, the game was used repeatedly and became a format for gradual exposure to material related to the violent death of a fellow student that had recently occurred. With repeated sessions, the group members created wax museums related to the themes of death, reporters, suicide, mental hospitals, rage, protection, and heaven.

Drama games such as these not only return children to their bodies, but also integrate kinesthetic experience with verbal and iconic learning. Drama builds the children's sense of competency by once again internalizing the locus of control (Macy, Macy, Gross, & Brighton, 2003). Role-play activities also provide a natural lead-in to teaching body-based self-regulation skills such as deep breathing, use of guided imagery, grounding oneself in the environment, and deep pressure/release self-touch, which can become easily incorporated into de-roling from dramatic scenes or closing rituals of the group session.

A Return to Connection

Although the drama therapy field is a young one, it is rooted in the ancient tradition of the theater, which dates back to early ancient Greece. Since its beginnings, the theater has been an art form based on community, in which people of all classes and backgrounds would gather to see life reflected on the stage. Some of the earliest recorded plays were tragedies, with traumatic events of grief, loss, murder, violence, and war an integral part of their narratives. Drama therapy is a natural extension of the Ancient Greek theater, drawing upon the power of representation, identification, and shared experience in connecting people.

For children who have been traumatized, this connection to a support network is essential (Pine & Cohen, 2002). Drama therapy targets the most basic components of connection: mirroring, validation, empathy, and universality. Macy and colleagues (2003) articulate the process in this way: "When a child moves to music, he experiences connection; when that same child moves to music and experiences peers mirroring that movement, affiliation is experienced; when vocalization accompanies the shared movement, integration may begin" (pp. 65–66).

Mirror exercises, in which one group member mirrors the movements and sounds of a partner or in which the group serves as a collective mirror for the expression of an individual, are powerful ways to forge that connection to others. There are many variations of mirror exercises that include having two children work together, each trying out being the leader and then the follower. In the warm-up to a group, I will sometimes have group members pass a movement around a circle. There are two components to this process: first, each member mirrors the movement that the child next to him has demonstrated; then he transforms that movement into a movement that is his own and passes it to the person next to him. As the movement goes around the circle, the group can witness the ways in which each person transforms it. As a facilitator, I often work with group members to be accurate mirrors of what they are to reflect, helping them to notice subtleties of expression and to accurately represent them, honoring the contribution of their fellow group members.

Objects can be used in the group to solidify connection. The passing of a ball or a toy from member to member not only engages the group members, but also makes the process of sharing focus tangible. I will verbalize this process by saying, "Throw the ball to someone you'd like to check in with," or "Pass the bear to someone who you think understands how you feel." In a group of very resistant teenagers, I once passed around a miniature toy version of Sigmund Freud. When the members received the toy, they were asked to identify the worst thing a therapist or adult had ever said to them. In residential settings, I often ritualize the beginning of the group by having the members send a greeting to someone in the circle, encouraging eye contact and authentic connection.

Finally, sociometric exercises that emphasize commonalities among group members are helpful in emphasizing that the group is an entity built on shared experience and emotions (Haen, 2005a). There are endless variations of these exercises, but they all involve performing an action that indicates similarities between members. For example, group members might be asked to cross from one side of the room to the other if they like pizza, to stand up from their seats if they have had nightmares, or to switch chairs if they sometimes cry when they think about their families. In each variation, the action is repeated: "Cross the room if you hate getting up in the morning. Now, everybody who thinks this group might be boring, cross the room." The expressions of connection are brief and nonverbal, allowing groups to take risks quickly. For example, I have been in groups where a member might say, "Cross the room if you have been raped." As members learn that exposure is minimal, they often take risks early on.

In another form of sociometry, children can be engaged in creating subgroups based on a specific criterion. For example, I sometimes establish different areas of the room—one corner might be for those who are angry, one for those who are sad, another for those who are scared, and another for those who are happy (Emunah, 1994). I then give a series of directions, such as, "Go to the corner that indicates how you feel about your family most of the time" and "Go to the area of the room that names a feeling you show other people a lot." Once in subgroups, the members can discuss why they placed themselves in that area.

Providing a sense of connection among members is one fundamental use of the group environment. Recently, as the result of research in the area of attachment, another important function of treatment has emerged. Carnochan (2004) wrote, "The capacity to think about self and others in a way that is affectively alive and that leads to an ability to learn from experience is a critical developmental achievement" (p. 84). Fonagy and colleagues use the term "mentalization" to refer to the ability to reflect on one's own thoughts and emotions as well as on the thoughts, feelings, desires, and beliefs of others (Fonagy & Target, 2003). Mentalization, or reflective function, is intimately tied to children's capacities to empathize, organize and regulate themselves, self-protect, articulate feelings, develop a sense of personal agency and an integrated sense of self, control impulses, and understand the impact of their actions upon others (Bateman & Fonagy, 2004; Fonagy & Target, 2000, 2003). Not surprisingly, exposure to trauma compromises mentalization in children, while a robust capacity to mentalize is thought to ameliorate some of the impact of trauma.

Attachment theorists believe that reflective function is developed in part through the process of pretend play (Bateman & Fonagy, 2004; Meares, 2005). During play, the child learns to link internal and external reality and to test out different possibilities (Irwin, 2005). Drama therapy can assist in reinvigorating this developmental milestone in traumatized children, particularly in a group setting (Barrat & Kerman, 2001). When children engage in dramatic play, they externalize aspects of the self so that they can be examined, organized, and understood (Bateman & Fonagy, 2004; Holmes, 2001). Similarly, when they engage in taking on roles, they are learning to take another's perspective and to reflect on others' thoughts, feelings, and intentions (Haen, 2005a).

Playback theatre, developed by Jonathan Fox, is a method in which a client tells a story and then witnesses it played back in action by a cast of actors (Salas, 2000). Variations of this process are useful for both the actor and the audience member. When children are asked to represent the feelings of another, a connection is forged that is supported by mentalizing activity. I might ask children to create a sculpture that represents something a group member has expressed or to act out another member's story using puppets. I often use the psychodrama technique of doubling (Hoey, 2005) to encourage reflective function. In doubling, group members are asked to speak as if they are another group member and to give voice to something he or she might be thinking or feeling but unable to express. For example, an avoidant child might say, "I'm not talking today." When group members double, with the permission of the child, they stand behind him or her and say things like, "I'm bored" or "I'm afraid to talk" or "I'm not sure if I like this group." The child is then encouraged to share with the group which member came closest to articulating his or her true feelings.

Mentalization can be encouraged through taking on roles that are distant from who the child is in real life. For example, a passive group member can be encouraged to play an authority figure, or an angry group member might be put in a scene in which his task is to keep an angry character calm. Finally, group members can be engaged in actively reflecting to a child the many aspects of him- or herself, as seen by the group. In an activity that I frequently use with hospitalized children (Haen, 2005a), the group members sculpt different aspects of one child, choosing a part of him or her to which they related. When tapped by the leader, they would say, "I am the part of Stephanie that feels insecure" or "I am the part of Stephanie that wants to beat everyone up."

When a traumatized child's system shuts down in order to protect him or her, it often cuts him or her off from the present moment. Trauma memories enter the mind without temporal anchoring; they are experienced as a reliving in the present rather than a remembering of the past (Stern, 2004; van der Kolk, 2003b). Children who have been exposed to trauma show impairment in their ability to be present, to take in new information, and to connect to what is happening around them from moment to moment (Drake, Bush, & van Gorp, 2001).

Stern (2004) has recently devoted a great deal of attention to the importance of the present moment in therapy. He cites the creative arts therapies, particularly those in which embodiment is central, as unique in their ability to focus the client in the present. He also hypothesizes that metaphor might bear the capability of both connecting the past to and separating it from the present, both crucially important skills for traumatized children. As an improvisational actor, I often felt a sense of heightened perception and connection when engaged fully in the experience of acting. In fact, the therapist's ability to stay focused and responsive to a client has many parallels to the skills needed for improvisation (Kindler, 2005).

Drama therapists frequently ask clients to reflect on their in vivo experience and to give it representation in metaphor or action. An often-used exercise involves asking group members to express a sound and movement to reflect how they are feeling in the present moment. I often begin groups with teenagers by asking them metaphorical questions, such as, "If how you are feeling inside today were a type of weather, what would be the forecast?" or "If you were a kind of food today, what kind would you be?" Similarly, I might call a client's attention to something his body is expressing but his words are not. A client who is saying he is happy while his hands are making fists might be asked to talk as if he were his fists. If I notice a client who is rocking in the group, I might ask the members to "try on" that rocking to see how it feels. They are then asked to give voice to that experience.

Improvisational exercises in which the group members must connect and respond to peers help focus them in the present, often without the intensity of experience that accompanies a focus on relationships in traditional verbal therapy. One such game involves getting two volunteers to begin a scene together. The key is spontaneity, so the actors must accept the given circumstances and keep the scene going. At any point, another group member can call out "Freeze!" and the actors must freeze their bodies in the scene. This group member then taps one of the two actors out, assumes his posture and begins a completely new scene. This process encourages the flow of ideas and staying engaged with another person, rapidly adjusting to new circumstances.

An additional way that therapists can encourage exploration of the present moment is through maximization (Hoey, 2005). "Maximization" refers to the group leader identifying an aspect of the client's expression that requires further exploration and amplifying it through dramatic action. For example, in a scene in which a group member confronts a bully, she might utter the line, "Leave me alone!" The leader, understanding that these are significant words, might intervene by having her repeat them several times, growing louder and stronger each time; the leader might also choose to have others in the group stand behind her and join her in saying the line. Another example of maximization occurs when the director freezes a scene and asks the actors to verbalize how the characters are feeling during a crucial moment of interaction. This intervention helps to connect here-and-now affect to language in a way that assists traumatized children in reflecting on and describing their internal, lived experience (Stern, 2004).

A Return to Self-Expression

Much has been written about the loss of voice that occurs as a result of trauma. This loss, often referred to as "speechless terror," has both psychological and biological origins (van der Kolk, 1994). Many traumatized children experience impairment not only in their ability to express emotions, but also in identifying and regulating them (Lubit & Eth, 2003). The loss of connection to and control over affect contributes to a diffuse sense of self and a general feeling of disempowerment.

Yet, even in the face of the silence that trauma renders, children seek opportunities to symbolically represent their stories. Coates, Schechter, and First (2003) wrote about the intense drive that many New York children had in the immediate aftermath of September 11, 2001, to draw, play about, and recreate the World Trade Center devastation. Even when children are able to use words to describe their memories, the words are often insufficient to capture the complexity of traumatic events. The unique ability to capture complexity and to play with time are two significant advantages that the arts hold over linguistic forms of representation used in traditional "talk therapy" (Bennett, 2005).

Drama, specifically, can act as an "emotional release valve" (Miranda, Arthur, Milan, Mahoney, & Perry, 1998) that assists a client in beginning to reclaim his or her voice through the safety of metaphor and character. I have witnessed this phenomenon time and again: children who cannot find their voice in discussion who begin to speak when handed a puppet or when given a character to play; kids who cannot talk about their past trauma but can represent it metaphorically in role play; adolescents who remain quiet and guarded until they are handed a prop microphone and asked to report on the events of the group. With self-expression, paced by an empathic, attuned therapist, comes the gradual "breathing out" of the trauma experience (Ziegler, Howe, & Pasternak, 2004, p. 165).

One exercise that I have adapted with success for groups of traumatized children was first articulated by Casson (2004). In this piece of dramatic work, children are asked to pretend to be pet owners in a veterinary office. Each is asked to create an imaginary pet who is sick and to bring the pet to the doctor's office. The kids talk to the doctor about the pet's physical sickness as well as its worries or feelings. The quality of the interaction between each child and pet is often tied to the amount and quality of caregiving that child has had in his or her own life. For example, in groups of children who have been abused, it is not uncommon for them to treat the pet abusively; however, when they articulate the pet's illness to the doctor, they frequently give voice to their own symptoms and worries. As the doctor, I (or my co-leader) engage the group members in identifying what the pet needs to feel better and, together, we try to provide the pet with what it needs to heal—an in vivo experience of active response to traumatic disempowerment.

Older children frequently enjoy role-playing a talk show or television interview on the topic of kids' fears (or a similar topic that provides appropriate distance from the direct experience). In a group for older children who had all experienced traumatic grief, each member worked with a partner to create a goodbye scene between two characters. Each pair was asked to role-play the scene with a different emotion attached to the goodbye—worry, anger, sadness, jealousy, and so on. Even the simple creation of family scenes without much prompting can yield surprisingly effective results.

A key element of any drama therapy process is the director's facilitation of the scene work: pausing the scene when the action becomes too intense; encouraging cognition if the scene is too affectively charged by asking for the characters' thoughts (or utilizing a similar intervention if the scene is too distant and requires a deeper exploration of affect); engaging the group in suggesting new directions or strategies for a character who is stuck; reversing roles if a client could benefit from exploring a new perspective or requires distance; suggesting multiple endings for a scene in order to play out different options the characters have; or projecting a scene into the past or future. The possibilities are numerous but require a skilled facilitator who is interested in the use of role play for more than didactic purposes and understands the multidimensional therapeutic benefits of the creative act. While the group leader is there to assist in providing direction, he or she must balance this duty with engaging the clients in collectively creating their own scenes and stories to return them to self-expression.

The act of creation is in direct opposition to the destruction that often results from trauma. Thus, engaging the group in creative tasks and purposeful action provides a sense of possibility and future that helps prevent retraumatization (Coates et al., 2003) and enlivens a collective sense of accomplishment. In Reisner's (2002) words, "to avoid trauma a person must react to the traumatic circumstance in an active way; a way in which previously held meanings are reasserted, energies are discharged, the social fabric is rewoven and belief systems and practices are reinforced" (p. 12).

In my drama therapy groups, children have collectively built a safe parent, safe school, safe boyfriend, ideal hospital, perfect town, and loving family when their experiences have been the opposite. In a boys' group in a residential facility, the members worked to create a video drama that articulated their experiences of mental illness and displacement from their families (Haen & Brannon, 2002). Even the act of creating a scene within the group can offer a sense of possibility when the members are all invested and engaged in its formation (Nash & Haen, 2005).

CLOSING THOUGHTS

Like trauma, the experience of acting somehow defies linguistic representation. It is difficult to capture in words all that happens when a child engages his or her imagination and steps into a role. It is an absorbing experience that can engage his or her ability to access possibility, indomitable spirit, and connection. Most drama therapists enter the field having felt the force of creativity during their own time as theater artists. Having recognized the resulting changes within themselves, they come with a wish to learn how to harness this force to help others.

Guided by research advances in parallel fields, the drama therapist can utilize what he or she knows intuitively—that working with children through their imagination provides a means to overcome the damage of the traumatic events that have been forced upon them (Weber, 2005). In the dramatic space, victims can become conquerors, midgets can become giants, and children who feel cornered can learn to see many pathways. Robert Edmond Jones, a theater artist, recognized the transcendent possibility of acting and articulated it in his 1941 book *The Dramatic Imagination*. In it, he wrote:

> These players became aware of the profound duality of life at the moment when they spoke their first lines on a stage, and thereafter all their acting was animated by it. They called it giving a good performance. But what they meant was that a spirit was present in them for a time, making them say things that they themselves did not know they

knew. . . . The thing that is absent from these records is the thing that never can be recorded, the emotion that these artists aroused in our hearts, the sense of triumph they gave us. Their peculiar power lay in this, that in their impersonations they could show us man's creating spirit, in action, before our eyes. They did not teach or preach about life or explain it or expound it or illustrate it. They created it—life itself, at its fullest and truest and highest (Jones, 1941/1995, pp. 156–157).

REFERENCES

Barrat, G., & Kerman, M. (2001). Holding in mind: Theory and practice of seeing children in groups. *Psychodynamic Counselling, 7*(3), 315–328.

Bateman, A. W., & Fonagy, P. (2004). *Psychotherapy for borderline personality disorder: Mentalization-based treatment.* Oxford: Oxford University Press.

Bennett, J. (2005). *Empathic vision: Affect, trauma, and contemporary art.* Stanford, CA: Stanford University Press.

Bloom, S. (2005). Foreword. In A. M. Weber & C. Haen (Eds.), *Clinical applications of drama therapy in child and adolescent treatment* (pp. xv–xviii). New York: Brunner-Routledge.

Bonne, O., Neumeister, A., & Charney, D. S. (2003). Neurobiological mechanisms of psychological trauma. In R. J. Ursano & A. E. Norwood (Eds.), *Trauma and disaster responses and management* (pp. 1–36). Washington DC: American Psychiatric Publishing.

Burmeister, J. (2000). Psychodrama with survivors of traffic accidents. In P. F. Kellermann & M. K. Hudgins (Eds.), *Psychodrama with trauma survivors: Acting out your pain* (pp. 198–228). London: Jessica Kingsley.

Carbonell, D. M., & Parteleno-Barehmi, C. (1999). Psychodrama groups for girls coping with trauma. *International Journal of Group Psychotherapy, 49*(3), 285–306.

Carnochan, P. (2004). Fantasy, symbol, and the development of thought. *Journal of Infant, Child, and Adolescent Psychotherapy, 3*(1), 82–91.

Casson, J. (2004). *Drama, psychotherapy and psychosis: Dramatherapy and psychodrama with people who hear voices.* New York: Brunner-Routledge.

Coates, S. W., Schechter, D. S., & First, E. (2003). Brief interventions with traumatized children and families after September 11. In L. Aaron & A. Harris (Series Eds.) & S. W. Coates, J. L. Rosenthal, & D. S. Schechter (Vol. Eds.), *September 11: Trauma and human bonds. Relational perspectives book series* (pp. 1–14). Hillsdale, NJ: Analytic Press.

De Bellis, M. D. (2001). Developmental traumatology: The psychobiological development of maltreated children and its implications for research, treatment, and policy. *Development and Psychopathology, 13*(3), 539–564.

De Bellis, M. D., Baum, A. S., Birmaher, B., Keshavan, M. S., Eccard, C. E., Boring, A. M., et al. (1999). Developmental traumatology. Part I: Biological stress systems. *Biological Psychiatry, 45*(10), 1259–1270.

Drake, E. B., Bush, S. F., & van Gorp, W. G. (2001). Evaluation and assessment of PTSD in children and adolescents. In S. Eth (Ed.), *PTSD in children and adolescents* (pp. 1–31). Washington, DC: American Psychiatric Association.

Emunah, R. (1994). *Acting for real: Drama therapy process, technique, and performance*. New York: Brunner/Mazel.

Fonagy, P., & Target, M. (2000). Mentalisation and the changing aims of child psychoanalysis. In K. von Klitzing, P. Tyson, & D. Bürgin (Eds.), *Psychoanalysis in childhood and adolescence* (pp. 129–139). Basel, Switzerland: Karger.

Fonagy, P., & Target, M. (2003). Evolution of the interpersonal interpretive function: Clues for effective preventive intervention in early childhood. In L. Aaron & A. Harris (Series Eds.) & S. W. Coates, J. L. Rosenthal, & D. S. Schechter (Vol. Eds.), *September 11: Trauma and human bonds. Relational perspectives book series* (pp. 1–14). Hillsdale, NJ: Analytic Press.

Fosha, D. (2001). Trauma reveals the roots of resilience. *Constructivism in the Human Sciences, 6*(1–2), 7–15.

Galatzer-Levy, R. M. (1991). Considerations in the psychotherapy of adolescents. In M. Slomowitz (Ed.), *Adolescent psychotherapy* (pp. 85–100). Washington, DC: American Psychiatric Association.

Haen, C. (2005a). Group drama therapy in a children's inpatient psychiatric setting. In A. M. Weber & C. Haen (Eds.), *Clinical applications of drama therapy in child and adolescent treatment* (pp. 189–204). New York: Brunner-Routledge.

Haen, C. (2005b). Rebuilding security: Group therapy with children affected by September 11. *International Journal of Group Psychotherapy, 55*(3), 391–414.

Haen, C. (2007). Fear to tread: Play and drama therapy in the treatment of boys who have been sexually abused. In S. Brooke (Ed.), *Creative therapies and trauma* (pp. 235–249). Springfield, IL: Charles Thomas.

Haen, C., & Brannon, K. H. (2002). Superheroes, monsters and babies: Roles of strength, destruction and vulnerability for emotionally disturbed boys. *The Arts in Psychotherapy, 29*, 31–40.

Hegeman, E., & Wohl, A. (2000). Management of trauma-related affect, defenses, and dissociative states. In R. H. Klein & V. L. Schermer (Eds.), *Group psychotherapy for psychological trauma* (pp. 64–88). New York: Guilford Press.

Hoey, B. (2005). Children who whisper: A study of psychodramatic methods for reaching inarticulate young people. In A. M. Weber & C. Haen

(Eds.), *Clinical applications of drama therapy in child and adolescent treatment* (pp. 45–65). New York: Brunner-Routledge.

Holmes, J. (2001). *The search for the secure base: Attachment theory and psychotherapy.* New York: Brunner-Routledge.

Irwin, E. (2005). Facilitating play with non-players: A developmental perspective. In A. M. Weber & C. Haen (Eds.), *Clinical applications of drama therapy in child and adolescent treatment* (pp. 3–23). New York: Brunner-Routledge.

Johnson, D. R. (1986). The developmental method in drama therapy: Group treatment with the elderly. *The Arts in Psychotherapy, 13*(1), 17–33.

Johnson, D. R., Lubin, H., James, M., & Hale, K. (1997). Single session effects of treatment components within a specialized inpatient posttraumatic stress disorder program. *Journal of Traumatic Stress, 10*(3), 377–390.

Jones, R. E. (1995). *The dramatic imagination.* New York: Theatre Art Books. (Original work published 1941)

Kellermann, P. F. (2000). The therapeutic aspects of psychodrama with traumatized people. In P. F. Kellermann & M. K. Hudgins (Eds.), *Psychodrama with trauma survivors: Acting out your pain* (pp. 23–40). London: Jessica Kingsley.

Kindler, R. (2005). Creative co-constructions: A psychoanalytic approach to spontaneity and improvisation in the therapy of a twice forsaken child. In A. M. Weber & C. Haen (Eds.), *Clinical applications of drama therapy in child and adolescent treatment* (pp. 87–103). New York: Brunner-Routledge.

Landy, R. J. (2003). Drama therapy with adults. In C. E. Schaefer (Ed.), *Play therapy with adults* (pp. 15–33). New York: Wiley.

Lindahl, M. W. (2002). Treatment strategies for traumatized children. In M. B. Williams & J. F. Sommer (Eds.), *Simple and complex post-traumatic stress disorder: Strategies for comprehensive treatment in clinical practice* (pp. 215–239). New York: Haworth.

Lubit, R., & Eth, S. (2003). Children, disasters, and the September 11th World Trade Center attack. In R. J. Ursano & A. E. Norwood (Eds.), *Trauma and disaster responses and management* (pp. 63–96). Washington, DC: American Psychiatric Association.

Macy, R. D., Macy, D. J., Gross, S. I., & Brighton, P. (2003). Healing in familiar settings: Support for children and youth in the classroom and community. *New Directions for Youth Development, 98*(Summer), 51–79.

Malchiodi, C. A. (2003). Expressive arts therapy and multimodal approaches. In C. A. Malchiodi (Ed.), *Handbook of art therapy* (pp. 106–117). New York: Guilford Press.

McKenna, P., & Haste, E. (1999). Clinical effectiveness of dramatherapy in the recovery from neuro-trauma. *Disability and Rehabilitation, 21*(4), 162–174.

Meares, R. (2005). *The metaphor of play: Origin and breakdown of personal being* (3rd ed.). New York: Routledge.

Miranda, L., Arthur, A., Milan, T., Mahoney, O., & Perry, B. D. (1998). The art of healing: The Healing Arts Project. *Early Childhood Connections, Journal of Music- and Movement-Based Learning, 4*(4), 35–40.

Mulkey, M. (2004). Recreating masculinity: Drama therapy with male survivors of sexual assault. *The Arts in Psychotherapy, 31*(1), 19–28.

Nader, K. (2004). Treating traumatized children and adolescents: Treatment issues, modalities, timing, and methods. In N. B. Webb (Ed.), *Mass trauma and violence: Helping families and children cope* (pp. 23–49). New York: Guilford Press.

Nash, E., & Haen, C. (2005). Healing through strength: A group approach to therapeutic enactment. In A. M. Weber & C. Haen (Eds.), *Clinical applications of drama therapy in child and adolescent treatment* (pp. 121–135). New York: Brunner-Routledge.

Perry, B. D. (2006). Applying principles of neurodevelopment to clinical work with maltreated and traumatized children: The neurosequential model of therapeutics. In N. B. Webb (Ed.), *Working with traumatized youth in child welfare* (pp. 27–52). New York: Guilford Press.

Pine, D. S., & Cohen, J. A. (2002). Trauma in children and adolescents: Risk and treatment of psychiatric sequelae. *Biological Psychiatry, 51*(7), 519–531.

Pitruzzella, S. (2004). *Introduction to dramatherapy: Person and threshold.* New York: Brunner-Routledge.

Reisner, S. (2002). Staging the unspeakable: A report on the collaboration between Theater Arts Against Political Violence, the Associazione Culturale Altrimenti, and 40 counsellors in training in Pristina, Kosovo. *Psychosocial Notebook, 3,* 9–30.

Rothschild, B. (2000). *The body remembers: The psychophysiology of trauma and trauma treatment.* New York: Norton.

Salas, J. (2000). Playback theater: A frame for healing. In P. Lewis & D. R. Johnson (Eds.), *Current approaches in drama therapy* (pp. 288–302). Springfield, IL: Charles Thomas.

Shapiro, F. (2001). *Eye movement desensitization and reprocessing* (2nd ed.). New York: Guilford Press.

Siegel, D. J. (2003). An interpersonal neurobiology of psychotherapy: The developing mind and the resolution of trauma. In M. F. Solomon & D. J. Siegel (Eds.), *Healing trauma: Attachment, mind, body and brain* (pp. 1–56). New York: Norton.

Silva, R., Cloitre, M., Davis, L., Levitt, J., Gomez, S., Ngai, I., et al. (2003).

Early intervention with traumatized children. *Pyschiatric Quarterly, 74*(4), 333–347.

Stern, D. (2004). *The present moment in psychotherapy and everyday life.* New York: Norton.

van der Kolk, B. A. (1994). The body keeps the score: Memory and the emerging psychobiology of posttraumatic stress. *Harvard Review of Psychiatry, 1,* 253–265.

van der Kolk, B. A. (2002). Beyond the talking cure: Somatic experience and subcortical imprints in the treatment of trauma. In F. Shapiro (Ed.), *EMDR as an integrative psychotherapy approach: Experts of diverse orientations explore the paradigm prism* (pp. 57–83). Washington, DC: American Psychological Association.

van der Kolk, B. A. (2003a). Neurobiological mechanisms of psychological trauma. In R. J. Ursano & A. E. Norwood (Eds.), *Trauma and disaster responses and management* (pp. 1–36). Washington, DC: American Psychiatric Association.

van der Kolk, B. A. (2003b). The neurobiology of childhood trauma and abuse. *Child and Adolescent Psychiatric Clinics of North America, 12*(2), 293–317.

van der Kolk, B. A. (2005, May). Attachment, helplessness and trauma: The body keeps the score. Paper presented at the Harvard Medical School conference on Attachment and Related Disorders, Boston, MA.

Weber, A. M. (2005). "Don't hurt my mommy": Drama therapy for children who have witnessed severe domestic violence. In A. M. Weber & C. Haen (Eds.), *Clinical applications of drama therapy in child and adolescent treatment* (pp. 24–43). New York: Brunner-Routledge.

Young, L. (1992). Sexual abuse and the problem of embodiment. *Child Abuse and Neglect, 16*(1), 89–100.

Ziegler, R. G., Howe, J., & Pasternak, G. (2004). Psychotherapeutic debriefing of children and adolescents after exposure to violence in home or community: Integrating narrative techniques. *Journal of Infant, Child, and Adolescent Psychotherapy, 3*(2), 163–184.

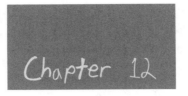

Chapter 12

A Group Art
and Play Therapy Program for
Children from Violent Homes

Cathy A. Malchiodi

Todd is an 8-year-old boy who recently witnessed the physical abuse of his mother by her boyfriend on several occasions. Previous to these incidents, Todd's biological father divorced his mother, Maria, after 3 years of verbally abusing Todd and battering Maria. At the age of 6, Todd attempted to intervene during one of his parents' violent episodes by contacting the police on his mother's cell phone. In response, his father punished him by locking him in a closet for 3 days. He and his mother are staying in a shelter for battered women and their children.

Shareesa is a 12-year-old girl who witnessed her stepfather beat her mother and her younger brother. Earlier in her life, her biological father physically and sexually abused her for 2 years until her mother decided to take her and seek refuge at a shelter for battered women and their children. Shareesa and her mother and younger brother are currently staying at a safe house for domestic violence survivors and will be moving to long-term housing for battered women in the next month.

Megan is a 10-year-old girl who witnessed her father beat her mother and threaten her with a gun and is a victim of physical abuse by her older brother. Megan also witnessed her father kill the family's dog during a particularly violent and prolonged episode. She is currently in foster care until her mother recovers from her injuries and is able to find a secure place for Megan and herself to live. Megan worries that if she tells anyone else about the abuse she has witnessed and experienced that she will be permanently taken away from her mother.

While each of these children has had numerous experiences that could be considered traumatic in nature, all have one experience in common—exposure to violence in their homes, also known as domestic violence. Domestic violence is defined as the use or threat of use of physical, verbal, emotional, or sexual abuse within an intimate relationship with the intention of creating fear, intimidation, or control (Groves, 1999). It is a serious problem in families and is a frequent source of trauma reactions in children.

For the most part, interventions have focused on women who have been victims of violence in the home. Over the past 20 years, the negative impact of domestic violence on child victims has been repeatedly acknowledged, but very few models of intervention have been developed to address these children's short- and long-term psychosocial needs (Groves, 1999; Malchiodi, 1997; Peled & Davis, 1995). In particular, structured group interventions for school-age children from violent homes have not been adequately identified and clarified. This chapter presents a brief description of the nature of domestic violence, its effects on school-age children (second grade through sixth grade), and an appraisal of the problems associated with children's exposure to violence in their homes. Finally, a model for structured intervention using a group format is proposed, based on available research and my clinical experiences with this population.

DOMESTIC VIOLENCE AND CHILDREN

Todd, Shareesa, and Megan are among the estimated 3 to 10 million children who may be exposed to domestic violence each year (Groves, 1999). Each has witnessed violence in their homes and seen their mothers beaten by an intimate partner or husband. Children may also be the direct recipients of physical and verbal assaults by family members in their homes. Child abuse is often a co-occurrence with domestic violence, and an estimated 30–60% of children who have experienced domestic violence have both witnessed and received maltreatment (Margolin & Gordis, 2000).

Because children can be witnesses and recipients of domestic violence, "exposure to domestic violence" is an inclusive description that covers the vast number of ways children experience violent behavior in their homes. Children's exposure to domestic abuse includes, but is not limited to, the following experiences (Gerwitz & Edleson, 2004; Groves, 1999; Margolin & Gordis, 2000):

1. Hearing an episode of violence.
2. Involvement as a witness.
3. Being used as part of the violence, such as a shield against an abusive parent or individual.
4. Intervening in an attempt to prevent family violence.
5. Experiencing repercussions of a violent episode.
6. Being forced to watch or participate in abuse or battering.
7. Being used as a pawn to convince an adult victim to return home or to a relationship.
8. Accidental harm during an attack on an adult victim.
9. Being coerced to remain silent about family violence and to maintain the family secret.

THE EFFECTS OF DOMESTIC VIOLENCE ON SCHOOL-AGE CHILDREN

Exposure to domestic violence can result in a wide range of emotional, psychological, cognitive, social, and behavioral problems for children. Research indicates that children who are exposed to domestic violence may incur any or all of the following problems (Groves, 1999; Malchiodi, 1997, 2003; Margolin & Gordis, 2000; McCloskey, Figueredo, & Koss, 1995).

1. *Emotional, social, and behavioral problems.* Children who are exposed to domestic violence may display more fear, anxiety, anger, low self-esteem, excessive worry, and depression than nonexposed children. They also may be more aggressive, oppositional in their

behavior, withdrawn, or lacking in conflict resolution skills and often have poor peer, sibling, and other social relationships. Children who have experienced domestic violence are often particularly watchful of others (hypervigilance) because events have led them to believe that people can be dangerous, volatile, or unpredictable. Others may have attachment difficulties throughout childhood, and many suffer from sleep, eating disorders, somatic symptoms, and/or bedwetting or other regressive behaviors. Children who come from violent homes are diagnosed more frequently with separation anxiety, obsessive–compulsive disorder, and conduct disorder than children who are not exposed to family conflicts. In brief, repeated exposure to domestic violence is well documented as having numerous negative effects on development and children's mental health.

2. *Cognitive problems.* Children exposed to family violence may perform poorly in school, have lower cognitive functioning, and have limited problem-solving abilities. They also may have difficulties in concentration and comprehension.

3. *Long-term problems.* As adolescents and adults, children exposed to domestic violence have more depression and trauma-related symptoms. They also may accept violence as normal to interpersonal interactions and may believe in gender stereotypes that support beliefs of male dominance in relationships. Studies of the intergenerational effects of domestic violence demonstrate that perpetrators of domestic violence who were abused as children are also more likely to maltreat their own children later in life.

The impact of domestic violence can be mediated by a number of factors, including type of experience with violence (witnessing, single direct assault, or multiple direct assaults), children's adaptive skills, age, gender, time elapsed since exposure, and exposure to other traumatic events. In recent years, there is a growing belief among both researchers and clinicians that many children who have been exposed to family violence experience posttraumatic stress disorder (PTSD) (Cohen, 1998). Three factors increase the likelihood of PTSD in children from violent homes: (1) severity of trauma, (2) parental or caregiver reactions to violent or abusive episodes and family coping skills, and (3) temporal proximity to family violence (Hamblen, 2006). Of these three factors, severity of trauma is generally considered to have the strongest relationship to PTSD in children who are exposed to violent family environments; in contrast, children who are physically farther away from family violence report less distress (Cohen, 1998; Groves, 1999). Finally, research also suggests that children who experience physical violence from family members are more likely to have PTSD than those who simply witness abusive events (Groves, 1999).

Children who have long-term exposure to domestic violence have striking similarities to children who survive wars and other conflicts. Unlike well-circumscribed traumatic events like automobile accidents or natural disasters, domestic violence (like war) encompasses a number of possible situations and outcomes. Interparental conflicts can wax and wane in their severity and can be sporadic or daily. Like children who are in the midst of wars, children from violent homes are witnesses and recipients of physical harm, unstable conditions, and volatile situations. There may be destruction of property, displacement, loss, and separation of family members. On occasion, children may be imprisoned or even held hostage. As a result, they develop thoughts, perceptions, and beliefs consistent with their experiences of conflict and react to disputes and disagreements between adults as stressful and possibly dangerous due to what they have learned from interactions between parents or caregivers.

Finally, despite exposure to domestic violence, some children are remarkably resilient and show few reactions as a result of their experiences. In other words, while some children react adversely to stressful circumstances, others recover quickly from exposure to violence when they return to safe living arrangements. Mediating factors for resilience to domestic violence include the level of exposure to violence, personal characteristics of the child, and the extent and quality of parental/adult support (Hughes, Graham-Bermann, & Gruber, 2001). Currently, there is limited data about what risk factors and protective aspects are most important in promoting resilience in children exposed to domestic violence.

PRESENTING PROBLEMS AND FOCUS OF INTERVENTION

Despite consistent recognition of the need for intervention with children from violent homes, relatively little has been written about models of treatment for this population. In part, this dearth is due to the multifaceted nature of children who have been exposed to family violence. Children such as Todd, Shareesa, and Megan have experienced a number of other traumas, including foster placement, physical and verbal abuse, and other emotionally disturbing events. In contrast to the treatment of single-incident traumatic events, intervention for domestic violence usually must address multiple crises and serious emotional disorders such as PTSD, depression, anxiety, and other stress-related problems. To some extent, the complexity of issues involved in work with children from violent homes has impeded the development of model programs for this population.

While children who have been exposed to domestic violence may have any number of emotional, cognitive, behavioral, and/or social problems, intervention usually attempts to address the following areas:

1. Expression of feelings about violence at home and its effects on the family.
2. Psychoeducation about the effects of exposure to family violence.
3. Provision of reassurance that what happened is not the child's fault.
4. Restoration of feelings of safety, including developing individual safety plans for the future.
5. Stress reduction strategies to address the physiological aspects of the traumatic stress of exposure to violence at home.

Intervention with children from violent homes may also include involving the nonabusive parent when feasible because domestic violence reaches beyond children and into family systems.

GROUP INTERVENTION WITH CHILDREN FROM VIOLENT HOMES

Group intervention is a popular strategy for addressing the trauma of school-age children's exposure to domestic violence (Peled & Davis, 1995). Group work reduces isolation, promotes corrective emotional experiences, and enhances interpersonal skills. In the case of children who have had traumatic experiences, it helps them realize that others have had the same or similar experiences and that they are not alone in their feelings of fear, anger, worry, sadness, or guilt. In general, groups have a number of curative aspects that are particularly helpful for children, including peer interaction and support, adult affirmation, and reinforcement of hope for the future (Connors, Schamess, &

Strieder, 1997). Because children who have been exposed to domestic violence often have confused generational boundaries, group intervention is particularly useful. Role reversals often occur, and children may act as "pseudoparents," taking care of other children or adults in the family system (Malchiodi, 1997; Roseby & Johnston, 1995). A group can help children redefine their identities within their families through activities designed to reinforce developmentally appropriate behaviors and roles.

Most groups for children exposed to domestic violence are time-limited and usually are 8 to 12 sessions. They often are structured and have psychoeducational components, including discussion of family violence, personal safety plans, and understanding feelings associated with trauma. Children who have serious emotional disorders, have witnessed a fatal domestic violence event, or are struggling with complicated bereavement may have severe trauma and are usually not good candidates for group treatment; these children may have problems that require long-term individual intervention (Klorer, 2000). Also, children who have experienced sexual abuse in addition to domestic violence may be uncomfortable with disclosure in a group setting and should be seen in individual treatment.

The optimal candidates for group intervention are children who share similar treatment histories and who have had some previous individual intervention. Individual work helps children address their specific problems and crises, prepares them for what to expect from a group setting, and can reduce some of their fears about attending a group. Additionally, children who are out of danger and have safe, consistent living arrangements are appropriate for group intervention because the nonabusive parent or caregiver is more likely to be emotionally and physically available and children themselves are stabilized. At the same time, it is important to realize that children like Megan, who is in short-term foster care and separated from her parent, can still benefit from group work in many cases.

ART AND PLAY THERAPIES WITH CHILDREN FROM VIOLENT HOMES

Art therapy and play therapy are two popular forms of treatment with children from violent homes (Gil, 1991; Klorer, 2000; Malchiodi, 1997; Webb, 2007). Any intervention with children who have been exposed to family violence has to provide positive, engaging sensory experiences and be developmentally appropriate to children's ways of learning. The program described below recommends using art and play interventions as a means of facilitating the work of the group because school-age children, particularly those who have been traumatized, prefer using nonverbal means of communication to initially express their experiences. Additionally, children who have been witnesses or recipients of abuse do not enjoy recalling trauma events; if traumas have been chronic, children may have spent a large part of their lives trying to forget these experiences. Art and play therapy allow memories and emotions to surface in ways that these children can tolerate and enable the use of make-believe toward therapeutic ends (Klorer, 2000; Malchiodi, 2003; Shirar, 1996).

School-age children who have been exposed to violence and abuse can benefit from cognitive and solution-focused approaches to art and play therapy (Berg & Steiner, 2003; Malchiodi, 2003; Selekman, 1997). Cognitive therapy has been widely and successfully used with individuals of all ages who have been traumatized and who may have stress-related symptoms or posttraumatic stress (Follette & Ruzek, 2006). Children also can become skilled at a number of solution-focused approaches, such as scaling, miracle questions, and exception-finding questions, through structured art and play and can learn through practice to apply activities to situations outside group treatment.

Finally, art and play are the natural activities of childhood. Unfortunately, domestic violence often robs young survivors of a normal childhood, taking away the very experience of being a child. Purposeful art and play activities can help these children reconnect with these experiences and restore the sense of spontaneity through providing opportunities for creative self-expression and imagination. Simply stated, intervention that is fun will help relax children so that they are more likely to be comfortable enough to participate and share feelings.

PLANNING AN ART AND PLAY THERAPY GROUP FOR CHILDREN FROM VIOLENT HOMES

This group is based on my interventions for traumatized children found in *Helping Children Feel Safe* (Steele, Malchiodi, & Klein, 2002) and is specifically designed for children who have already disclosed information about the extent of their exposure to domestic violence.

The group consists of six to eight participants and is designed to meet for 12 90-minute sessions, although it can be adjusted to 8 sessions if necessary. Group members should be of the same gender if possible and roughly the same age (maximum 3-year difference in age). In a school-age group, large differences in skills and abilities make it difficult to apply interventions in a developmentally appropriate way. The overall goal is to establish a group in which all members will feel comfortable and to help the group develop cohesion.

In working with children from violent homes, it is important to get a commitment in writing from parents or caregivers that children will regularly attend weekly group sessions. This commitment can be obtained at the same time parents and children sign an informed consent statement in order to participate in the group. Children's groups often are held at the same time as groups for mothers to increase commitment and attendance. This children's group works best with this arrangement because the final stages of the group involve parental attendance and participation.

Items that are helpful to have in a group art and play therapy group of this nature include the following:

1. Tables and comfortable chairs for children.
2. Pillows and floor mats for relaxation activities.
3. Art materials (paper, posterboard, oil pastels, felt-tip markers, collage materials, child-safe scissors, stapler, tape, white glue, clay, tempera paint, and brushes).
4. Puppets (multicultural family puppets, assortment of animal puppets, finger puppets, and rescuer puppets such as police, doctors, or other first-responders).
5. Children's books for quiet reading time and for therapeutic storytelling.
6. Board games for recreation and therapeutic games for group work (such as Ungame or the Talking, Feeling, and Doing Game).
7. Building blocks or Legos for construction.
8. Snacks for breaks and stickers or other tokens as treats.

Generic play materials and toys are preferable to figures that are associated with story characters from movies or cartoons because they allow children to use their imaginations to project their own experiences. The group art and play room should not be overstimulating in terms of supplies or toys. Because children who have been exposed to abuse or violence may have difficulties with concentration, it can be countertherapeutic to have too many elements in the room.

PHASES OF GROUP INTERVENTION

Judith Herman (1992), a well-known expert on the trauma of abuse and domestic violence, describes a three-part trauma recovery model that is applicable to developing group intervention with children from violent homes. Her model includes (1) establishing safety, (2) telling the trauma story, and (3) restoration of connection between trauma-tized individuals and their communities. With slight modification, Herman's model provides a relevant structure for group intervention with child survivors of domestic violence.

While the structure and format of the art and play therapy group is designed for small groups of school-age children who have been exposed to domestic violence, it can also be applied to individual and residential group work with adaptation. For example, children who reside in safe houses and who are residents for 2 to 3 months can bene-fit from the same sequence of interventions. Additionally, therapists can apply the program's principles to children who may have problems that prohibit group participation, such as sexual abuse or aggressive behavior. In the case of children with serious emotional problems, each phase of intervention may require additional time, and therapists may have to adapt interventions to months or even years.

Phase I: Establishing Safety (Weeks 1–3)

The first phase of group intervention emphasizes trust and safety. Children who come from violent homes often are fearful or anxious about the environment and unfamiliar children and adults, including the therapist. No child who has come from an abusive situation, whether a victim of physical assault or a witness, will be able to recover from trauma, be comfortable with self-disclosure, or learn new skills without first feeling secure. In beginning a group of this nature, it is important to address safety because it sets the stage for future work by creating a sense of trust.

It is imperative to discuss confidentiality during initial interviews for entry into the group and during the first several group meetings. Children should know and understand that the therapist will not repeat their words to parents or caregivers without their permission but that the therapist will keep them informed about what issues children are working on in therapy and children's general progress. Children should also know and understand that certain disclosures that come up in the group, such as intent to self-harm, threat of harm from others, or threat of harm to others, cannot be kept confidential.

During the initial session, group rules are introduced. In general, children are wondering what will happen, who is in charge, and who will take care of them. Rules are important because they establish safety through limits on behavior, consistent routines, and unconditional acceptance of feelings.

In work with children from violent homes, it is imperative to discuss rules about physical contact and to state clearly that hitting or other forms of physical assault and verbal abuse (name calling, bullying, and insults) are not acceptable. Confidentiality (with the exception of abuse or self-harm) and respect for group members' feelings, opinions, and personal space are also important to establish. These rules can be placed on a colorful poster, signed by the children to reinforce the group's contract, and displayed in the group meeting room. It is also critical to convey that it is acceptable to talk about violence and abuse, that abuse is not okay, and that it is important to value the expression of emotions and experiences.

Activities during the first several sessions of the group include:

1. "Getting to know you" by creating name tags and participating in games that help group members learn more about each other.
2. Reading the story of Brave Bart, a cat who is traumatized and participates in a group for other traumatized cats.
3. Creating a safe place for a small toy animal using art materials.
4. Creating a "safety hand," with names and contact information of people to call in case of emergency or danger of violence.
5. Making a drawing of a worry and learning to use scaling techniques such as a "feelings thermometer" or "how big is my worry" to identify how bad the worry is.
6. Making an "abuse is not okay" poster.
7. Practicing several relaxation activities such as deep breathing and yoga poses.
8. Free drawing and play during each session to allow for spontaneous expression.

In brief, activities during this phase provide experiences that address personal care and safety and provide opportunities for expression of feelings about events associated with violence or abuse. The focus is on supporting children's abilities to learn self-care through identifying resources, situations that create worry or anxiety, and strategies for reducing stress when uncomfortable feelings arise. Psychoeducation on domestic violence is introduced to help participants understand that physical and verbal abuse is not okay under any circumstances and that children are not at fault when violence happens in their homes. Overall, it is important to support group members' needs for safety and control in choosing what to talk about in the group in order to build trust.

Telling the Trauma Story (Weeks 4–8)

The second phase of the group, telling the trauma story, involves activities to encourage sharing personal experiences and self-disclosure. During these sessions, children are encouraged to talk about how domestic violence has affected them if they feel comfortable doing so. The overall goal during this stage is to help children address the trauma of violent events and to begin to regain their abilities to experience and enjoy life even though bad things have happened. James (1989) states, "The goal is to have traumatized children reach the point where they can say something like, 'Yes, that happened to me. That's how I felt and how I behaved when it happened. This is how I understand it all now. I won't really forget that it happened, but I don't always have to think about it either'" (p. 49).

Structured interventions during this phase include:

1. Creating a magazine picture collage of what it feels like to be powerful and powerless.
2. Drawing a picture of "your family."
3. Reading therapeutic storybooks about domestic violence.
4. Draw something about "what happened" (domestic violence, abuse, or other traumatic events) and draw "what would make what happened get better."
5. Drawing "who/what makes me worried (afraid or angry) since it happened."
6. Making "how hands can help or hurt" posters.
7. Learning about negative and positive self-talk and practicing

simple cognitive-behavioral techniques to reduce negative thinking.

8. Practicing scaling techniques such as feelings thermometers and "success towers."

9. Free drawing and play during each session to allow for spontaneous expression.

10. Relaxation and stress reduction activities and identifying where worries or other uncomfortable feelings are in one's body.

During this phase, the therapist verbally models how to be supportive of group members, reassures group members that domestic violence is not their fault, and acknowledges each child's unique contributions to the group. Because discussing traumatic events or feelings can produce anxieties or trigger stress reactions, free time to draw and play becomes particularly important during these sessions. Children need to release tension accumulated after disclosing or discussing abuse or may simply require time to relax after talking about uncomfortable experiences or recalling traumatic memories.

Returning to the Community (Weeks 9–12)

Herman (1992) notes that the final stage of trauma recovery involves restoration of connections with important people in the individual's life. In the case of children who have been exposed to domestic violence, nonabusive parents or caregivers are the most important connection and are central to the child's current and future emotional reparation and recovery. For some group members, foster parents, other caregivers, or even teachers may be important to children's current and future well-being.

In the final phase of the group, nonabusive parents or caregivers are asked to participate in the group alongside the children in two sessions. In a practical sense, this participation gives the therapist the opportunity to help parents learn additional information about maintaining a safe and stable home environment for themselves and their children. As long as exposure to violence or lack of safety at home continues, children cannot begin the process of reparation from the trauma of exposure to domestic violence. Many of the activities used during the first phase of the group to help children feel safe and secure can be adapted or repeated in child–parent sessions.

Child–parent sessions strengthen connections, attachment, and bonding between parents and children through inviting them to engage in creative activities together. During these joint sessions, it is important to let children take the lead by encouraging them to share accomplishments and achievements. Because of their previous experiences with the group, child participants are also "experts" on art and play therapy. They are the authorities on their experiences within the group, and this status can be a source of self-esteem and pride.

The final several sessions of the group focus on termination— preparing to say goodbye to the other participants and the therapist and to end the group. Endings can be particularly difficult for children from violent homes because of previous negative experiences of separation or abandonment by parents, caregivers, or other family members. Therefore, termination should be carefully and sensitively planned so that children understand not only its significance, but also that, despite the group's ending, no one will be abandoned and support is available if needed in the future.

Interventions during this final phase include:

1. Sharing of self-selected artwork, skills learned, and accomplishments from previous sessions by children with parents.
2. Child–parent dyad work such as co-creating drawings or collages or engaging in structured play activities together.
3. Child–parent co-created "safety hands" to reinforce and rehearse plans for emergencies or dangerous situations and/or a co-created "escape route" picture.
4. Child–parent digital photographs to be included in co-created collages.
5. Child-created drawing or collage about the "past, present, and future," summing up the progress made during the group.
6. Termination activities, including group photos and creating goodbye cards for participants.
7. Drawing worries and using scaling techniques to compare current worries to those expressed in early sessions.
8. Reviewing and practicing relaxation skills.
9. Having a group celebration during the final session and receiving portfolios of artwork, photos of group members, goodbye cards, and a certificate of completion.

EXPECTED OUTCOMES

While it is difficult to predict how children like Todd, Shareesa, and Megan will progress in any form of treatment, the interventions described in this chapter address the needs of children who have experienced domestic violence and other traumatic events. Actual outcomes of group treatment are best evaluated by pre- and post-evaluations such as checklists of trauma symptoms and parent, social worker, teacher, and/or foster care pre- and posttherapy surveys of behavior. If possible, an additional individual session with parent and child can help identify future needs for individual, group, or family therapy. It is also useful to have child participants use scaling techniques to describe how they felt at the beginning versus the end of the group.

If intervention is successful, children will experience one or more of the following changes, posttreatment:

1. An increased knowledge of the emotional and physical effect of family violence.
2. An understanding that violence to a parent or themselves is not their fault and is not okay.
3. A reduction in stress-related or posttraumatic stress symptoms.
4. An increase in skills to reduce stress-related symptoms.
5. A decrease in negative self-talk.
6. An improvement in identification of feelings.
7. An improvement in communication of feelings with peers and adults.
8. An increased sense of social support from other group members and the therapist.
9. A stronger connection with the nonabusive parent or caregiver.
10. An improvement in personal skills and resilience to cope with future crises.

A short course of group art and play therapy will not result in complete recovery from exposure, but it can establish the foundations necessary to reduce stress-related symptoms. For some children from violent homes, positive changes will occur relatively easily and will be noticeable to parents, teachers, and helping professionals. For others, behavioral changes occur slowly and are more difficult to identify. For these children, group intervention is a significant step along a longer journey toward healing. In all cases, individual personalities, personal histories, parental support, and the availability of additional intervention will affect each child's potential for emotional reparation and recovery.

REFERENCES

Berg, I. K., & Steiner, T. (2003). *Children's solution work*. New York: Norton.

Cohen, J. (1998). Practice parameters for the assessment and treatment of children and adolescents with posttraumatic stress disorder. *Journal of the American Academy of Child and Adolescent Psychiatry, 37*, 10–15.

Connors, K., Schamess, G., & Strieder, F. (1997). Children's treatment groups: General principles and their application to group treatment with cumulatively traumatized children. In J. Brandell (Ed.), *Theory and practice in clinical social work* (pp. 288–314). New York: Free Press.

Follette, V., & Rusek, J. (Eds.). (2006). *Cognitive-behavioral therapies for trauma*. New York: Guilford Press.

Gewirtz, A., & Edleson, J. L. (2004). Young children's exposure to adult domestic violence: The case for early childhood research and supports (Series Paper #6). In S. Schechter (Ed.), *Early childhood, domestic violence, and poverty: Helping young children and their families* (pp. 1–18). Iowa City, IA: University of Iowa School of Social Work.

Gil, E. (1991). *The healing power of play*. New York: Guilford Press.

Groves, B. (1999). Mental health services for children who witness domestic violence. *The future of children: Domestic violence and children, 9*(3), 122–132.

Hamblen, J. (2006). *PTSD in children and adolescents: A National Center for Posttraumatic Stress Disorder fact sheet*. Retrieved from *www.ncptsd. va.gov/facts/specific/fs_children.html*.

Herman, J. (1992). *Trauma and recovery*. New York: Basic Books.

Hughes, H., Graham-Bermann, S., & Gruber, G. (2001). Resilience in children exposed to domestic violence. In S. Graham-Bermann & J. Edleson (Eds.), *Domestic violence in the lives of children: The future of research, intervention, and social policy* (pp. 67–90). Washington, DC: American Psychological Association.

James, B. (1989). *Treating traumatized children*. New York: Free Press.

Klorer, P. (2000). *Expressive therapy with troubled children*. Northvale, NJ: Aronson.

Malchiodi, C. A. (1997). *Breaking the silence: Art therapy with children from violent homes* (2nd ed.). New York: Brunner-Routledge.

Malchiodi, C. A. (2003). *Handbook of art therapy*. New York: Guilford Press.

Margolin, G., & Gordis, E. (2000). The effects of family and community violence on children. *Annual Review of Psychology, 51,* 445–479.

McCloskey, L., Figueredo, A., & Koss, M. (1995). The effects of systemic family violence on children's mental health. *Child Development, 66,* 1239–1261.

Peled, E., & Davis, D. (1995). *Group work with children of battered women.* Thousand Oaks, CA: Sage.

Roseby, V., & Johnston, J. (1995). Clinical interventions with latency-age children of high conflict and violence. *American Journal of Orthopsychiatry, 65*(1), 48–59.

Selekman, M. (1997). *Solution-focused therapy with children.* New York: Guilford Press.

Shirar, L. (1996). *Dissociative children: Bridging inner and outer worlds.* New York: Norton.

Steele, W., Malchiodi, C. A., & Klein, N. (2002). *Helping children feel safe.* Grosse Pointe Woods, MI: National Institute for Trauma and Loss in Children.

Webb, N. B. (Ed.). (2007). *Play therapy with children in crisis* (3rd ed.). New York: Guilford Press.

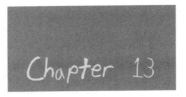

Interventions for Parents of Traumatized Children

William Steele
Cathy A. Malchiodi

Parents often do not know how to help their children following the children's exposure to a potentially traumatizing incident. Generally, education focuses on what parents can say to their children rather than what activities might help their children find relief from overwhelming and terrifying responses to trauma. Following exposure to trauma, efforts to assist children verbally in making sense of trauma fall short because trauma is not initially a cognitive experience but an experience felt in the body. Therefore, parents need to be educated about the sensory experience of trauma to appreciate that what they *do* for their children can be far more helpful than what they *say* to them. This chapter describes what parents need to know about the effects of trauma and outlines approaches and activities to help parents assist their children during trauma recovery.

PARENTS' REACTIONS
TO CHILDREN'S TRAUMA

When children have been traumatized, their parents are likely to experience extreme distress and worry at a time when children need them to be emotionally supportive and confident in their responses to their fears and confusion. Following World War II, studies found that the level of upset displayed by the adult in a child's life, not the war itself, was the single most important factor in predicting the emotional well-being and recovery of the child (Byers, 1996). Increasingly, research demonstrates the importance of parents' calm response when their children are exposed to extreme distress (Siegel & Hartzell, 2003; Williams, 2005). Even the most emotionally stable parents, however, are likely to feel unable to help their traumatized children when they have no information about trauma or the way children may be experiencing traumatic events.

Questions commonly asked by parents about their children after trauma provide a window to understanding parents' anxieties, confusion, and lack of confidence about how to help their children. Some of these questions include:

- What do I tell my child when I am scared too?
- Can I say too much?
- Are there things I should be doing or not doing?
- How do I know how serious this may be for my child?
- How do I know if my child is getting worse?
- How do I know if what I am seeing and hearing from my child is normal?
- Is there anything as a family we should or should not be doing?
- What if my child does not want to talk about what happened?
- Can my child really understand what happened?
- What do I tell the rest of the family?
- Everyone is telling me to keep up our routine. Is that enough?
- What if my child does not want to do the things he or she used to do before all this happened?
- What if my child wants to keep telling me what happened?
- Someone told me things have to get worse before they get better. Is that true?
- Can talking about what happened make things worse?

- Are there any indicators that will tell me my child is doing better?
- How do I handle my worry that something else might happen?
- People tell me I need closure, that I need to put this behind me and move forward. How do I do that?
- What can I do now to make it easier for my child should something else happen?

Answers to these questions and others can lessen parents' anxieties about their children's experiences. Therapists can help parents by providing trauma-specific information, modeling effective responses, and offering structured activities to use with children. Appropriate information about trauma helps parents begin to make sense of what happened and restores parents' sense of competency as caregivers. The remainder of this chapter addresses many of these common questions and suggests activities that not only teach parents about trauma responses, but also provide them with "what to do."

WHERE TO BEGIN WITH PARENTS

As practitioners, we are expected to inform parents about trauma in a way they can easily understand but also in a way that allows them to immediately use the information presented. The following section contains responses to typical parents' questions, worries, and concerns about their traumatized children.

"What do I tell my child when I am scared too?" Therapists frequently hear this question from worried parents, but they do not always answer it in a way that helps parents understand that engaging in activities to help restore their child's sense of safety is often far more important and powerful than what they might say to their child. If asked this question, the initial response should be, "I am sorry, but I do not know what to tell you because I do not know how your child is actually experiencing the situation." Parents will be surprised by this response but must learn that how a child experiences a trauma may be quite different than how adults think that child is reacting. The parent should be informed that in order to know what their child may need, they first need to know how their child may be processing, thinking, and feeling about his or her trauma experience. To accomplish this, parents are encouraged to ask their child, "Since this happened, what is your biggest worry?"

Inform parents to be ready to be surprised by the child's response. It would not be unusual to hear a child reply, "Does this mean we can't go on our school field trip?" Obviously, this child is not consumed by his or her experience, whereas another child exposed to the same situation may respond, "Is Mommy going to die too?" This child is clearly worried, maybe even terrified. Parents' responses to this child should be far different than their responses to the other child.

Asking the child to describe or, better yet, draw his or her biggest worry since the traumatic event is a simple, yet powerful device, as it gives the child the opportunity to make parents witnesses of the experience. There are several questions that can help a parent better appreciate how the child is experiencing that situation and what the child is thinking and feeling as a result of his or her traumatic experience. These questions include, "What is the worst part for you now? What helps you (or might help you) feel a little better? What or who makes you (or might help you) feel really safe right now?" Again, these questions are designed to help the child teach parents not only what the experience is like now, but also communicate what the child needs to feel better. If the child likes to draw, parents can ask that he or she draw the answers to these questions.

Therapists should help parents learn this valuable lesson: it is not the situation itself that creates trauma but the child's level of vulnerability at the time of the situation that determines whether the situation will be traumatic. Certainly, the child who is worried about his or her mother dying is far more traumatized than the child who is worried about missing a field trip. How a child experiences a potentially trauma-inducing situation can be far different than how adults think he or she might be experiencing that situation. This lesson is very important for parents and practitioners.

HELPING PARENTS LEARN ABOUT TRAUMA

It is important that parents understand trauma as an experience rather than a set of reactions or diagnostic criteria. This understanding of trauma establishes the foundation for the acceptance of the interventions suggested in this chapter. For example, the words "intrusive memories" mean very little to parents, but describing trauma as an experience of feeling totally unsafe and powerless to do anything about a situation gives parents a much more meaningful understanding of their child's struggles. It also helps parents determine what can help their child feel safe, empowered, and capable once again.

Therapists should teach parents the basic differences between grief and traumatic responses. Parents must appreciate that grief produces an overwhelming sense of sadness and longing for the person who has died but that it does not leave us feeling unsafe and powerless. In contrast, trauma is a terrifying experience that weakens or destroys our sense of safety and power. Every instinctive survival response to trauma is an attempt to regain that sense of safety and power. Only after safety and a sense of control are restored will grief emerge.

It is helpful to provide parents with an example of how trauma consists of an experience in which individuals feel totally unsafe and powerless. Following September 11, 2001, many children (as well as parents) momentarily experienced the absence of a sense of safety. The children in Lower Manhattan had a much more intense level of terror and understandably felt more powerless and unsafe than those farther away from the scene. Six months later, initial research (Gil-Rivas, Holman, McIntosh, Poulin, & Silver, 2002) demonstrated that thousands of children were experiencing posttraumatic stress disorder (PTSD). The most common reaction was agoraphobia (fear of open places), which may also have represented the simple need to feel safe. Those children in Lower Manhattan who saw people jump from the World Trade Center and who were in the middle of the chaos and confusion were terrified. Once at home, their safe place, many feared going back outside, anticipating experiencing more chaos and terror. They felt safest remaining at home.

After relating this example, ask parents to recall a time when they felt unsafe about anything. Give them a moment to think about it and then ask what they did to feel safe again. This experience will help them understand why their child may be acting in specific ways since being exposed to a traumatic incident.

HELPING PARENTS UNDERSTAND TRAUMA AS A SENSORY EXPERIENCE

When a child is upset, parents naturally want to give verbal reassurance that all will be fine in a few days or weeks. Parents hope that a few gentle, comforting words will be all that is needed. During a trauma event and shortly after, words bring little comfort because many survivors do not feel safe. If children do not feel safe, all the cognitive reassurance in the world will fail to alter their lost sense of safety. Their terrified bodies seek out the sensory experience that best calms them or relieves them of fear.

Therapists can ask parents to think about the last time they were really stressed. Ask them, "Did you go home and try to talk your way out of that stress?" In most cases, they will report that they went home and did something they had done in the past that brought them emotional and physical relief. They exercised, ate, slept, or read a good book; most important, they physically did something to calm themselves and to forget their fear for a while. Parents can support children by allowing them to do those things that help calm them—eating, playing, or engaging in familiar routines.

Providing parents with information as to the way memory processes trauma helps them better understand the sensory needs of the traumatized child. "Explicit memory," discussed in Chapter 1 in this volume and sometimes referred to as declarative memory, refers to the cognitive awareness of facts or events. In explicit memory, we have words to describe what we are thinking and feeling. We can communicate to others our thoughts and feelings, and we can take in information and process it to determine what we may need to do (van Dalen, 2001). Explicit memory allows us to make sense of what is happening.

Trauma is experienced at the "implicit" level for the majority of people. Implicit memory refers to how an event is remembered by the body and central nervous system (van der Kolk, McFarlane, & Weisaeth, 1996; Rothschild, 2000; Squire, 1994). There is no language in implicit memory, no words to describe what is being experienced. We remember and define our experience through our senses: what we saw and heard, the sounds and sights that remind us of what happened.

Parents need to understand that comfort food and stuffed animals really do help and that doing something that helps restore the child's sense of safety and power is initially far more helpful than cognitive reassurances. The child is living traumatic experiences at the sensory level, not the cognitive level. Parents should be asking themselves, "What can I do to help my child feel safe?" They can begin this process by asking their child what helps him or her feel just a little better (e.g., foods, activities, games, familiar people).

Finally, therapists should educate parents about the arousal response and the role it plays in behavior as well as cognitive impairments due to trauma. Arousal refers to those physiological and neurological reactions of the brain (right hemisphere) activated by trauma. Understanding this concept will help parents become less frightened by their child's behavior and more tolerant of any cognitive problems that might result from exposure to trauma (e.g., difficulty attending, focusing, retaining, recalling).

Explain to parents that, in the face of trauma, their child's brain becomes very aroused, ready to do what is needed to help the child survive. In the first few minutes, the brain decides what to do and, during this time, we really do not make a conscious decision as to what we do. This information is important for parents to hear because children will often feel ashamed or guilty about what they did or did not do in the first few moments of the traumatic experience and will rarely tell others. Parents need to hear that it is not uncommon in these situations to lose control of one's bladder, vomit, freeze, or cry out; these are the body's ways of marshaling all the resources needed for survival. Months later, it is not uncommon for child survivors to ask, "Why did I run? Why didn't I call for help?" Parents need to help their child understand that these reactions are normal when first exposed to trauma. It is acceptable to say to children, "I wouldn't be surprised if you wet yourself or pooped on yourself or just didn't know what to do." These statements can help alleviate any shame and guilt over what happened or did not.

SUGGESTED ACTIVITIES

This section describes specific activities parents can use to help calm their child and begin to restore some sense of safety and power to him or her. This first section provides some general concepts that therapists can offer parents of traumatized children.

- Remember, children may have difficulty processing what is said because of the cognitive dysfunction temporarily brought on by the experience of trauma. It is important to be patient if they do not "get it."
- Let children know that the thoughts, feelings, and physical reactions they are having are very normal and will lessen in time.

Encourage children to talk about those thoughts or feelings or ask questions. Be patient. Children may ask the same questions repeatedly because they need to hear the answer several times for it to take hold.

• Use simple, concrete words when giving information. It is always better for parents to be the initial source of information as this allows children to trust them. After giving details, redirect children into an activity.

• Ask children what will help them feel just a little bit better and try to provide it.

• Allow yourself to be curious by asking questions, "What are some of the other kids saying?" (if others are involved); "What do you think most about since this happened?"; "What is your biggest worry?"; "What has been the worst part of what has happened?"

• Children need to feel that their parents are in control. If the situation has created intense worry for you, talk to someone so that personal worries do not frighten them. It is okay to be sad and even to say, "I'm not sure what will happen next, but what I am sure about is I will be with you and we will get through this together." Follow this with a hug.

• Return to family routines as quickly as possible; familiarity supports a sense of safety and control. Give children choices in some of their activities to help restore some sense of power and control and reduce fear.

• If children return to behaviors that they engaged in when younger, be patient; those behaviors are likely to be self-soothing and calming.

• Protect children from exposure to other frightening situations, news about what happened, and reminders of what happened.

• Avoid unnecessary separations between children and family for 2 or 3 weeks, if possible.

The following activities are directed specifically at what therapists can tell parents to do to help restore their children's sense of safety and power. All activities are written in language that most parents can easily comprehend, addressing parents as "you," as previously in this chapter. Keep in mind that these activities may be difficult for some parents because their children's trauma has triggered memories of their own trauma histories. These parents may need trauma intervention for themselves before they feel comfortable with or capable of helping their child. At the same time, some parents who have been traumatized find these activities nonintrusive, or even soothing and comforting to themselves.

These activities and suggestions are directed at restoring the child's sense of safety and power and diminishing the fear and terror created by trauma. Should a child's reactions persist 6 to 8 weeks after parents' attempts to help, a more intense, trauma-specific, structured sensory intervention may be needed (Steele & Raider, 2001).

All activities are listed by chronological age; however, appreciate that some older children will enjoy activities for 3-, 4-, or 5-year-olds. Any of the activities presented can be adjusted to meet a particular child's age or developmental needs. For example, singing for very young children might include teaching songs like "The Itsy Bitsy Spider." If a parent is working with a teenager, he or she may ask the teenager to sing a favorite song or, if too embarrassed, to write out or say the lyrics of a favorite song.

Before starting an activity, tell your child that you have a number of activities for the two of you to try to help him or her feel a bit better. Tell the child that some activities may work and others may not and that sometimes it takes time to find what helps the most.

Infant to 3 Years Old

Safety, Security, and Feeling (adapted from Konarz, 2003)

When trying to create safety and security with children, keeping a daily routine in place is very helpful. To make your child feel safe and secure you can:

- Make regular eye contact.
- Hold your child often and plan for "snuggle time" before bed or naps. Rocking in a chair can be very comforting.
- Engage in smiling and laughter with your child.
- Play games such as patty-cake and peek-a-boo while holding your child.
- Swing your child in a blanket while singing a favorite song.
- Read a book or watch a short video together on the sofa.
- Crawl with your toddler; be excited when he or she crawls toward you.

- Talk to your child often; voice recognition is very calming for infants.
- If your child enjoys water, play with water in the sink or a small tub.
- Let your child help you make his or her favorite food. Remember, comfort foods can be very comforting to any children under stress.

To reinforce attachment and establish a sense of connection, try the following activity. Hold your child on your lap in front of a mirror. Demonstrate facial expressions while you encourage your child to join you. Say, "I feel surprised!" with exaggerated facial expression. Then, calling your child by name, say, "[Child's name] feels surprised!"

Continue with "I feel sad."
"[Child's name] feels sad."
"I feel lonely."
"[Child's name] feels lonely."
"I feel excited."
"[Child's name] feels excited."
"I feel happy!"
"[Child's name] feels happy!"

Repeat this activity regularly, even after your child can easily copy your expressions. Try different feelings and expressions, always beginning and ending with positive ones. These exercises allow your child to begin to understand and manage deep feelings while feeling safe and secure on your lap.

3 to 6 Years Old

Memories

Gently suggest that your child tell you about his or her best memories by drawing a picture or finding one in a magazine that reminds him or her of a good memory. Young children can show you how they are remembering by their selection of colors and the lines in their drawings.

Encourage your child to think about what she remembers smelling and hearing and how her body felt at the time of her good memory. Listen to and respect her memories. After discussing several positive memories over several weeks, suggest that she think about her saddest memory, following the same routine and comforting her. End by talking about her good memory again. Remind her that sad feelings are like a rainstorm; they can always come back but never stay very long. Tell her that she can have happy and sad feelings together and that it is okay to have fun and laugh at times when sad things happen. Finish by having her tell you in detail about one of the funniest times she remembers.

How Big Is Your Hurt?

Tell your child that you know he has been hurt on the inside by this incident. Tell your child that you care about how he feels. Ask your child, "How big is your hurt today?" As a way of measuring the severity of the hurt, ask your child to stretch out his arms as wide as the hurt is big. Take a wide ribbon, measure the length of the child's arms (this equals the amount of hurt), and cut the ribbon. Put the ribbon in an envelope and decide together where to keep the envelope.

Tell your child that in a few weeks you will measure his hurt again and that hurt always gets smaller. For example, you could say, "It is like when you fall down and scrape your knee. At first you have a really big cut or scrape, and it hurts a lot. Then, after a little while, it starts to go away. It gets smaller and smaller until finally it does not hurt anymore."

Reflect the following with your child:

• Is it okay to feel hurt? Of course it is. We all feel hurt sometimes. Even grown-ups feel hurt sometimes.
• Does the hurt stay forever? No. It goes away, just like when it's cloudy and raining outside, it does not rain forever. The sunny, happy, hopeful days come out and stay for a while. It is also like when we blow bubbles; the bubbles get big, but then they pop and go away. They do not last forever, just like the hurt does not last forever.
• It is okay to cry when we feel hurt.
• It helps to talk about our hurt to other people. Who can we tell when we feel hurt?

- Family member (Mom, Dad, Grandma, Grandpa, etc.)
- Friend, schoolmate
- Teacher, counselor, bus driver

End this activity on a positive note. Have a snack together, read a book, or play outside with your child.

Later, ask your child how big (or little) his hurt is now by having him hold out his arms as wide as the hurt is now. With a new ribbon, measure how big or little the hurt is now. Take out the ribbon from the envelope and compare the measurement of the two ribbons. Hopefully, your child's hurt will be lessened and the ribbon will be smaller. If so, ask your child about how much less hurt he is feeling now or reinforce that in time his hurt will get smaller and go away. Even if it takes a long time, remind him there are things he can do to stay safe and have fun. If the hurt is as big as it was earlier, it may be time to seek help. Always end on a positive note after this activity; if the hurt is smaller, emphasize how much has been accomplished. If the hurt is bigger, communicate to your child that you will be there as a support and that other help is available, too.

Play Activities

- All young children find relief from stress through water play. When they are out of sorts and nothing seems to comfort them, encourage them to play at the kitchen sink while standing on a chair. A slow stream of water, a plastic bowl, and small plastic cups work wonders. Bubbles can add to the joy.
- Have children run, hop, somersault, and skip back and forth between parents while parents encourage and compliment children upon arriving at each adult.
- Sing songs that are fun for the child. Singing communicates a sense of comfort, security, and happiness.

5 to 11 Years Old

Rainstorms

Rainstorms (adapted from Klein, 2001) is an activity is designed to help children express their feelings and increase their ability to cope with their fears as well as diminish the stress and anxiety such fears can induce. Provide your child with drawing paper, crayons, and a pencil for this activity,

The purpose of this activity is to help your child understand the process of grieving. To introduce this activity, explain to your child that, when we lose someone, we may feel really sad. After a while, our feelings of sadness may come more slowly and less often, yet at unexpected moments, a sudden rainstorm of feelings may blow in and take us by surprise. Even long after an event of trauma, death, or loss has occurred, we may sometimes experience surprising and strong feelings. What might make us think about the trauma/death/loss again? Using examples such as the game Chutes and Ladders or Candy Land may help your child understand this concept. In these games, when you think that you are making forward progress, you may land on a square that sends you backward.

Your child may respond, "Sometimes I feel like I am the only person who is still crying." Or, "What if I cannot stop crying?" Let her know that crying is normal and not to be afraid of pouring out feelings. Let her know that other people may be crying at times and places where you do not notice their tears or sadness. Tell her not to worry about making others feel worse if she expresses her feelings. If she is worried or concerned about crying, tell her to talk to an adult who can help her understand her feelings.

Ask your child to draw a picture of a stormy day with big raindrops falling from a cloud. In some of the raindrops, have her draw a picture of and/or write about the feelings that she has when she cries. Point out that positive things occur that strengthen us and give us encouragement. Help her see that where there are clouds, there are also rainbows, and where there are tears, there may also be laughter.

Cut out some of the raindrop tears from the original activity. Have your child color a new picture of something hopeful that has happened since the loss. Glue the tears above the new picture to demonstrate that we can find things to be thankful for even as we are experiencing sadness, fear, anger, or loneliness.

Safety Hand

Safety hand (Klein, Malchiodi, & Steele, 2002) is another simple activity to help children take self-empowering actions to defuse feelings of anxiety, fear, worry, and anger. Although the age range for this activity is second through sixth grade, it is also appropriate for older children to make a list of people they can call on for help and a safety plan.

Ask your child to put his hand on an 8½" × 11" piece of paper and spread his fingers. Then ask him to trace his handprint. On the fingers of the handprint, ask him to write the names and phone numbers of people he can call for help should he need it. On another piece of paper, help your child make a safety plan. Have him write down all the things he can do to feel safe—how to run to a neighbor's house or dial 911—in case of danger, violence, or stressful feelings.

This activity can be creative, and many children enjoy coloring the image; however, its purpose is to identify resources for children, such as people who could be called upon to help if violence recurs or if children feel unsafe in their home or neighborhood. Younger children may need help identifying phone numbers, but try to help your child list as many people as possible.

12 Years Old and Older

Journals

Encourage your child to journal or draw about the following situations. Ask him or her to include what the child or animal in the story or picture does to feel better and/or what he or she would do to make the animal or child feel better.

- A lonely, lost kitten that is wet, cold, and hungry.
- A doll or baby that cannot stop crying.
- A strong lion that is chased away from the family he grew up in.
- A magical bandage that could heal any hurt it was used for—how and where might your child use it?
- An imaginary suitcase where a child could pack away all hurting memories or problems. What would be placed there?

It is very important that you never make comments or corrections on the drawings or to the writing. The memories expressed, even bad ones, belong to your child. Anxious children can get emotional relief by expressing these memories on paper because it allows them to begin to control or manage the memory, rather than the memory controlling them. Only your child can decide what he or she would like to do with the drawings or writings.

Road Map Activity (Kordas & Steele, 1998)

This activity is best for adolescents, although younger children may be able to participate with extra guidance. Ask your child to draw a road on an 18" × 24" piece of paper and to put her current age at one end and her birth date at the other end. Explain that the space on the right side of the road is for places lived or visited, schools attended, or other important places. The space on the left side is for the bad and good things that have happened along the way. For instance, if the first destination is going to school and something bad (a divorce, death, etc.) or something good (learning to ride a bike or winning a competition) happened at that time, then have her write or draw them on the road map. Talk with your teenager to help generate some ideas and memories of what might be included on the road.

Help your teen only if she is having a hard time getting started. She may not remember things that happened in preschool and before. Ask your teenager to focus on the good things (getting a bike, riding without training wheels, winning a competition, being praised for special projects in school, making a new friend, being promoted to the next grade, a new addition to the family), but do not neglect the bad things that happened.

After the road map is filled in, help your teenager see how the trauma is just one part of life and that good things have happened, too. Despite the trauma in her life, she continues to move forward and accomplish new things. There is a part of your child that is a survivor, and you should stress that part to your child. Point out that, in life, we keep moving forward, driving down the road to the future. Every now and then there are some spots that slow us down, just like when there is construction work on the expressway, but we keep moving forward to the next destination, getting further away from some of the bad things that have happened, and we gain more and more experience at surviving the hard times.

Explain that, when something traumatic happens, it is like construction crews have put up a "Road Closed" or a "Detour" sign. The detour is not easy; the road is full of potholes, and there are usually only two lanes. Your teen cannot pass the car in front of her and has to go at the traffic's pace. A trauma can push us off the road, and there can be so many obstacles that we lose our sense of direction. Sometimes we forget where we wanted to go, or we may feel it is best to stay off the main road and not worry about going anywhere because it is too dangerous. Many people who have experienced a trauma think a lot of other horrible things are going to happen to them or others close to them if they keep going.

Finally, ask your teen to extend the road past the present to include a destination. The destination can be graduation, going to college, a holiday, or a family vacation. Emphasize that there is something to look forward to (the destination) and that sometimes trauma distracts us from our destinations, but it is important to keep sight of them. A destination acts like a magnet that keeps us moving forward even where there are detours. Destinations can always change, but when we do not have one in front of us, trauma keeps us from moving forward to find out what makes us hopeful and happy.

CONCLUSIONS

Trauma is a sensory experience of terror in which we feel unsafe and powerless to do anything about our situation. It is this terror and lack of security and control that teaches us what behaviors can help us feel safe and in control again. By helping parents understand the nature of trauma and implicit memory and how to respond to their children's traumatic experiences, therapists can assist both parents and children in regaining a sense of safety and normalcy. More important, providing practical information, appropriate responses, and activities to parents strengthens the bonds between parents and their children and empowers families to participate in their recovery from trauma.

REFERENCES

Byers, J. (1996). Children of the stones: Art therapy interventions in the West Bank. *Art Therapy: Journal of the American Art Therapy Association*, 13, 238–243.

Gil-Rivas, V., Holman, E. A., McIntosh, D. N., Poulin, M., & Silver, R. C. (2002). Nationwide longitudinal study of psychological responses to September 11. *Journal of the American Medical Association*, 288(10), 1235–1244.

Klein, N. (2001). *Healing images with children*. Watertown, WI: Inner Coaching.

Klein, N., Malchiodi, C. A., & Steele, W. (2002). *Helping children feel safe*.

Grosse Pointe Woods, MI: The National Institute for Trauma and Loss in Children.

Konarz, R. (2003). *Recognizing and responding: Infant and toddler grief.* Grosse Pointe Woods, MI: The National Institute for Trauma and Loss in Children.

Kordas, P., & Steele, W. (1998). *What color is your hurt?* Grosse Pointe Woods, MI: The National Institute for Trauma and Loss in Children.

Rothschild, B. (2000). *The body remembers.* New York: Norton.

Siegel, D., & Hartzell, M. (2003). *Parenting from the inside out: How a deeper self-understanding can help you raise children who thrive.* New York: Tarcher/Penguin.

Squire, L. R. (1994). *Memory and brain.* New York. Oxford University Press.

Steele, W., & Raider, M. (2001). *Structured sensory intervention for children, adolescents, and parents (SITCAP).* New York: Mellen Press.

van Dalen, A. (2001). Juvenile violence and addiction: Tangled roots in childhood trauma. *Journal of Social Work Practice in the Addictions, 1,* 25–40.

van der Kolk, B. A., McFarlane, A. C., & Weisaeth, L. (Eds.). (1996). *Traumatic stress: The effects of overwhelming experience on mind, body, and society.* New York: Guilford Press.

Williams, M. (2005). When children's parents are traumatized. In D. Catherall (Ed.), *Family stressors: Interventions for stress and trauma* (pp. 55–76). New York: Brunner-Routledge.

ADDITIONAL RESOURCES FOR PARENTS

Answering Difficult Questions
www.pbs.org/parents/issuesadvice/talkingwithkids/war/questions.html

Children and Fear of War and Terrorism: Tips for Parents and Teachers
www.nasponline.org/NEAT/children_war_general.html

General Parenting Articles
www.kidsource.com/kidsource/pages/parenting.general.html

http://www.zerotothree.org

Gift from Within
www.giftfromwithin.org and *www.anothersgrief.com*

An international nonprofit organization dedicated to those who suffer from and are at risk for PTSD and those who care for traumatized individuals.

Life Challenges
www.lifechallenges.org

Parents Trauma Resource Center
www.tlcinstitute.org

Guidelines, activities and information for parents to help their grieving traumatized child.

Positive Parenting
www.cwla.org/parenting/default.htm

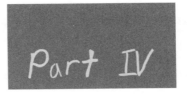

CREATIVE INTERVENTION
AS PREVENTION

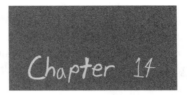

Chapter 14

Resilience and Posttraumatic Growth in Traumatized Children

Cathy A. Malchiodi
William Steele
Caelan Kuban

What are the best ways to help children become more resilient to the effects of trauma? Are there strategies that support emotional growth, posttrauma, in children who have experienced trauma? The answers to these questions have to do with resilience and posttraumatic growth, terms used to describe the experience of positive coping following adversity. Resilience and posttraumatic growth represent two different responses to the stress of traumatic events. In brief, resilience is generally defined as the ability to "bounce back" or return to prior functioning, while posttraumatic growth implies that functioning is improved in one or more aspects posttrauma (Ungerleider, 2003).

Research indicates that children who are resilient will have some transient reactions, but very few will develop posttraumatic stress disorder (PTSD) (Bonanno, Papo, & O'Neill, 2004). Children who experience posttraumatic growth have personal characteristics that are somewhat different from those found in resilient children. These characteristics allow them to cope more effectively than other individuals (Tedeschi & Calhoun, 2004; Wiesel & Amie, 2004).

This chapter explains resilience and posttraumatic growth and their importance in work with traumatized children. It also presents strategies to enhance resilience in children and to encourage posttraumatic growth in children who are recovering from traumatic events. Finally, practical activities that support resilience and posttraumatic growth are described to help therapists address both intervention and prevention in their work with child survivors of trauma.

RESILIENCE

Resilience in children exists prior to exposure to trauma or adversity and has been described as the ability to recover or return to pretrauma levels of functioning following minimal reactions to exposure (Bonanno, Papa, & O'Neill, 2001). Resilient individuals may experience transient challenges to normal functioning (e.g., several weeks of sporadic preoccupation or restless sleep) but generally exhibit healthy functioning over time and a capacity for positive emotions. The following factors are associated with resilience in children (Cloitre, Morin, & Linares, 2005; Rice & Groves, 2005):

- Above-average verbal communication skills, cognitive abilities, and problem-solving abilities.
- Positive beliefs about self and the future.
- Talents, hobbies, and/or special skills.
- Ability to self-regulate behavior.
- Ability to ask for help from adults.
- Stable, nurturing parent or caregiver and extended family and supportive, positive school experiences.
- Consistent family environment, such as family traditions, rituals, and/or structured routines.
- Strong cultural connections and cultural identity.

Cloitre et al. (2005) note that a number of factors affect resilience in children. Overall, resilient children are more able to cope with trauma. Proximity to the traumatic event, relationship to victims, and amount of emotional suffering (fear or panic) will challenge even the most resilient children during the short term; however, resilient children will do better than children who do not have resilient character-istics.

Genetics may play a role in ability to adapt in resilient children, but family characteristics are also often a strong influence. For exam-ple, children who have parents who model positive reactions to trau-ma do better than those children who do not. Children with strong community support in the form of extended family, friends, religious groups, or cultural groups are generally more resilient.

Finally, developmental factors influence resilience, and resilient behaviors are demonstrated differently in young children, children, and adolescents. For example, resilient school-age children who talk about upsetting experiences can practice positive self-talk and ask oth-ers for help. Resilient adolescents have these skills too, but they also can understand the feelings of others and express interest in the future.

IDENTIFYING RESILIENCE IN TRAUMATIZED CHILDREN

It is important to keep in mind that some young victims, even those who are resilient, may benefit from early intervention. For many, the simple passage of time provides the opportunity for resilience to emerge and trauma-specific intervention is unnecessary. Those with preexisting risk factors such as previous trauma, arousal, dissociative reactions, and lack of social support are in need of both intervention and activities to support the development of resilience. Helping pro-fessionals need to screen all children for these possible risk factors as well as for their abilities to manage traumatic experience with limited intervention.

The following questions may help provide some sense of how chil-dren perceive a traumatic event, how they are experiencing it, and how resilient they are after. These questions are appropriate for school-age children and adolescents, and their responses to these ques-tions should be considered along with other behavioral observations to determine how they are coping from day to day.

- With all that has happened, what makes you smile, even just a little?
- Despite all that has happened, have you been able to laugh a little when things strike you as funny?

- On a scale of 1 to 10, with 10 being the most positive, how positive do you feel after this difficult crisis? [With younger children, it is helpful to use a feelings thermometer or other visual tool to convey the idea of scaling.]
- On a scale of 1 to 10, with 10 being the most stressful, where would you rate the stress you are experiencing?
- Do you believe you will bounce back from this? Have you already begun to do so?
- Have your plans for the future changed since this happened or not?
- Do you find that you push most of what happened out of your mind?

Creative expressions can also provide a window to resilience in children. In talking with children about their drawings of a traumatic event, it is important to explore and discuss whether or not elements of rescue, caregiving, or protection are included. Children who have hope for the future generally include one or more of these elements in their art expressions. For example, a child who survived the tsunami in southeast Asia depicted a scene in which a number of adult caregivers and rescue vehicles such as aircraft carrying food and first aid appear (Figure 14.1). In a similar manner, a child who was displaced after Hurricane Katrina included themes of rescue in his drawing (Figure 14.2). These are visual indications of resilience in children who have an internal sense that they will be supported and that life will improve despite adverse circumstances.

SUPPORTING RESILIENCE IN CHILDREN EXPOSED TO TRAUMA

Recently, there has been an increased focus on encouraging and enhancing resilience in children, particularly those who have been traumatized. Research on resilience has demonstrated that it is especially important to identify and observe children who quickly return to pretrauma levels of functioning so that programs to encourage resilience in high-risk children can be developed and enhanced. As a result of this research, the following factors are believed to promote resilience in children (American Psychological Association, 2004a, 2004b):

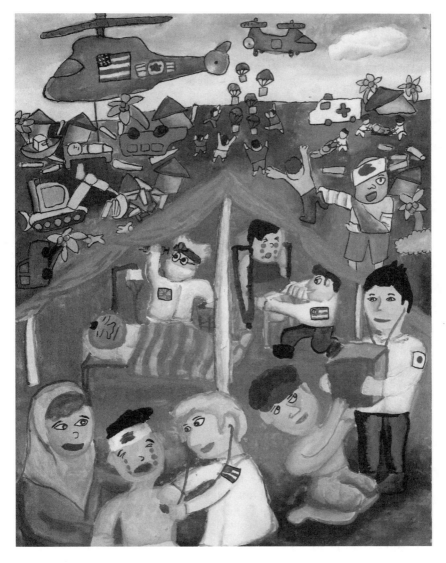

FIGURE 14.1. *After Tsunami*, painting by an adolescent boy. Courtesy of International Children's Art Foundation at *www.icaf.org*.

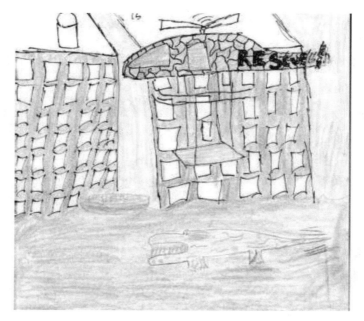

FIGURE 14.2. Drawing of rescue efforts after Hurricane Katrina by 16-year-old boy. Courtesy of Katrina's Kids Art Project, *www.katrinaskidsproject.org*.

- Providing perceptions of safety and security.
- Providing the opportunity to discuss feelings and concerns to correct any misperceptions and to offer reassurance.
- Providing predictable activities and normal routines to enhance a sense of safety and security.
- Providing and maintaining interpersonal connections such as friendships and social activities.
- Encouraging healthy behaviors such as exercise, sleep, and proper nutrition.
- Educating and encouraging parents or caregivers to model positive coping skills (nurturing behaviors, consistency, and clear limits) to children and help children practice these skills.
- Reducing children's exposure to events that increase stress (for example, viewing repeated images of disaster or terrorist acts) and encouraging them to participate in other activities (games, reading, creative expression, or athletics).
- Having response plans that address psychological impact in the case of mass trauma (terrorism or natural disaster).

Overall, the relationship between a parent or caregiver and a child is considered the strongest factor for resilience in children and is a significant factor in how well children do after a trauma (Siegel, 1999). Riley (2001), an art therapist and marriage and family therapist, underscores the importance of using sensory modalities such as drawing, play, and music to enhance relationships and attachment between parent and child. Riley observes that shared sensory activities not only support parent–child attachment, but also may "reprogram" behavior, reinforcing successful and positive bonding experiences and the child's resilience. Steele and Raider (2001) discuss the importance of intervening with distressed, terrified, traumatized children through implicit, sensory activities that focus on restoring a sense of safety and power. They observe that trauma interventions that only engage cognitive processes and explicit memories are less likely to be effective because traumatized children are in a high state of arousal. Steele and others agree that children must reexperience a sense of safety from and control (regulation) over those reactions induced by trauma before they can engage the explicit processes needed for cognitive restructuring (i.e., the reordering of the experience in a way they can now manage makes this memory a resource rather than a memory to be avoided). The creative interventions that follow are examples of implicit, sensory activities that can assist in the development of resilience in children.

CREATIVE INTERVENTIONS TO PROMOTE RESILIENCE IN CHILDREN

In brief, creative interventions to support and enhance resilience should capitalize on the factors relevant to resilience, including the parent–child relationship; the child's feelings of capability, personal safety, and self-esteem; and positive memories, despite the experience of trauma and loss. The presence of a stable, nurturing parent or caregiver who provides consistency in family values, routine, and discipline can instill resilience in infants and toddlers and help children and adolescents feel safe. Early experiences of attachment during everyday moments such as diapering, feeding, holding, bathing, eye contact, gentle touch, reciprocal smiling, and talking form the basis for resilience in later life. A child whose interactions are meaningful and safe will learn trust, connection, pleasure, and contentment. For children who have not had these experiences, activities that approximate positive relationships, attachment, and trust strengthen children's abilities to cope with stress; these experiences support the development of healthy neural connections (Siegel, 1999).

Interventions with parents and younger children (ages 3 to 6 years) emphasize enjoying activities together to reinforce attachment through joint sensory experiences. Suggested activities include but are not limited to the following:

1. *Two-way scribble drawing.* In this activity, parent and child create a scribble together on one large piece of paper with crayons, felt-tip markers, or chalk pastels. This activity can also be made into a game by instructing the parent and child to take turns being the leader in a scribble chase across the paper. For example, if the child is the leader, then the parent follows the child's scribble on the paper. To supplement the activity, music can be used to add to the sensory experience. When the scribbles are complete, the parent and child can find shapes or images within the lines and add additional colors and details.

2. *Exploring art and play materials together.* Drawing materials, finger paint, clay, small toys, or a sandtray can be offered to stimulate interaction between parent and child.

3. *Co-creating an environment for a favorite character or toy.* If a child has a favorite animated or storybook character or figure, it can be used as the inspiration for this activity. The child and parent are asked to co-create an environment or world for the figure where the figure can feel happy, cared for, and safe. Three-dimensional materials such as a shoebox or other small container for the figure, clay, and collage material can be used to create the environment. What is important about this activity is the dyadic work involved and the themes of nurturance, comfort, and security, all of which are important to the development of resilience.

4. *Singing songs.* In resilient children, singing is often a self-affirming, spontaneous form of self-expression. With traumatized children, therapists can use familiar songs to enhance interpersonal relationships and attachment; music contributes to the process of engagement between children and helping professionals. Lullabies, for example, naturally recreate the experience of bonding because of their comforting, rhythmic, and soothing tones and words. Calming music also provides a sense of containment and reassurance, building feelings

of trust and reducing hyperarousal and generalized fears and anxieties. Choosing songs known to both the therapist and the child can instill a sense of safety and a starting point for beginning reparative experiences during the course of intervention. For young children who have experienced physical or emotional neglect or abuse, the sound and words of familiar songs can provide the sensation of nurturance, positive attachment, and relaxation through singing or listening.

Interventions with parents and older children (ages 7 to 12 years) emphasize enjoying activities together to reinforce attachment and can introduce specific themes to enhance or develop resilience. In brief, interventions should encourage self-awareness, particularly recognition of emotions, communication, and self-regulation. They should also help develop social awareness and interaction, empathy, appreciation of individual differences, and collaboration. Finally, interventions should enhance abilities to solve problems and make decisions and develop flexibility and personal strengths.

Suggested activities include but are not limited to the following:

1. *Co-creating with parent a picture or making a collage of a positive memory.* Trauma work often involves the exploration of negative, intrusive, or recurring memories about what happened. While traumatic events include unhappy feelings and experiences, it is important to remind children that there are good memories that can be enjoyed. Experiencing these good memories in the form of a drawing, collage, or other creative experience can be a tangible statement that life has not always been sad, hopeless, or discouraging and crises can be overcome. For example, in the case of traumatic loss, this picture can be about a positive memory of the deceased or what has been lost, such as a home, to recall positive experiences that may be temporarily forgotten because of worries or fears about the future. Instead of a drawing, the therapist may ask children or adolescents to create a collage of personal photos that have good memories or a collection of songs that encourage positive thoughts.

2. *Co-creating with parent a collage or drawing about the child titled "the good things about me."* Using collage materials, colored pencils, or oil pastels, the parent and child can work together to co-create art to represent "good things" about the child. The therapist may prompt discussion by asking questions such as "What is one good thing you do at school?" or "What is one thing that makes you a good friend?"

Asking questions about different aspects of the child's life such as school, home, friends, sports, or church may help the child recall positive aspects of him- or herself. The prompting can also focus on the positive ways the child handled a traumatic situation or loss. Hearing the parent give praise and creating an image of the good things about him- or herself can be a sensory experience that identifies capabilities, self-esteem, and personal contributions in addition to reinforcing attachment.

This activity can be easily adapted to a children's trauma or loss group. For example, children in the group may be asked to write a few words about or make a picture of a good thing about each group member. The child participants then use the words or images to create individual collages about their positive characteristics.

3. *Creating an invention to solve a problem or situation.* The Israel Psychotrauma Center encourages the development of resilience in children and parents in its ongoing trauma intervention programs with survivors of terrorism and war. Children are asked to focus on their strengths while expressing their experiences of bombings and life-threatening circumstances. Group leaders have initiated a number of resilience-building activities for participants, including one activity that directed children to invent a device to deal with rocket bombings. In Figure 14.3, the "rocket pump" sucks the missile up and sends it back to where it came from. In another drawing, a child depicts a "hiding house" that can go underwater so that missiles will not be able to find it (Figure 14.4). The goal of this particular intervention is to enhance the sensory experience of personal empowerment through active, hands-on participation.

POSTTRAUMATIC GROWTH

While many children exhibit resilient responses to traumatic events, others may have a different type of posttrauma experience. Tedeschi and Calhoun (2004) refer to this experience as "posttraumatic growth" and suggest that it develops as a result of lessons learned from exposure to trauma or crisis. Posttraumatic growth is a relatively new area of study that differs from resilience and is manifested in several clearly defined behaviors and thought patterns not necessarily present prior to exposure (Turner & Cox, 2004). Research on adults indicates that

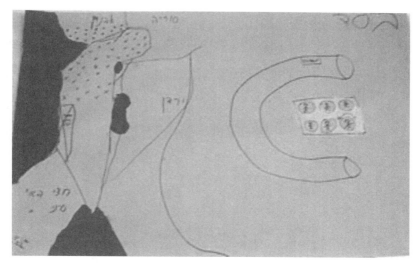

FIGURE 14.3. "Rocket pump." Courtesy of Israel Psychotrauma Center, *www.traumaweb.org/au060801.html.*

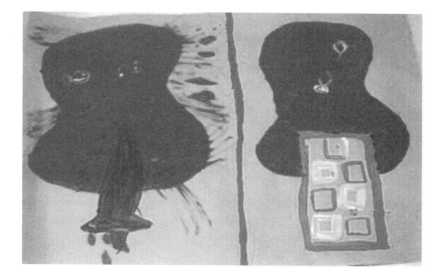

FIGURE 14.4. "Hiding house." Courtesy of Israel Psychotrauma Center, *www.traumaweb.org/au060801.html.*

posttraumatic growth includes greater appreciation for life, an increased sense of personal strength, realization of new possibilities, and improved interpersonal relationships. In other words, the experience of trauma produces valuable psychological and interpersonal gains in some individuals.

Experiences that children and adolescents may have that are associated with posttraumatic growth include (Tedeschi & Calhoun, 2004; Ungerleider, 2003):

- Feeling more compassion and empathy for others after personal trauma or loss.
- Increased psychological and emotional maturity when compared to similar-age peers.
- Increased resiliency.
- A more complex appreciation of life when compared to similar-age peers.
- A deeper understanding of personal values, purpose, and meaning in life.
- A greater value placed on interpersonal relationships.

It is possible for children to display resilience (a high level of coping after a trauma) and not exhibit posttraumatic growth. Additionally, it is possible for children who experience posttraumatic growth to display several of the characteristics mentioned above, yet not be resilient in the true sense of the word.

IDENTIFYING POSTTRAUMATIC GROWTH IN TRAUMATIZED CHILDREN

As with resilience, asking children questions may be useful in exploring and determining if they have experienced posttraumatic growth. These questions are based on the available literature about how individuals express posttraumatic growth after a crisis or loss.

- Would you be willing to tell me of the details of what happened?
- What is it that you now will no longer take for granted?
- What do you appreciate now more than before this happened?

- Would you say you are the kind of person who never gives up and will not give up even with all that has happened?
- On a scale of 1 to 10, with 10 being the highest value, where would you put your value for family and friends since this event happened?
- Do you believe that you could be of help to others who have faced a similar situation?
- Would you say you have the same or greater appreciation for life since this happened?
- Since this happened, are you doing more or doing less?

ENCOURAGING POSTTRAUMATIC GROWTH IN TRAUMATIZED CHILDREN

Research remains sparse on how to promote posttraumatic growth in children who have experienced adversity. Most of the current literature on posttraumatic growth focuses on children who have survived cancer or serious illness; less is known about those children who have experienced trauma from violent environments or abuse, family dysfunction, natural or manmade disasters, or mass trauma. There is, however, a growing body of research on children's recovery from trauma and interventions used to reduce posttraumatic stress. Several authors observe that service programs and interventions that reduce posttraumatic stress may help encourage posttraumatic growth. These interventions may include but are not limited to the following:

- Social support from significant others (family, friends, other survivors, and support groups) during trauma recovery.
- Developing a cohesive trauma narrative (telling one's story, being heard, and being validated).
- Understanding that one is not to blame for what happened.

Most important, researchers concur that providing opportunities early in treatment help children develop an understanding of the traumatic event and their feelings and responses and help integrate the experience of trauma into their lives in ways that allow them to better manage that experience (Calhoun & Tedeschi, 1999; Tedeschi & Calhoun, 2004; Turner & Cox, 2004).

CREATIVE INTERVENTIONS TO ENCOURAGE POSTTRAUMATIC GROWTH

Creative activities can be used as opportunities to help children not only express "what happened," but also to explore what they have learned since the traumatic event. While it is important to provide children with the opportunity to communicate their memories of and feelings about what happened, it is equally important to ask them to explore how the experience may have helped them to become stronger or discover new things. Otherwise, they are left with the sensory aspects of the trauma and have not identified how they have changed for the better in some cases since the crisis or loss occurred.

The following activities introduce children to some of the concepts associated with posttraumatic growth. While not all children will experience posttraumatic growth as a result of these interventions, they help children identify their own resources for adaptive coping, explore the meaning of what has happened, and, with the help of a therapist, reflect on what they have learned from traumatic events.

1. *Creating a "powerful and powerless" collage.* This activity is for older children and adolescents who can understand the concepts of what makes one feel powerful and powerless. The activity can be redirected, if appropriate, to create a collage about "when you felt powerful or powerless" since the traumatic event happened. Situations that may have caused feelings of powerlessness can be explored to help the child understand that he or she is not at fault for what happened.

2. *Personal or power shield.* This activity for older children can be accomplished on 8½" × 11" paper with a simple drawing of a shield on it or on a full-size shield that can be created out of posterboard or cardboard. Children are asked to decorate the shield with images or words that answer the following questions: What makes you feel powerful or strong? What is one thing you learned from what happened? Since the trauma happened, what makes you happy? The goal is to create a shield that contains experiences and feelings that help child survivors recognize what they have learned, how they have grown since the traumatic event, and what helps them deal with life's adversities.

3. *Photo collage of "my support group."* This activity works best if children can collect and photocopy photographs of loved ones, friends, and/or caregivers who assisted them during a trauma or loss. If

possible, it is useful to make this activity special by helping children frame or laminate their creations so that they can hang their photo collages and regularly recall positive memories of helpers. Those children who attend a medical support group, such as a pediatric cancer group, can make a collage of fellow participants from whom they received support and encouragement during their treatment. This image can be a powerful source for exploration and development of empathy for others who have been through similar experiences.

4. *Butterfly life cycle.* This activity is useful with younger children but can be applied to individuals of all ages who have experienced a life-changing traumatic loss. It uses the metaphor of a caterpillar changing into a butterfly as a way to demonstrate how things eventually change after a crisis. For the youngest children, butterfly and caterpillar puppets and a paper bag (the cocoon) can be used as props to tell the following story (adapted from Goffney, 2002):

> "Going through a loss is like the birth of a butterfly. Before the butterfly is ready to fly free in the world, it has to go through many changes as a caterpillar. While all these changes happen, the caterpillar stays safe in its cocoon [keep the caterpillar in a paper bag].
>
> "When people go through a bad event or have someone they love die, it hurts them. Sometimes the only way we can feel better is to stay in our cocoons for a while. While we are in our cocoons, we have many different thoughts and feelings. Grieving is about having many different thoughts and feelings while protecting ourselves for a little while as if we were in a safe cocoon.
>
> "As time goes by, we do not need that cocoon as much as we did at first. We eventually want to spread our wings and fly again [have the caterpillar break out of the cocoon and become the butterfly]."

For group participation, children can make butterflies out of colored paper, caterpillars from the fingers of old gloves, and cocoons from brown paper bags. This activity can also be adapted to other expressive techniques such as dance/movement, dramatic role play, creative play, and storytelling. For example, the therapist can tell the story of the caterpillar's transformation and facilitate children's spontaneous movement either individually or as a group activity.

CONCLUSIONS

Lew (2002) summarizes the basic needs that all children have after a traumatic event and require for emotional well-being: to connect, to feel capable, to count, and to have courage. These needs are relevant to trauma intervention because they encompass the principles of relationship, a positive sense of self, and the ability to overcome adversity. A feeling of connection to others who care, recognition of personal capabilities and contributions, and an internal sense of control form the foundations of resilience and posttraumatic growth in individuals of all ages.

Research continues to expand the existing knowledge about resilience and posttraumatic growth in children who have experienced trauma. While resilient behavior may exist in many children pre-trauma, both resilience and posttraumatic growth can be developed in children to prepare them better for future exposure or adversity. Fortunately, many of the psychological factors that contribute to resilient behaviors and posttraumatic growth have been identified, providing directions for helping professionals cultivate these characteristics in children. These characteristics can be cultivated early in life to help reduce and even prevent the negative impact of traumatic exposure and following traumatic exposure as the focus of intervention.

REFERENCES

American Psychological Association. (2004a). *The road to resilience*. Retrieved February 4, 2006, from *www.apahelpcenter.org/featuredtopics/feature.php?id=6*.

American Psychological Association. (2004b). *Resilience guide for parents and teachers*. Retrieved February 4, 2006, from *www.apahelpcenter.org/featuredtopics/feature.php?id=39*.

Bonanno, G. A., Papa, A., & O'Neill, K. (2001). Loss and human resilience. *Applied and Preventive Psychology, 10*, 193–206.

Calhoun, L., & Tedeschi, R. (1999). *Facilitating posttraumatic growth: A clinician's guide*. Mahwah, NJ: Erlbaum.

Cloitre, M., Morin, N., & Linares, O. (2005). *Children's resilience in the face of trauma*. New York: New York University Child Study Center.

Goffney, D. (2002). Seasons of grief: Helping children grow through loss. In J. Loewy & A. Hara (Eds.), *Caring for the caregiver: The use of music and music therapy in grief and trauma* (pp. 54–62). Silver Spring, MD: American Music Therapy Association.

Lew, A. (2002). Helping children cope in an increasingly threatening world. *The Family Journal, 10*(2), 134–138.

Rice, K. F., & Groves, B. M. (2005). *Hope and healing: A caregiver's guide to helping young children affected by trauma.* Washington, DC: Zero to Three Press.

Riley, S. (2001). *Group process made visible.* New York: Brunner Routledge.

Siegel, D. (1999). *The developing mind.* New York: Guilford Press.

Steele, W., & Raider, M. (2001). Structured sensory intervention for traumatized children, adolescents, and parents. *Trauma and Loss: Research and Interventions, 1*(2), 5–10.

Tedeschi, R. G., & Calhoun, L. G. (2004). Posttraumatic growth: Conceptual foundations and empirical evidence. *Psychological Inquiry, 15*(1), 1–18.

Turner, D., & Cox, H. (2004). Facilitating posttraumatic growth. *Health and Quality of Life Outcome, 2*, 43.

Ungerleider, S. (2003). Posttraumatic growth: Understanding a new field of research. *The Prevention Researcher, 10*, 1–3.

Wiesel, R., & Amie, M. (2004). Posttraumatic growth among holocaust survivors. *Journal of Loss and Trauma, 8*, 229–237.

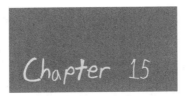

Chapter 15

Ready . . . , Set . . . , Relax!

Relaxation Strategies
with Children and Adolescents

Roger J. Klein

"Every night I sit and weep. I hear them yell, I do not peep. First they argue, then they scream. . . . BOOM. . . . then dad slams the screen. I race to my window to see him walk . . . walk to his car. . . . I do not talk. John and I go downstairs. Mom looks like she's been fighting off millions of bears. We quietly raced back up to our rooms. Then he comes home. You can tell . . . BOOM. Then mom leaves, he comes upstairs and we fear for . . . oh gasp!!!! John is screaming . . . oh hear [sic] he comes!"—Aaron, grade 6

"I have a sister who is 10 years old. She has Tourette's syndrome. She throws things at me; she bites me; she swears at me and then sometimes I'll call her names and my mom yells at me and blames me and I get sent to my room. I feel worried a lot."—Sue, grade 7

"Every time I try and fall asleep I get really scared and then I can't fall asleep so that's why I go to my mom and dad's room."—Amber, grade 3

"I'm totally stressed by school and friends and not getting along with my mom. . . . that's why I smoke pot. It settles me down and then I don't have to feel so stressed out."—Bill, grade 9

These students' self-reports typify the stresses of childhood. Children who have been traumatized like Aaron or are prone to anxiety like Amber benefit from techniques that help them develop problem-solving response sets and self-soothing techniques. This chapter outlines the use of progressive relaxation, guided imagery, and positive self-talk as ways to help children overcome stress and develop an internal locus of control.

Children face more and more stress, and most never learn effective coping strategies. Video games, the Internet, television, homework, and practice, lessons, and competitions often replace nature's cure of creative play as a way of reducing the negative effects of stress and trauma. In the past, most attention in the field of stress research has been directed toward adults, with little attention paid to stress as it affects children.

The violent events perpetrated by children and adolescents in the late 1990s drew much attention to the need to understand what is happening in children's lives. These events, coupled with September 11, 2001, the ongoing threat of terror, and parents' fears of letting their children play unsupervised, has led to acknowledgment of the need for ways to help children cope with stress.

A look at the societal changes over the past several decades reveals the difficult challenges our children now face. The average elementary school child watches 3 hours of television a day and spends 3 more hours playing video games and using computers (Baron, 2000). Prekindergarten educational programs for children as young as 3 years old emerged in the late 1980s (Fiske, 1986). As children advance in school, pressures increase. The difficulty and amount of homework, competition for grades, fear of not being promoted due to high-stakes state testing programs, and peer pressure are a few of the many things that can add to a child's level of stress. Berliner and Amrein (2003) research points out the flaws in the No Child Left Behind policy and has shown that the higher the stakes, the less well children tend to perform because of the extreme anxiety produced by these types of tests.

I and many other mental health professionals have observed that the number and severity of child and adolescent stressors has increased dramatically in the past two decades. A report completed in 2000 by the National Institutes of Health (U.S. Public Health Service, 2000) reported that one in every five children was suffering from mental illness. Those of us who work daily with children know they are experiencing a great deal of stress. They have many fears and anxieties and worry more than most adults might suspect. Stress also contributes to physical complaints by children (Rutter, 1998). Research supports specific psycho–physiological patterns occurring in children with a variety of presenting physical problems including anxiety disorders, headaches, sleep disturbance, attention-deficit/hyperactivity disorder (ADHD), and elimination disorders (Culbert, Reaney, & Kohen, 1994; Gagnon, Hudnell, & Andrasck, 1992; Murphy, 1992).

The traditional therapy-only approach is an inadequate model to deal with the large numbers of children suffering from stress-related problems. Even if there were adequate numbers of trained therapists, only the most severe cases are generally offered therapeutic intervention. Of those cases, many parents refuse or are hesitant to become involved in the mental health care system. The high numbers of children under stress and the severity of their problems convinced me to redirect my energy into a primary stress prevention program built on a foundation of teaching muscle relaxation skills and using imagery to facilitate learning positive self-talk.

METHODS OF RELAXATION

According to Selye (1956), stress results when our bodies react in a "general adaptation syndrome." This syndrome consists of three stages: an alarm reaction, the resistance stage, and the exhaustion stage. In the first stage, the body reacts to the stressor and causes the hypothalamus to produce a biochemical "messenger" that causes the pituitary gland to secrete adrenocorticotropic hormone (ACTH) into the blood (Selye, 1956). This hormone causes the secretion of adrenaline and other corticoids, which causes shrinkage of the thymus and a concomitant influence on heart rate, blood pressure, respiration rate, etc. In the second stage, resistance develops. This process is called a "fight or flight" response and was first described as an emergency reaction by Walter Cannon (1914). This process was helpful to ancient man, who often needed to prepare for physical action during the hunt or in confrontations with an enemy. These same physiological responses occur now, regardless of the stressful conditions, most of which are emotional rather than physical. The third stage, exhaustion, occurs if there is continuous exposure to the same or similar stressors.

Benson's (1976) research indicated a variety of techniques that can be used to quiet the aroused sympathetic nervous system.

> Each of us possesses a natural and innate protective mechanism against "overstress," which allows us to turn off harmful bodily effects, to counter the effects of the fight-or-flight response. This response against "overstress" brings on bodily changes that decrease heart rate, lower metabolism, decrease the rate of breathing, and bring the body back into what is probably a healthier balance. This is the Relaxation Response. (p. 250)

Benson suggests that evoking the relaxation response is extremely simple if the following four essential elements are included: (1) a quiet environment, (2) a mental device such as a word or a phrase repeated in a specific fashion over and over again, (3) the adoption of a passive attitude, and (4) a comfortable position.

Currently, there are a number of proven techniques that elicit the relaxation response. These include biofeedback, meditation, yoga, hypnosis, systematic desensitization, autogenic training, music, imagery, and progressive muscle relaxation (PMR). A review of the literature of large-group interventions suggests that the most effective of these techniques, when considering cost and ease of implementation, are imagery, PMR, behavioral relaxation, and music.

Imagery

The key concept of imagery is the belief that when people imagine themselves successfully performing a certain behavior, the likelihood of actually doing so increases (Anderson, 1983; Klein, 2001; Sherman, Cialdini, Schwartzman, & Reynolds, 1985). The use of imagery by psychologists has been making a comeback in popularity during the last 25 years. Psychologists and others have long noted the mind's ability to mimic internally the possible motions and transformations of objects in the external world (Shepard & Cooper, 1982).

The power of imagery was noted as early as the 18th century by David Hume (1748/1907), who wrote that to "join incongruous shapes and appearances costs the imagination no more trouble than to conceive the most natural and familiar objects. . . . This creative power of the mind amounts to no more than the faculty of comprehending, transposing, augmenting, or diminishing the material afforded us by the senses and experience" (p. 253).

The study of imagery has always been a part of the science of the mind. During the dominance of Watson and behaviorism, imagery was studied as "conditioned hallucinations" (Selye, 1956, p. 14). Today, imagery is a well-documented and successful technique not only to influence behavior, but also to enhance physical healing (Anbar, 2001; NewsRx.com, 2004) and children's motor performance (Afremow & Overby, 2001).

Progressive Muscle Relaxation

Jacobson (1944) developed the technique of PMR, which is still the muscle relaxation technique referred to most often in the literature and probably the one that has had the most widespread application. In this technique, the individual concentrates on progressively relaxing one muscle group after another while comparing the difference between tension and relaxation in each muscle group. The use of PMR is prevalent in the literature as a means of reducing anxiety. Relaxation techniques like PMR have been used to help children become more focused and receptive to subsequent imagery scripts.

According to Chang and Hiebert (1989), PMR at the elementary school level has been used primarily with children diagnosed as hyperactive and/or having learning and academic problems. These authors cite a number of studies that report encouraging results using PMR as a behavior management strategy with hyperactive children. Loffredo, Omizo, and Hammett (1984) provided three 15-minute PMR training sessions on a biweekly basis to 16 hyperactive boys of average intelligence, 5 to 7 years old. Mothers, who participated in group relaxation separately from their sons, were requested to cue their children to relax prior to situations where they might become anxious or agitated. They were also requested to practice relaxation at home with them. Porter and Omizo (1984) trained two groups of 11 hyperactive first- and second-grade boys in relaxation and stretching. Parents of the children in the second treatment group were requested to encourage them to practice relaxation daily at home, but no evidence was given to indicate that they actually did so. Both treatment groups improved their scores as compared to a control group on a locus of control scale. In addition, Chan (2002) reported that parents often seek alternative treatments such as PMR when addressing the needs of children with ADHD.

Behavioral Relaxation

One does not necessarily have to tense and relax muscle groups to achieve deep muscle relaxation. Imagining one's muscles tense and then consciously releasing tension can achieve the same results. Sometimes termed behavioral relaxation (Schilling & Poppen, 1983), this form of relaxation simply requires the subject to progressively let go of the tension in each muscle group rather than first tensing the group and then releasing the tension. A 1998 study (Rasid & Parish) compared 18 high school students in a behavioral relaxation group, 20 students in a PMR group, and 17 students in a no-treatment control group. All training was done for the first and second groups via videotaped instructions of the appropriate relaxation technique. Both groups completed four 20-minute training sessions in 2 weeks. The day after the last treatments were administered to the relaxation groups, all three groups were asked to complete the State–Trait Anxiety Inventory. The findings indicated that the state anxiety scores for the first and second groups did not vary significantly from one another but were both significantly lower than the state anxiety scores for the students in the control group. These findings indicate that both behavioral relaxation and PMR are capable of helping high school students reduce their state anxiety. Two other studies with high school students as subjects indicated that they are less likely to practice PMR because of the effort it takes to tense muscles (Field, Grizzle, Scafidi, & Schanberg, 1996). The teenagers in these two studies both commented that PMR was hard work.

My own experience in working with both behavioral relaxation and PMR reinforces these findings. I often use PMR with young children and switch to behavioral relaxation with teens. Both procedures are combined in a stress management program I helped design for elementary school children called Ready . . . , Set . . . , R.E.L.A.X. (Relax, Enjoy, Learn, Appreciate, eXpand) (Allen & Klein, 1996). The first part of the program teaches children to use PMR to achieve the relaxation response. After adequate practice with PMR, the children in the study were able to achieve the relaxation response using behavioral relaxation in the form of stories that incorporated both behavioral relaxation and imagery. The 123 children in the original study outperformed the control group on the Metropolitan Achieve-ment Tests and achieved significantly lower scores on self-report mea-sures of depression and anxiety. In addition they had a significant increase in their self-report of self-concept as measured by the Piers–Harris Self-Concept Scale.

Another effective muscle relaxation strategy is called the fast/slow technique. It is particularly useful with preschool and early elementary school-age children. It requires the child to follow the directions of the facilitator, who asks the child to move various body parts as fast as possible and then as slow as possible. Some hyperactive children who rarely move slowly begin to understand the concept of "slow down" when they pair those words with the muscle memory of moving vari-ous muscle groups slowly.

In addition to the above techniques, I often teach a simple, fast way to relax, which is used after the child or teen has mastered pro-gressive relaxation. On the count of 1, I ask children to shift their gaze to the ceiling without moving their neck; on 2, they are instructed to close their eyes and take a deep breath; and on 3, to let go of the breath, bow their heads gently forward, and release all tension in their muscles while saying the words calm and relax. "Calm" and "relax" are the key words that have been learned from the previous relaxation practices. When saying "calm" and "relax," the child is asked to imag-ine one hand or the other to begin to feel very light and buoyant, as if a group of helium balloons were attached to the arm. With each slow breath the suggestion is given that the hand and arm get lighter and lighter until the hand begins to slowly rise (the child can be asked to gently lift the arm if it does not begin to rise on its own). The higher the arm raises, the deeper the relaxation. The goal is to have the hand reach the child's face, at which time a very deep relaxed state has been achieved. The child then repeats whatever positive image or phrase has been practiced.

Music and Stress Reduction

The ancient schools of music believed that it was the bridge linking all things. Therapeutic use of music has its roots in primitive times, when it was used during incantations to ward off spirits. During the 16th and 17th centuries, music was used to treat depression or effect behavior change (Rolla, 1993). Following the ideas of Pythagoras, the classical music era composers built a sacred canon of specific harmonies, inter-vals, and proportions into their music. These ideas became the basis of baroque music, which was supposed to affect the listener by aligning, harmonizing, and synchronizing mind and body to more harmonious patterns (Ostrander & Schroeder, 1979). Sedative music, such as the baroque, has been found to be effective in stress reduction as measured by physiological changes such as galvanic skin response (Peretti & Swenson, 1974), heart rate (Landreth & Landreth, 1974), pulse rate and blood pressure (Webster, 1973), respiration rate (Webster, 1973), electromyogram (Prager-Decker, 1979), and electroencephalogram (Furman, 1978).

Reynolds (1984) compared the efficacy of five relaxation-training procedures, four of which employed electromyographic auditing feedback: (1) biofeedback only (BFL), (2) autogenic training phrases (ATP), (3) music (MU), (4) autogenic training phrases and music (ATP & MU), and (5) a control group. The purpose of the study was to develop self-regulation of a "cultivated low arousal state" as a countermeasure to tensed muscular reaction to stressful imagery. After eight training sessions, the MU and ATP & MU groups achieved highly significant differences when compared with the control group. The ATP & MU group attained the lowest postbaseline arousal level as measured by the electromyogram.

Wesecky (1986) suggests that the reactivity for rhythm and melodies must be located within a primitive region of the hierarchical structure of the brain because even severely retarded children respond to music. He demonstrated that music therapy could bring about at least a temporary cessation of the stereotyped movements in children with Rett syndrome.

With the advent of New Age music in the late 1970s and early 1980s, along with compositions designed to induce relaxation versus excitation states, music therapists expanded their repertoires of musical selections that would induce effective changes (Logan & Roberts, 1984). Smith and Joyce (2004), however, provided evidence that classical music is more effective than New Age music in promoting the relaxation response.

SCHOOL-BASED INTERVENTION USING RELAXATION TECHNIQUES

Although anxiety disorders represent the primary reason children and adolescents are referred for mental health services, children showing symptoms of these disorders are often not identified (Tomb & Hunter,

2004). School psychologists and school counselors are in a unique position to help identify as well as provide preventative measures to combat the development of anxiety disorders; this identification is critical because greater resources and attention are given to children with disruptive disorders (e.g. hyperactivity, conduct problems, and oppositional behavior) than disorders like depression and anxiety that present with internalizing symptoms. Greenberg, Domitrovich, and Bumbarger (2001) state, "It is clear that to reduce levels of childhood mental illness, interventions need to begin earlier, or ideally, preventive interventions need to be provided prior to the development of significant symptomology" (p. 3).

Matthews (1989) cites teaching relaxation skills to children and adolescents as a key element in developing an effective comprehensive school health program. Matthews trained 10-to-18-year-old students in relaxation techniques and found that: (1) relaxation training decreases arousal, with high-anxious persons more capable of change than low-anxious persons; (2) students evoke the relaxation response easily but have difficulty evoking arousal; (3) all training techniques are suitable, with cognitive relaxation methods more effective with extended practice; (4) practice creates an incremental effect; (5) personal training is more effective than recorded programs; and (6) biofeedback instrumentation enhances measurement of relaxation states. Relaxation training improved students' self-management skills, decreased state anxiety, increased girls' social interaction skills, improved self-concept, reduced test anxiety, and raised test scores and achievement.

Forman and O'Malley (1985) stress that attitudes and perceptions of self are formed early in life and remain with us as memory traces and influences on our behavior. Adults must do everything possible to ensure that children have an opportunity to develop positive attitudes and perceptions of themselves. Children who are given positive messages at home benefit from reinforcement of those messages at school, while children who receive negative messages at home need exposure to positive messages. Skill in stress management is also an important factor in a child's personal development. Numerous studies have shown that various measures of anxiety can be lowered as a result of the use of relaxation procedures (Allen & Klein, 1996; Barrett & Turner, 2001) or imagery techniques (Speidel & Troy, 1985).

The literature supports the idea of a relatively long program (at least 6 weeks) as opposed to the introduction of relaxation training in a short time frame. Cauce, Conner, and Schwartz (1987) determined positive, long-term effects of a systems-oriented school program to prevent mental illness. Prior to this study, it was unclear whether preventative efforts had detectable long-term effects, even though their short-term effects were reasonably well established by earlier studies (Levine & Perkins, 1980; Rappaport, 1979).

Another important factor in determining success rate is how a stress reduction program is delivered. Because of the techniques and/or standardization requirements for research, many of the researchers were directly involved. Herzog (1982) maintained that children appear more able to relax in an environment that does not include strangers. Therefore, a program that teachers themselves could administer should yield more optimal results (Cowen, 1982).

READY . . . , SET . . . , R.E.L.A.X.

My personal interest in school-based relaxation programs began with a self-designed stress-reduction program for high school varsity athletes using PMR, success imagery, and sedative (baroque or New Age) music once per week during 10 hour-long sessions. Pre- and posttesting using self-report inventories showed promising results in decreasing self-report of anxiety and depression and increasing self-report of self-concept. Following this program, I used the same methods in an attempt to increase the musical skills of sophomore band students. A relaxation training session was held for 10 consecutive weeks during which time the experimental group was led through a relaxation and success imagery exercise. Self-report inventories of anxiety and depression generally decreased while self-reported self-concept increased. The participants in both these groups frequently stated that the techniques used would be beneficial to all students. This feedback, coupled with the knowledge of the damaging effects of stress and anxiety in children, led me to consider a schoolwide intervention program. The concept of a primary prevention program was appealing from the standpoint of its potential to have a positive impact on large numbers of children. There is a critical need to teach relaxation skills at all levels of education. The goal of the program, called Ready . . . , Set . . . , R.E.L.A.X., was to provide a tool for children to use in a variety of settings to combat the negative effects of stress and anxiety.

The elementary school level was chosen for several reasons. First, children of this age tend to be more receptive to new experiences and would be more likely to be cooperative subjects. Second, the elementary school schedule is more flexible than that of a secondary school setting and lends itself to an available block of time for a schoolwide intervention. Finally, the hope was to provide a program that students would incorporate into their lives throughout the year by making it a part of their daily school lives.

The Ready . . . , Set . . . , R.E.L.A.X. program uses sedative music as an adjunct to muscle relaxation training and imagery. Interestingly, very few reports of combining these three techniques can be found in the literature. Not only is the use of such music supported by the literature, but my experience using music with my own children and with students in school, at workshops, and in groups gave evidence of its benefits. Children who do not actively take part in PMR or imagery are at least exposed to a passive form of relaxation. An additional benefit is the opportunity to develop an appreciation for an enriching form of music.

One of the reasons to use a multimethod intervention is the belief that each person has his or her own style of seeing the world (Folkman & Lazarus, 1985). For some children, change is accomplished through behavior, which in turn affects cognition and feeling. For others, the key to change is cognition, which in turn affects feelings and behavior. Theoretically, then, some students may benefit more directly from the use of PMR while others may benefit more from a cognitive-based success imagery technique. Children usually use several types of coping behavior in virtually every type of stressful encounter, including coping directed at solving or managing the problem that is causing distress (problem-focused coping) and coping directed at regulating the distress itself (emotion-focused coping) (Folkman & Lazarus, 1985).

It is important to try to teach children how to select the most appropriate mode of coping. For example, if a problem is not solvable (disliking one's teacher), continuing to engage in problem-focused behavior becomes counterproductive. Likewise, the same is true for engaging in emotion-focused coping when direct action and problem solving will resolve the conflict. Therefore, an important component of any intervention program is teaching children how to realistically appraise what must be done in a specific situation to cope. The Ready . . . , Set . . . , R.E.L.A.X. program provided this component by having the children imagine resolving problem-oriented issues. Additionally, suggestions were given to the classroom teacher for a brief follow-up discussion of the topic for the day. Included in the program was an opportunity for the students to repeat a positive self-statement. The purpose of these self-statements was to have the children develop a problem-solving response set. Self-regulated, private speech can function as an instructional cue that guides one's thoughts, feelings, and behaviors. Self-instructions have an influence on one's appraisal, attention processes, and physiological reactions (Meichenbaum, 1977). Folkman and Lazarus (1985) believe that stress management procedures can be effective only when they stimulate new ways of appraising and coping with potentially stressful conditions.

INDIVIDUAL INTERVENTION

Relaxation techniques are invaluable in the treatment of a variety of diagnoses, especially with trauma, depressive, and anxiety disorders. When treating children or adolescents with these disorders, it is important to provide them with tools that they can use not only to soothe themselves, but also to help them develop healing positive self-talk statements. First, it is important to lay some groundwork to enlist their cooperation and belief in the techniques you will be using to help them heal. Within the first sessions I introduce some of the basic tenets of cognitive-behavioral therapy (CBT). I always use two specific demonstrations to help demonstrate the power of thoughts. The first requires a small metal washer (about 1" in diameter) tied to the end of a string about 18" to 24" long. Instruct the client to hold the end of the string between her pointer finger and thumb (emphasize squeezing hard) and hold it in front of her body with her lower arm parallel to the ground. Then give the following instructions: "Keep your hand and arm perfectly still and simply think about your washer moving left to right across the front of your body. That's right; just think the thought of moving the washer and picture in your mind the washer moving on its own." With this instruction, the washer will begin to move in the direction requested. Next, use the same instructions and ask the child to imagine that the washer is moving forward and backward or toward her body and away from her body. Finally, ask the child to look at you and not to think anything; then, give her this instruction: "Now I want you to clear your mind of all thoughts and just listen to my words. Without your even thinking about it your washer will begin to move in a circle, round and round, in a nice circle." Ask her to look down at the washer, and it will be moving in a circle.

I follow this activity with the arm strength demonstration. Simply ask the child to raise one arm or the other straight out from his shoulder (arm parallel to the floor) to the side of his body. Then say, "I want to test your arm strength, so I'm going to push down on the middle of your arm, and I want you to resist. [pause] Now I want you to think the word 'strong,' and say out loud, 'I am strong.'" I again push down on his arm. [pause] Now I want you to try and keep your arm up, but I want you to think the word 'weak' and say 'I am weak' to yourself." I then push down on his arm. With this last suggestion the child finds either an inability to keep his arm up or a noticeable diminishing of his strength. Both of these demonstrations can then be used to explain the power of our thoughts and words. This mind–body connection is the basis for the study of psychoneuroimmunology and the powerful effects our thoughts have on our bodies and our behavior (Klein, 2001).

The next step is to generate a list of positive self-statements enlisting suggestions from the child and parents. I also suggest using statements that are goal behaviors the child may not yet be experiencing or believing (e.g., I feel happy; I am worthwhile and important; I always try my best; I listen to my parents, etc.). For good examples of positive self-statements check the table of contents in the book *Ready, Set, R.E.L.A.X.* (Allen & Klein, 1996). Part of the child's homework assignment is to read this list out loud every day. I then begin to teach him or her PMR and send him or her home with the CD *Ready, Set, Release* (Allen & Klein, 2000) to practice at home. What I like most about these techniques is the generalization effect. I have had numerous children stay in touch with me and continue to report using their relaxation and positive self-talk list years after therapy ended. They feel empowered and have been able to apply the techniques learned in therapy to new problems and stress in their lives.

CASE EXAMPLES

Emily

Emily was 8 years old when I first saw her in my private practice. She was fearful of sleeping in her room and awakened her parents nightly, wanting to sleep with them. Bedwetting was also a major problem. Adding to her stress was difficulty in school due to a learning disability. Emily came from an intact, caring family. There was a history of depression on the maternal side of her family. My screenings using standard evaluations supported a diagnosis of anxiety disorder. After spending two sessions with Emily establishing rapport and teaching her the basic principles of CBT, I led her through a relaxation exercise using one of the scripts from the *Ready, Set, R.E.L.A.X.* book. She took home a *Ready, Set, Release* CD and practiced relaxation daily. She was instructed to listen to the CD before she left her room to go to her parents' bedroom.

After 2 weeks of practice she was able to calm herself and was no longer leaving her room. We next addressed the enuresis. A complete physical exam by her pediatrician ruled out any physical problem causing her bedwetting. I showed Emily a picture of the bladder and the urethra. I next had her draw her bladder and urethra. I then asked her to draw a line across the bottom of her bladder, separating it from the urethra. I told her to imagine that this line was a gate. I led her through a PMR exercise and asked her to imagine her bladder and urethra and then to imagine a gate closing off the urethra. I asked her to keep a chart of her dry nights so we could track her progress. She continued practicing relaxation daily; each night before bed, she did a relaxation exercise and imagined a gate closing off her bladder. The frequency of her dry nights increased immediately, and within a month she stayed dry nightly.

Troy

I have used this same technique of systematic desensitization with a 13-year-old boy who had a storm phobia. Four years prior to our therapy he had witnessed a tornado in the distance. His fear of that tornado hitting his house was very real and cemented in his mind the memory of the radio and television storm warnings, the panic and rush of his family calling him inside to the basement, the ominous dark clouds, the thunder and lightning of the rainstorm that preceded his sighting of the tornado, and the feeling of the heat and humidity. Subsequent to this storm he began sleeping on the floor, as he was afraid to be too close to his bedroom wall in case a tornado struck in the middle of the night. In addition he refused to go outside if there was even a severe thunderstorm watch and became nervous on hot and humid days. Whenever traveling in a car he insisted that all the windows be closed because the sound of the wind when the windows were open caused the same intense anxiety responses. In the initial stage of treatment he was very intrigued by the washer and arm strength demonstration and enjoyed the feeling of being relaxed. We developed a list of triggers of his fear and continued to practice relaxation paired with my description of impending storms beginning with a storm in a neighboring state. He used Klein and Klein's (1997) CD *Relaxation and Success Imagery* to practice the same visualizations at home between sessions. I saw him five times over the course of 2 months. Coincidentally there was a storm warning issued the day of his fifth session. I reframed this warning as a perfect opportunity for him to practice his breathing and relaxation "in vivo." When he came in for his sixth session both he and his mother reported that his fear was completely gone. He was sleeping in his bed, riding in the car with the windows open, and stayed outside to watch the approaching thunderstorm that hit shortly after he left his fifth session.

These same techniques can be applied to most phobic behaviors with good success and provides the therapist with a proven way of helping children and teens overcome fears that interfere with what should be a relatively carefree time in their lives.

CONCLUSIONS

The use of relaxation strategies incorporating muscle relaxation, music, and imagery have been incorporated in numerous studies and programs intended to help therapists, physicians, educators, and parents enhance the physical and emotional well-being of children and adolescents. Those of us who use these techniques in our own practices know that they work. In most cases, the techniques are eagerly learned by young people and easily administered. Given the solid research base, it amazes those of us who are actively using these strategies with children that this valuable treatment and prevention tool is too often overlooked. It is my hope that if you are not using these strategies in your practice, you will try them in the near future. If you need convincing, take Emily's advice. Near the end of her treatment she said, "Dr. Klein, why doesn't everyone learn how to do this?" To her credit, she introduced relaxation training to her classmates and her teacher, who has set aside time on a daily basis to practice what Emily preaches.

REFERENCES

Afremow, J., & Overby, L. (2001). Using mental imagery to enhance children's motor performance. *Journal of Physical Education, Recreation and Dance, 72*(2), 19.

Allen, J., & Klein, R. (1996). *Ready, set, R.E.L.A.X.: A resarch based program of learning and self-esteem for children.* Watertown, WI: Inner Coaching.

Allen, J., & Klein, R. (2000). *Ready, set release: Music and relaxation exercises for children.* Watertown, WI: Inner Coaching.

Anbar, R. (2001) Self-hypnosis for the treatment of functional abdominal pain in childhood. *Clinical Pediatrics, 40*(8), 447.

Anderson, C. A. (1983). Imagination and expectation: The effect of imagining behavioral scripts on personal intentions. *Journal of Personality and Social Psychology, 45,* 293–305.

Baron, M. (2000). The effects of television on child health: Implications and recommendations. *Archives of Disease in Childhood, 83,* 289–292.

Barrett, P. M., & Turner, C. (2001). Anxiety disorders of childhood and adolescence: A critical review. *Journal of the American Academy of Child and Adolescent Psychiatry, 30,* 519–552.

Benson, H. (1976). *The relaxation response.* New York: Avon Books.

Berliner, D., & Amrein, A. (2003). The effects of high-stakes testing on student motivation and learning. *Educational Leadership, 60*(5) 32–38.

Cannon, W. B. (1914). The emergency function of the adrenal medulla in pain and major emotions. *American Journal of Physiology, 33,* 356–372.

Cauce, A. M., Conner, J. P., & Schwartz, D. (1987). Long term effects of a systems-oriented school prevention program. *American Journal of Orthopsychiatry, 57*(1), 127–131.

Chan, E. (2002). The role of complementary and alternative medicine in attention-deficit hyperactivity disorder. *Journal of Developmental and Behavioral Pediatrics, 23*(Suppl.), 837–845.

Chang, J., & Hiebert, B. (1989). Relaxation procedures with children: A review. *Medical Psychotherapy, 2,* 163–176.

Cowen, E. L. (1982). Primary prevention: Children and the schools. *Journal of Children in Contemporary Society, 14,* 56–58.

Culbert, T., Reaney, J., & Kohen, D. (1994). Cyberphysiologic strategies with children: The clinical hypnosis/biofeedback interface. *International Journal of Clinical Experiential Hypnosis, 42,* 97–117.

Field, T., Grizzle, N., Scafidi, F., & Schanberg, S. (1996). Massage and relaxation therapies' effects on depressed adolescent mothers. *Adolescence, 31*(9), 903.

Fiske, E. B. (1986, April). Early schooling is now the rage. *New York Times,* pp. 24–30.

Folkman, S., & Lazarus, R. (1985). Methodological issues in stress research. In A. Eichler, D. Silverman, & H. Pratt (Eds.), *How to define and research stress* (pp. 95–104). Washington, DC: American Psychiatric Press.

Forman, S., & O'Malley, P. (1985). A school-based approach to stress management education of students. *Special Services in the Schools, 1,* 61–71.

Furman, C. E. (1978). The effect of musical stimuli on the brainwave production of children. *Journal of Music Therapy, 15,* 108–117.

Gagnon, D., Hudnell, L., & Andrasck, F. (1992). Biofeedback and related procedures in coping with stress. In A. La Greca, L. Siegell, J. Wallander, & E. Walker (Eds.), *Stress and coping in child health* (pp. 303–326). New York: Guilford Press.

Greenberg, M. T., Domitrovich, C., & Bumbarger, B. (2001). The prevention of mental disorders in school-age children: Current state of the field. *Prevention and Treatment, 4,* Article 1 (Online serial). *www.journals. apa.org/prevention* Directory: volume4/pre0040001a.html

Herzog, S. (1982). *Joy in the classroom.* Boulder Creek, CA: University Press.

Hume, D. (1907). *An inquiry concerning human understanding.* Chicago: Open Court. Reprinted from 1748.

Jacobson, E. (1944). *Progressive relaxation.* Chicago: University of Chicago Press.

Klein, N. (2001). *Healing images for children: Guiding families facing childhood cancer and other serious illnesses.* Watertown, WI: Inner Coaching.

Klein, R., & Klein, N. (1997). *Relaxation and success imagery: Using the power of the mind–body connection.* Watertown, WI: Inner Coaching.

Landreth, J. E., & Landreth, H. F. (1974). Effects of music on physiological response. *Journal of Research in Music Education, 22,* 4–12.

Levine, M., & Perkins, D. V. (1980). Social setting intervention and primary prevention: Comments on the report of the task panel on prevention to the President's Commission on Mental Health. *American Journal of Community Psychology, 8,* 147–157.

Loffredo, D. A., Omizo, M., & Hammett, V. L. (1984). Group relaxation training and parental involvement with hyperactive boys. *Journal of Learning Disabilities, 17,* 210–213.

Logan, T. G., & Roberts, A. R. (1984). The effects of different types of relaxation music on tension level. *Journal of Music Therapy, 21,* 177–183.

Matthews, D. (1989). Relaxation theory for rural youth. *Research Bulletin 46.* Orangeburg: South Carolina State College.

Meichenbaum, D. (1977). *Cognitive behavior modification: An integrative approach.* New York: Plenum Press.

Murphy, J. (1992). Psychophysiological responses to stress in children and adolescents. In A. La Greca, L. Siegel, J. Wallander, & E. Walker (Eds.), *Stress and coping in child health* (pp. 45–71). New York: Guilford Press.

NewsRx.com. (2004, October 19). Pain medicine: Imagery reduces children's postoperative pain. *Life Science Weekly*, 1049.

Ostrander, S., & Schroeder, L. (1979). *Super learning*. New York: Dell.

Peretti, P. O., & Swenson, K. (1974). Effects of music on anxiety as determined by physiological skin responses. *Journal of Research in Music Education, 22*, 278–283.

Porter, S. S., & Omizo, M. M. (1984). The effects of group relaxation training/large-muscle exercise, and parental involvement on attention to task, impulsivity, and locus of control among hyperactive boys. *Exceptional Child, 31*, 54–64.

Prager-Decker, I. J. (1979). The relative efficacy of progressive muscle relaxation, EMG biofeedback, and music for reducing stress arousal of internally vs. externally controlled individuals. *Dissertation Abstracts International, 7*, 3177.

Rappaport, J. (1979). *Community psychology: Values, research, and action*. San Francisco: Jossey-Bass.

Rasid, Z. M., & Parish, T. S. (1998). The effects of two types of relaxation training on student's level of anxiety. *Adolescence, 33*, 99–101.

Reynolds, S. B. (1984). Biofeedback, relaxation training, and music: Homeostasis for coping with stress. *Biofeedback and Self-Regulation, 9*(2), 169–179.

Rolla, G. (1993). *Inner music: Creative analysis and music memory*. Wilmette, IL: Chiron.

Rutter, M. (1998). Stress, coping and development: Some issues and some questions. In N. Garmezy & M. Rutter (Eds.), *Stress, coping and development in children* (pp. 1–42). Baltimore: Johns Hopkins University Press.

Schilling, D. J., & Poppen, R. (1983). Behavioral relaxation training and assessment. *Journal of Behavior Therapy and Experimental Psychiatry, 14*, 99–107.

Selye, H. (1956). *The stress of life*. New York: McGraw-Hill.

Shepard, R. N., & Cooper, L. A. (1982). *Mental images and their transformations*. Cambridge, MA: MIT Press.

Sherman, S. J., Cialdini, R. B., Schwartzman, D. F., & Reynolds, K. D. (1985). Imagining can heighten or lower the perceived likelihood of contracting a disease: The mediating effect of ease of imagery. *Personality and Social Psychology Bulletin, 11*, 118–127.

Smith, J., & Joyce, C. (2004). Mozart versus New Age music: Relaxation states, stress, and ABC relaxation theory. *Journal of Music Therapy, 14*(3), 215.

Speidel, G. E., & Troy, M. E. (1985). The ebb and flow of mental imagery in education. In A. A. Sheikh & S. Sheikh (Eds.), *Imagery in education* (pp. 11–38). Farmingdale, NY: Baywood.

Tomb, M., & Hunter, L. (2004). Prevention of anxiety in children and adolescents in a school setting: The role of school-based practitioners. *Children and Schools*, 26, 87.

U.S. Public Health Service. (2000). *Report of the surgeon general's conference on children's mental health: A national action agenda.* Washington, DC: Department of Health and Human Services.

Webster, C. (1973). Relaxation music and cardiology: The physiological and psychological consequences of their interrelation. *Australian Occupational Therapy Journal*, 20, 9–20.

Wesecky, A. (1986). Music therapy for children with Rett syndrome. *American Journal of Medical Genetics*, 24, 253–257.

Index

"f" following a page number indicates a figure;
"t" following a page number indicates a table.

Accidents
  interventions with survivors of, 117–
    129, 119f, 120f, 122f, 123f, 124f,
    126f, 128f
  medical settings and, 113–114
  overview, 112–113, 129
  types of traumatic injuries, 115–117
Acculturation, degree of, 27
Action therapies, 15. See also *individual
    approaches*
Adolescents, music therapy and, 73–75,
    77–78
Adoption, narrative therapy and, 215–220
Adrenaline, stress and, 304–305
Affect regulation, 18
Aggression. See also Bullying behavior;
    Violence
  domestic violence and, 249–250
  scratchboard medium and, 94–95
  social information processing, 137
Agoraphobia, parents of traumatized
    children and, 268
American Art Therapy Association
    (AATA)
  ethical standards of, 23
  neurological factors and, 57
American Dance Therapy Association
    (ADTA), 23
American Music Therapy Association
    (AMTA), 23, 62–63
Amygdala, 7

Anchoring, temporal, 237
Anger
  domestic violence and, 249–250
  parents of traumatized children and,
    276–277
Anti-bullying programs, 132–133, 147–
    148
Anxiety. See also Anxiety disorders
  bibliotherapy and, 177–178
  bullying behavior and, 133
  crisis intervention and, 203–204
  domestic violence and, 249–250
  mandala projects and, 129
  overview, 302–304
  parents of traumatized children and,
    276–277
  relaxation and, 310
  sensory-based methods and, 36, 127
Anxiety disorders. See also Anxiety
  relaxation and, 309–310
  stress and, 304
Arousal reduction, 18
Arousal response, parents of traumatized
    children and, 270
Art materials, cultural competence and,
    28
Art therapy
  accident survivors and, 117–129, 119f,
    120f, 122f, 123f, 124f, 126f, 128f
  affect regulation and, 18
  attachment and, 17

Art therapy (cont.)
  best practices in creative arts therapies and, 27
  case examples, 53–56, 55
  crisis intervention and, 198–199
  cultural competence and, 28
  domestic violence and, 253–256, 261–262
  ethical practice and, 23–25
  Journeys Program of Valley Home Care and, 87–108, 91f, 92f, 94f, 98f, 100f, 101f, 102f, 103f, 104f, 106f, 107f
  medical settings and, 113–114
  to minimize the impact of bullying, 146–159, 149f, 154f, 155f, 158f
  music therapy and, 68–69
  neurological factors and, 57
  overview, 11, 13
  posttraumatic growth and, 298–299
  posttraumatic play and, 35
  posttraumatic stress disorder (PTSD) and, 27
  relaxation response and, 18
  resilience and, 291–294
  sensory processing and, 15
  treating grief and trauma in children and, 86–87
  World Trade Center attacks and, 87–108, 91f, 92f, 94f, 98f, 100f, 101f, 102f, 103f, 104f, 106f, 107f
Assessments
  bridge drawings and, 121, 125
  music therapy and, 65
Assimilation, art therapy and, 91–92
Association for Play Therapy (APT), 23
Attachment
  adoption and, 215–220
  brain development and, 46–50
  case examples, 53–56
  clinical implications, 52–53
  defining, 44–45
  domestic violence and, 250
  drama therapy and, 236
  overview, 16–18, 56–57
  parents of traumatized children and, 273
  resilience and, 291–292, 293
  safety and, 230
  sensory-based methods and, 37–38
  storied life and, 211–212
Attachment theory, 16–17

Attention-deficit/hyperactivity disorder (ADHD)
  bullying behavior and, 136–137
  stress and, 304
Avoidance, 5

B

Before and after drawings, 95, 104–105, 104f
Behavioral problems, domestic violence and, 249–250
Behavioral relaxation, 307–308
Bereavement, bibliotherapy and, 178–182
Bereavement goals, 96–105, 98f, 100f, 101f, 102f, 103f, 104f
Bereavement groups
  case examples, 75–78
  domestic violence and, 253
  music therapy and, 65–66, 67–71
  session planning example for, 71–75
Best practices in creative arts therapies, 26–27
Bibliotherapy
  bullying behavior and, 153
  case examples, 169–171
  death and bereavement and, 178–182
  discussing stories, 182–183
  guidelines for, 171–173
  music therapy and, 69–70
  overview, 12, 167–169, 183
  as trauma intervention, 173–178, 174f
Blame, posttraumatic growth and, 297
Bodywork
  drama therapy and, 232–234
  treating grief and trauma in children and, 87
Brain development, 45–47
Brain functioning. See also Physiology of trauma
  attachment and, 17–18
  clinical implications, 52–53
  hemispheric activity and, 51–52
  overview, 56–57
  research on, 43
Brain stem, physiology of trauma and, 7–9, 8f
Breathing techniques, crisis intervention and, 203–204
Bridge drawings, 121, 125

Broca's area, memory and, 10
Bullying behavior
    defining, 134–136
    gender differences in, 140–145
    impact on the school environment,
        133–134
    interventions to minimize the impact
        of, 146–159, 149f, 154f, 155f, 158f
    overview, 132–133, 159
    psychological implications of, 136–137
    theoretical perspectives of, 137–140
    victims of, 145–146
Burns, 117

C

Call-and-response drumming, 67–68
CD cover creation, 69
Characteristics seen in traumatized
    children, 4–6
Child abuse, domestic violence and, 249
Cognitive approach. See also Cognitive-
    behavioral therapy (CBT)
    domestic violence and, 254
    integrating creative therapies into, 13
Cognitive-behavioral therapy (CBT). See
    also Cognitive approach
    as an evidence-based practice, 26
    music therapy and, 64–67
    relaxation and, 313–314
Cognitive impairments, attachment and,
    48
Cognitive problems, domestic violence
    and, 250
Cognitive reframing, bullying behavior
    and, 147–148
Collage creation
    domestic violence and, 258
    Journeys Program of Valley Home Care
        and, 93–94, 94f, 101f
    narrative drawing and, 121
    posttraumatic growth and, 298–299
    resilience and, 293–294
Collage materials, cultural competence
    and, 28
Comfort boxes, 89–90
Community support, resilience and, 287
Compassion, posttraumatic growth and,
    296
Competency, drama therapy and, 233–234

Conduct disorders
    bullying behavior and, 133–134
    domestic violence and, 250
Confidentiality
    domestic violence and, 257
    group intervention and, 257
Conflict resolution skills, domestic
    violence and, 250
Connection
    domestic violence and, 259–260
    drama therapy and, 234–238
    parents of traumatized children and, 273
Coping
    art therapy and, 90–91
    mask projects and, 93, 125
    Ready . . . , Set . . . , R.E.L.A.X
        program and, 312–313
    resilience and, 290
Cortex
    attachment and, 17–18
    overview, 45–46
    physiology of trauma and, 7–9, 8f
Craft materials, cultural competence and,
    28
Creative arts therapies, 11–12. See also
    individual approaches
Creative expression
    art therapy and, 18
    cultural competence and, 29
    ethical practice and, 23–25
    free drawing and, 118
    mass terrorism and, 83
    sensory-based methods and, 37–38
Creative interventions in general. See also
    individual approaches
    characteristics of, 13–18
    overview, 10–13, 19
Crisis, 192–193
Crisis intervention
    challenges of, 190–192
    concept of crisis, 192–193
    overview, 191, 193–195, 207
    recommended creative interventions,
        196–207, 200f, 202f
    resources for, 209–210
Cultural competence, 22–23, 27–30
Cultural factors, narrative therapy and,
    213
Cultural identity
    overview, 27–28
    resilience and, 286

D

Dance/movement therapy
  ethical practice and, 23–24
  overview, 11–12, 13
  posttraumatic growth and, 299
  relaxation response and, 18
Death, bibliotherapy and, 178–182
Department of Education, bullying
    behavior and, 133
Depression
  bullying behavior and, 133
  domestic violence and, 249–250
Development, language. See also
    Developmental factors
  brain development and, 46
  characteristics of creative interventions
    and, 13
  memory and, 10
  physiology of trauma and, 7
Developmental approach, integrating
    creative therapies into, 13
Developmental factors
  bibliotherapy and, 172
  bullying behavior and, 142–143
  cultural competence and, 27
  death and bereavement and, 178
  drama therapy and, 232
  language development, 7, 10, 13, 46
  medical settings and, 114
  music therapy and, 65
  parents of traumatized children and,
    272–279
  play therapy and, 28
  treating grief and trauma in children
    and, 86–87
Developmental theory of aggression,
    bullying behavior and, 139–140
*Diagnostic and Statistical Manual of Mental
    Disorders* (DSM-IV-TR), 44–45
Directive approach, cultural competence
    and, 29–30
Disaster diary intervention, 199, 201
Disasters, natural and manmade, 176
Displacement, bibliotherapy and, 177
Diversity
  cultural competence and, 27–28
  play therapy and, 28
Domestic violence
  art and play therapies and, 253–256,
    261–262
  children and, 248–251

  effects of, 249–251
  group intervention and, 252–253, 254–262
  overview, 247–248, 261–262
  presenting problems and, 251–252
Doubling technique, 236–237
Drama therapy
  efficacy of, 227–228
  overview, 11, 225–227, 241–242
  posttraumatic growth and, 299
  via group treatment, 228–241
Dramatic play, 236. See also Drama
    therapy; Play therapy
Drumming, 67–68
Dynamic posttraumatic play, 34–35, 34t
Dysregulation, internal, 229

E

Early intervention, resilience and, 287
Elimination disorders, stress and, 304
Emotion regulation
  crisis intervention and, 202–205
  mask projects and, 125
  resilience and, 293
Emotional brain, 7. See also Limbic system
Emotional problems, domestic violence
    and, 249–250
Empathy
  posttraumatic growth and, 296
  resilience and, 293
Ethical practice, 22, 23–25
Ethnicity, cultural competence and, 27
Events, types of, 4–6
Evidence-based practice, 25–27
Explicit memory, 9–10
Exploding Red Light, Green Light game, 233
Expression, creative
  art therapy and, 18
  cultural competence and, 29
  ethical practice and, 23–25
  free drawing and, 118
  mass terrorism and, 83
  sensory-based methods and, 37–38
Expressive therapies. See also *individual
    approaches*
  interventions with survivors of
    accidents and, 117–129, 119f, 120f,
    122f, 123f, 124f, 126f, 128f
  overview, 11–12
  posttraumatic play and, 35
  sensory processing and, 15–16

Externalization
  art therapy and, 91–92, 151
  drama therapy and, 226–227
  overview, 14
Eye movement desensitization and
  reprocessing (EMDR)
  drama therapy and, 231
  overview, 57
  with survivors of accidents, 127

F

Family, death and bereavement and, 179–
  180
Family factors
  crisis intervention and, 193–194
  cultural competence and, 27
  domestic violence and, 252
  resilience and, 286–287
  traumatic brain injury, 115–116
Family history, narrative therapy and, 219
Family portrait intervention, 231
Family therapy sessions
  domestic violence and, 252, 259–260
  mask projects and, 126
  music therapy and, 66
Fantasies, drama therapy and, 231
Fear
  bullying behavior and, 133
  domestic violence and, 249–250
  Journeys Program of Valley Home Care
    and, 89–90
  parents of traumatized children and,
    276–277
Fight or flight response
  physiology of trauma and, 6–10, 8f
  stress and, 304–305
Flexibility, art therapy and, 91
Fragmentation, art therapy and, 90
Free drawing, with survivors of accidents,
  118, 119f, 120f
Free expression. See Creative expression

G

Games, drama, overview, 232–234
Gender factors
  bullying behavior and, 140–145
  cultural competence and, 27
  play therapy and, 28

General adaptation syndrome, 304–305
Genetics, resilience and, 287
Glasgow Coma Scale, 115
Goals, bereavement. See Bereavement
  goals
Grief camps, music therapy and, 65–66
Grief work, bibliotherapy and, 178–182
Grief work, music and
  case examples, 75–78
  overview, 62–67, 78
  session planning example for, 71–75
  techniques used in, 67–71
Grief work, World Trade Center attacks
  and
  Journeys Program of Valley Home Care
    and, 87–108, 91f, 92f, 94f, 98f, 100f,
    101f, 102f, 103f, 104f, 106f, 107f
  overview, 83–85
  treating grief and trauma in children
    and, 85–87, 86f
Group approaches
  art and play therapies and, 254–256
  bullying behavior and, 152–159, 154f,
    155f, 158f
  case examples, 75–78
  domestic violence and, 252–253, 254–
    262
  drama therapy and, 228–241
  mask projects and, 126
  music therapy and, 65–66, 67–71, 71–
    75, 75–78
  phases of, 256–260
  posttraumatic growth and, 299
  session planning example for, 71–75
Group projects, bullying behavior and,
  157
Growth, posttraumatic
  encouraging, 297–299
  identifying in traumatized children,
    296–297
  overview, 285–286, 294–296, 295f, 300
Guided imagery, 12–13

H

Heart-box collage technique, Journeys
  Program of Valley Home Care and,
  101f
Helplessness
  mask projects and, 125
  medical settings and, 113

Hemispheric activity, 51–52
Hermeneutic approach, 214–215
Hippocampus
    development of, 50
    overview, 7
Humanistic approach, integrating creative
    therapies into, 13
Hyperarousal
    drama therapy and, 229
    overview, 5
    sensory-based methods and, 36
Hypervigilance, domestic violence and,
    250
Hypothalamus, 7

I

Iconic symbolization, 16
Imagery. *See also* Relaxation techniques
    art therapy and, 90–91
    Journeys Program of Valley Home Care
        and, 102–104, 103*f*
    overview, 305–306, 316
    Ready . . . , Set . . . , R.E.L.A.X
        program and, 312
    sleep disturbances and, 102–104, 103*f*
Imagination
    bibliotherapy and, 172–173
    drama therapy and, 231, 241–242
    sensory processing and, 16
Implicit experiences, 37
Implicit memory
    overview, 9–10
    parents of traumatized children and,
        269
    sensory processing and, 15–16
Improvisational exercises, 238
Indirect aggression, 142. *See also* Bullying
    behavior
Information processing
    memory and, 9–10
    parents of traumatized children and,
        270
Inhibition, social, 152
Integrative approaches to expressive
    therapies, 12
Interactive bibliotherapy, 168–169
Internal dysregulation, drama therapy and,
    229
Internal regulation, drama therapy and,
    230–231

Intimidation, bullying behavior and, 133
Isolation
    bibliotherapy and, 175
    as a form of bullying behavior, 136

J

Journaling, parents of traumatized children
    and, 277
Journey drawings, 100, 101
Journeys Program of Valley Home Care,
    87–109, 91*f*, 92*f*, 94*f*, 98*f*, 100*f*, 101*f*,
    102*f*, 103*f*, 104*f*, 106*f*, 107*f*

K

Knowledge, social constructionist stance
    and, 214–215

L

Language development. *See also*
    Developmental factors
    brain development and, 46
    characteristics of creative interventions
        and, 13
    memory and, 10
    physiology of trauma and, 7
Learning disability (LD), bullying
    behavior and, 136–137
Limbic system
    physiology of trauma and, 7–9, 8*f*
    sensory processing and, 15–16
Location (rural or urban), cultural
    competence and, 27
Loss
    bibliotherapy and, 178–182
    posttraumatic growth and, 296, 299
LUV (Listen, Understand, and Validate)
    approach, 194–195
Lyrics, 70–71

M

Magic box intervention, 231
Magic shop intervention, 231–232
Maltreatment, severe. *See* Severe
    maltreatment

Mandalas, with survivors of accidents, 127, 129
Mask projects
  Journeys Program of Valley Home Care and, 90–91, 91f, 92f, 93
  with survivors of accidents, 125–126, 126f
Materials in creative approaches
  crisis intervention and, 191, 201–202, 202f
  domestic violence and, 255–256
  music therapy and, 67
  narrative therapy and, 215
  resilience and, 292
  titration and, 36–37
Maturity, posttraumatic growth and, 296
Maximization, 238
Meaning making, crisis intervention and, 198–202, 200f, 202f
Media
  cultural competence and, 29
  World Trade Center attacks and, 85
Medical settings, 113–114
Meditation, 12–13
Memorial projects, Journeys Program of Valley Home Care and, 105–106, 106f
Memory
  drama therapy and, 230–231
  externalization in therapy and, 14
  Journeys Program of Valley Home Care and, 90, 95–96
  overview, 9–10
  parents of traumatized children and, 269, 273–274
  posttraumatic play and, 30–35, 32f, 33f, 34t
  resilience and, 293
  sensory-based methods and, 36
Mentalization, drama therapy and, 236, 237
Metaphor
  drama therapy and, 237–238
  posttraumatic growth and, 299
  trauma narratives and, 92
Mimicry, art therapy and, 18
Mind–body connection, physiology of trauma and, 9
Mirror exercises, drama therapy and, 234–235
Movement therapy. See Dance/movement therapy

Moving, bibliotherapy and, 177
Muscle relaxation
  overview, 306–308, 316
  Ready . . . , Set . . . , R.E.L.A.X program and, 312
Music therapy
  case examples, 75–78
  crisis intervention and, 204–205
  ethical practice and, 23–24
  grief work and, 64–67, 78
  overview, 11, 13, 62–64
  Ready . . . , Set . . . , R.E.L.A.X program and, 312
  relaxation and, 18, 308–309, 316
  resilience and, 292–293
  session planning example for, 71–75
  techniques used in, 67–71

N

Narrative approach. See also Trauma narratives
  adoption and, 215–220
  bullying behavior and, 147–148
  case examples, 220–221
  domestic violence and, 258–259
  integrating creative therapies into, 13
  Journeys Program of Valley Home Care and, 92–93, 92f
  narrative drawing, 119–121, 122f–124f
  overview, 222–224
  play therapy and, 213–214
  posttraumatic growth and, 297
  social constructionist stance, 214–215
  storied life and, 211–213
  toys and, 215
  treating grief and trauma in children and, 87
National Association for Poetry Therapy (NAPT), 23
National Child Traumatic Stress Network (NCTSN), 27–28
National Education Association, 133
National Institute of Child Health and Human Development, 133
National Threat Assessment Center, 133
Neurological factors. See also Physiology of trauma
  brain development and, 45–50
  case examples, 53–56
  clinical implications, 52–53

Neurological factors (*cont.*)
  hemispheric activity and, 51–52
  overview, 56–57
  research on, 43
Neurological model, 17–18. *See also*
  Physiology of trauma
Neurons, 45–46
9/11 attacks. *See* World Trade Center
  attacks
No Child Left Behind policy, stress and, 303
Nondirective approach, cultural
  competence and, 29–30
Nonverbal learning disability (NVLD),
  bullying behavior and, 136–137
Nonverbal therapies, 13
Normalizing thoughts, feelings and
  reactions, 270–271
Numbing, emotional
  Journeys Program of Valley Home Care
    and, 96
  sensory processing and, 16

O

Object relations theory, brain
  development and, 47–50
Obsessive–compulsive disorder (OCD)
  bullying behavior and, 157–159, 158*f*
  case examples, 157–159, 158*f*
  domestic violence and, 250
Oppositional behavior, domestic violence
  and, 249–250

P

Parent–child relationship. *See also* Parents
  of traumatized children; Relationship
  patterns
  attachment and, 17
  domestic violence and, 259–260
  resilience and, 291
Parents of traumatized children. *See also*
  Parent–child relationship
  activities parents can use, 270–279
  helping to learn about trauma, 267–268
  including in therapy, 259–260
  overview, 264, 279
  questions of, 265–267
  reactions of to children's trauma, 265–
    266

  resources for, 280–281
  sensory experiences and, 268–270
  where to begin when working with,
    266–267
Peer questioning, bullying behavior and, 155
Peers. *See also* Bullying behavior;
  Relationship patterns
  cultural competence and, 27
  domestic violence and, 250
  posttraumatic growth and, 296
Pervasive developmental disorder (PDD),
  bullying behavior and, 136–137
Pet, death of, 180–181
Photo collage materials, cultural
  competence and, 28
Physiology of trauma
  attachment and, 17–18
  brain development and, 45–50
  case examples, 53–56
  clinical implications, 52–53
  drama therapy and, 232–234
  hemispheric activity and, 51–52
  overview, 6–10, 8*f*, 56–57
  parents of traumatized children and,
    270
  research on, 43
  stress and, 304–305
Placebo affect, art therapy and, 18
Play, parents of traumatized children and,
  275
Play, posttraumatic, 30–35, 32*f*, 33*f*, 34*t*
Play therapy
  adoption and, 216
  attachment and, 17
  crisis intervention and, 201–202, 202*f*
  cultural competence and, 28
  domestic violence and, 253–256, 261–
    262
  drama therapy and, 236
  ethical practice and, 23–24
  medical settings and, 114
  narrative drawing and, 120–121
  narrative therapy and, 213–214
  overview, 12
  posttraumatic growth and, 298–299
  resilience and, 291–294
Playback theatre method, 236–237
Poetry therapy
  ethical practice and, 23–24
  overview, 12
Political factors, cultural competence and,
  27–28

Posttraumatic growth
  encouraging, 297–299
  identifying in traumatized children,
    296–297
  overview, 285–286, 294–296, 295f, 300
Posttraumatic play, 30–35, 32f, 33f, 34t
Posttraumatic stress disorder (PTSD)
  best practices in creative arts therapies
    and, 27
  brain development and, 49–50
  bullying behavior and, 147–148
  domestic violence and, 250–251
  memory and, 10
  overview, 5–6
  parents of traumatized children and, 268
  resilience and, 285–286
  school-based approaches and, 147–148
  sensory processing and, 16
  World Trade Center attacks and, 85
Presenting problems, domestic violence
  and, 251–252
Products created in therapy, 24–25
Professional organizations, ethical
  standards of, 23–24
Progressive muscle relaxation
  overview, 306–308, 316
  Ready . . . , Set . . . , R.E.L.A.X
    program and, 312
Psychodynamic approach, integrating
  creative therapies into, 13
Psychoeducation
  domestic violence and, 252, 258
  parents of traumatized children and,
    267–268
Psychotherapy approaches
  bullying behavior and, 133
  free drawing and, 118
  integrating creative therapies into, 13

R

Rancho Los Amigos Scale, 115
Reactions to trauma, physiology of trauma
  and, 6–10, 8f
Reactive attachment disorder, 44–45
Reactive bibliotherapy, 168–169
Ready . . . , Set . . . , R.E.L.A.X
  program
  case examples, 314–316
  individual intervention, 313–314
  overview, 311–313

Reassurance, domestic violence and, 252
Record keeping
  art therapy and, 24–25
  ethical practice and, 24–25
Reexperiencing of trauma
  overview, 5
  through play, 30–35, 32f, 33f, 34t
Reexposure to traumatic memories
  bullying behavior and, 147–148
  parents of traumatized children and, 271
Reflective function, drama therapy and,
  236–237
Regionalization, cultural competence and,
  27
Relational aggression, 141–143. See also
  Bullying behavior
Relationship patterns. See also Parent–
  child relationship; Peers
  attachment and, 17
  domestic violence and, 250
  posttraumatic growth and, 296
Relaxation techniques. See also Imagery;
  Stress reduction methods
  bibliotherapy and, 177–178
  case examples, 314–316
  individual intervention, 313–314
  methods of, 304–309
  overview, 12–13, 302–304, 316
  Ready . . . , Set . . . , R.E.L.A.X
    program, 311–313
  school-based approaches and, 309–311
Religious affiliation, cultural competence
  and, 27
Repetition in play or art, narrative
  drawing and, 121
Resilience
  art therapy and, 90–91
  crisis and, 192–193, 195
  crisis intervention and, 206
  identifying in traumatized children,
    287–288
  overview, 285–287, 300
  posttraumatic growth and, 296
  promoting via creative interventions,
    291–294
  supporting, 288–291, 289f, 290f
Response plans, resilience and, 290
Rhythmic improvisation, 68
Rituals, narrative therapy and, 217–218
Role play
  bullying behavior and, 155–156
  drama therapy and, 237, 240

Role play (cont.)
    mask projects and, 126
    posttraumatic growth and, 299
Romanian orphan research, brain
        development and, 47–49
Routines
    parents of traumatized children and,
        271, 272
    resilience and, 286
Rural location, cultural competence and, 27

S

Safe spaces, drama therapy and, 230
Safety boxes, 89–90
Safety, feelings of
    domestic violence and, 252, 256–258,
        259–260
    drama therapy and, 228–232
    group intervention and, 256–258
    Journeys Program of Valley Home Care
        and, 89–90, 108–109
    parents of traumatized children and,
        272–273, 276–277
    sensory-based methods and, 37–38
    sensory experiences and, 269
    treating grief and trauma in children
        and, 85–87, 86f
Safety planning
    domestic violence and, 252
    treating grief and trauma in children
        and, 86–87
Safety, restoring feelings of, 18
Sandplay therapy, 12
School-based approaches
    bullying behavior and, 133, 147–148
    music therapy and, 66–67
    relaxation and, 309–311
School environment, bullying behavior
        and, 133–134
School phobia, bullying behavior and, 148
Scratchboard medium, 94–95
Sculptures, body, 233
Self-awareness
    bullying behavior and, 152
    resilience and, 293
Self-care, narrative therapy and, 218–219
Self-concept
    mask projects and, 125
    treating grief and trauma in children
        and, 86–87

Self-esteem
    bullying behavior and, 133, 146, 152
    domestic violence and, 249–250
    sensory-based methods and, 37–38
Self-expression
    cultural competence and, 28–29
    drama therapy and, 239–241
    externalization in therapy and, 14
    posttraumatic play and, 35
    resilience and, 292–293
Self-management, treating grief and
        trauma in children and, 86–87
Self-portraits, 106
Self-regulation, resilience and, 293
Self-soothing
    art therapy and, 18
    parents of traumatized children and,
        271
    posttraumatic play and, 35
    sensory-based methods and, 37–38
Self-talk, domestic violence and, 258–259
Sensory-based method
    overview, 35–38
    with survivors of accidents, 127, 128f
Sensory experiences
    bibliotherapy and, 172–173
    domestic violence and, 253–254
    memory and, 10
    overview, 9
    parents of traumatized children and,
        268–270, 279
Sensory processing, 15–16
Separation anxiety
    bibliotherapy and, 175
    domestic violence and, 250
Separations, parents of traumatized
        children and, 271
Session planning, music therapy and, 65–
        66, 71–75
Severe maltreatment, defining, 44–45
Sexual abuse, bibliotherapy and, 172
Sibling relationships, domestic violence
        and, 250
"6-R" tasks of bereavement, treating grief
        and trauma in children and, 87
Sleep, distinguishing from death, 72–73
Sleep disturbances, 102–104, 103f
Social aggression, 142. See also Bullying
        behavior
Social awareness, resilience and, 293
Social blindness model of bullying, 137,
        138

Social constructionist stance, narrative therapy and, 214–215
Social Experience Questionnaire, 142
Social information processing, bullying behavior and, 137–138, 138–139
Social inhibition, bullying behavior and, 152
Social injustice, as a form of bullying behavior, 136
Social intelligence model of bullying, 137, 138–139, 140
Social problems, domestic violence and, 249–250
Social skills, bullying behavior and, 139
Social skills deficit model of bullying, 137, 138
Social support, posttraumatic growth and, 297
Socioeconomic status (SES), cultural competence and, 27
Sociometric exercises, drama therapy and, 235
Solution-focused approach
    domestic violence and, 254
    integrating creative therapies into, 13
Spinal cord injuries, 116–117
Spiritual affiliation, cultural competence and, 27
Split-brain studies, 51–52
Stability, sensory-based methods and, 37–38
Stagnant posttraumatic play, 34–35, 34t
Storied life. See also Narrative approach
    overview, 211–213, 222–224
    "The Seven Sons of Morrison in Cold Winters When the Ice Was Thick" story, 212–213
    "The Three Brothers" story, 222–224
Story reading. See also Bibliotherapy
    music therapy and, 69–70
    overview, 182–183
Storymaking, toys and, 215
Stress
    bibliotherapy and, 177
    overview, 302–304
    resilience and, 290
Stress reduction methods. See also individual approaches; Relaxation techniques
    bibliotherapy and, 177–178
    domestic violence and, 252, 261
    overview, 12–13, 18

Suicide, bullying behavior and, 133
Symbolism, art therapy and, 90–91
Symptoms
    bibliotherapy and, 175–176
    domestic violence and, 250
    posttraumatic stress disorder (PTSD) and, 5–6
    sensory-based methods and, 36
Synapse, 45–46
Systems-based approach
    crisis intervention and, 193–194
    integrating creative therapies into, 13

T

Task-oriented approach, 86–87
Tasks of bereavement, treating grief and trauma in children and, 87
Temperament, bullying behavior and, 146
Temporal anchoring, drama therapy and, 237
Termination, domestic violence and, 260
Terrorism, mass. See also World Trade Center attacks
    overview, 81–83
    treating grief and trauma in children and, 85–87, 86f
"The Seven Sons of Morrison in Cold Winters When the Ice Was Thick" story, 212–213
"The Three Brothers" story, 222–224
Theory of mind model of bullying, 137, 139
Therapeutic relationship, art therapy and, 90
Thinking brain, 7. See also Cortex
Time-limited approaches, music therapy and, 66–67
Timelines, 121, 125
Tissue paper collage technique, 93–94, 94f
Titration, 36–37
Touch in therapy
    ethical practice and, 24
    play therapy and, 24
Toy selection
    cultural competence and, 28
    sensory-based methods and, 37–38
    storymaking and, 215
Trauma, defining, 4–6
Trauma-focused cognitive-behavioral therapy (TF-CBT), 26

Trauma in general, compared to crisis,
    192–193
Trauma narratives. *See also* Narrative
        approach
    bullying behavior and, 147–148
    domestic violence and, 258–259
    Journeys Program of Valley Home Care
        and, 92–93, 92*f*
    overview, 37
    posttraumatic growth and, 297
    treating grief and trauma in children
        and, 86–87
Trauma, physiology of. *See* Physiology of
        trauma
Traumatic brain injury, 115–116
Traumatic events, types of, 4–6
Traumatic injuries. *See* Accidents
Treatment planning, music therapy and,
    65–66
Trust, art therapy and, 91
Types of traumatic events, 4–6

U

Urban location, cultural competence and,
    27

V

Verbal therapies, externalization in
        therapy and, 14
Violence, 134. *See also* Aggression;
        Bullying behavior; Domestic violence
Visualization
    overview, 12–13
    treating grief and trauma in children
        and, 87
Vulnerability, art therapy and, 90

W

Wax Museum game, 233
Well-being, relaxation response and, 18
Withdrawn behavior, domestic violence
    and, 250
Workplace violence, bullying behavior
    and, 134
World Trade Center attacks. *See also*
        Terrorism, mass
    bibliotherapy and, 169–171, 176
    drama therapy and, 226, 239
    Journeys Program of Valley Home
        Care and, 87–108, 91*f*, 92*f*, 94*f*, 98*f*,
        100*f*, 101*f*, 102*f*, 103*f*, 104*f*, 106*f*,
        107*f*
    music therapy and, 78
    overview, 81–83, 83–85
    parents of traumatized children and,
        268
    treating grief and trauma in children
        and, 85–87, 86*f*, 87
Worldviews of children
    cultural competence and, 28
    treating grief and trauma in children
        and, 86–87
Worry
    domestic violence and, 249–250
    parents of traumatized children and,
        276–277

Y

Yoga, 12–13

Z

Zero-tolerance policy, 132–133, 147–148